D1095711

# Hospitals, Doctors, and
# The Public Interest

# Hospitals, Doctors, and The Public Interest

EDITED BY

John H. Knowles, M.D.

*General Director of
the Massachusetts General Hospital*

HARVARD UNIVERSITY PRESS

CAMBRIDGE, MASSACHUSETTS

1 9 6 6

# PREFACE

In 1948, Dr. Nathaniel W. Faxon, then Director of the Massachusetts General Hospital, published a series of lectures sponsored by the Lowell Institute and given by members of the staff of the M.G.H., entitled "The Hospital in Contemporary Life." In his preface to the lectures Doctor Faxon stated, "This book endeavors to tell the layman something of what he should know about the past history, present operation, and future possibilities of hospitals . . . It is presented in the hope that it will promote a fuller understanding of the place of the modern hospital in the life of today and of the layman's responsibility for keeping it there."

Fifteen years later it seemed a good time to review the problems of hospitals and medicine and for the very same reasons — with the additional emphasis that the medical profession also needs a fuller understanding of the hospital, an incredible blind spot in the physician's intellectual equipment. The lectures were once again sponsored by the Lowell Institute in the public interest and were held weekly at the Massachusetts General Hospital in the late winter and early spring of 1963 under the title, "The Hospital's Responsibility to the Community." An attempt was made to consider the role of the hospital as a social instrument, the socioeconomic issues of medical care, the educational responsibility of the hospital, and finally, the present and future role of the hospital in the community. The lectures were well attended by an interested public and were reported faithfully by an enlightened press.

This book is intended for laymen, medical students, the medical profession, for those in the field of politics, and for the experts of other disciplines in the hopes that it will increase understanding and lead to considered and constructive action on all sides. Better understanding of the hospital, its historical evolution, its present problems, and its obligatory role as a social, as well as an educational and scientific instrument is necessary if the medical profession wishes to keep the use of this instrument in its own hands, and if the community wishes to see the best reflection of its humanitarian efforts.

I would like to record my sincere thanks and those of the Massachusetts General Hospital to the Lowell Institute and its Trustee, Mr. Ralph Lowell. Both have never failed the best interests of Boston. Also, Curator of the Lowell Institute, Dean Richard Gummere was always helpful, always "there." I am grateful too for the thoughtfulness of the Sagamore Foundation, which helped defray the expenses of the lectures and provided for informal "seminars" following the lectures. Mr. George Jacobsen, the Editor of the *M.G.H. News,* helped with some of the editing. An enlightened press interviewed each lecturer and accurately reflected the content of his talk. Mr. Herbert Black, medical reporter of the Boston *Globe,* must be singled out for his vital contribution and generally his untiring efforts to report accurately, completely, and fairly the successes and failures and the problems of medicine and hospitals. He is a public servant in the finest sense. The Boston *Herald* also gave complete coverage with a number of excellent reporters. I am indebted to the *New England Journal of Medicine* for permission to republish "The Balanced Biology of the Teaching Hospital."

It is a pleasure to work with Mr. Joseph D. Elder and Miss Virginia Wharton of Harvard University Press and I am indebted to them for their patient help. I am grateful to my secretary, Miss Joan Bloch, who has exercised her usual equanimity and intelligence while making this task an easier one for me. My wife and six children provide the best setting and the best stimulus to productive and enjoyable work.

John H. Knowles, M.D.

*Massachusetts General Hospital*
*Boston, 1965*

# CONTENTS

■ THE TEACHING HOSPITAL: HISTORICAL PERSPECTIVE AND
A CONTEMPORARY VIEW     I

John H. Knowles, M.D., General Director, Massachusetts General Hospital; Lecturer on Medicine, Harvard Medical School

■ THE BALANCED BIOLOGY OF THE TEACHING HOSPITAL     22
John H. Knowles, M.D.

■ THE NATURE OF A TEACHING HOSPITAL AND ITS RELA-
TIONSHIP TO CHANGES IN THE COMMUNITY     47

Ellsworth T. Neumann, M.D., Administrator, Massachusetts General Hospital

■ STUDIES IN THE EVALUATION OF HOSPITAL FUNCTION:
SOME EXAMPLES OF THE CONTRIBUTION OF THE BEHAV-
IORAL SCIENCES TO MEDICINE     64

George G. Reader, M.D., Professor of Medicine and Director, Comprehensive Care and Teaching Program, New York Hospital–Cornell Medical Center

■ THE HOSPITAL AS A SOCIAL INSTRUMENT: RECENT EX-
PERIENCES AT MONTEFIORE HOSPITAL     93

Martin Cherkasky, M.D., Director, Montefiore Hospital, New York City

■ THE PROBLEMS OF MAINTAINING QUALITY IN HOSPITALS     III

Ray E. Trussell, M.D., Commissioner of Hospitals, New York City

■ GOVERNMENT AND HOSPITALS     125

Jack Masur, M.D., Assistant Surgeon General and Director, Clinical Center, National Institutes of Health, Public Health Service, Department of Health, Education and Welfare, Bethesda, Maryland

■ MEDICAL CARE RESEARCH: COUNTERBALANCE TO OPINION
AND HABIT 147

Osler L. Peterson, M.D., Visiting Professor in Preventive Medicine, Harvard Medical School

■ THE VOICE OF THE CONSUMER: COST, QUALITY, AND ORGANIZATION OF MEDICAL SERVICES 167

Jerome Pollack, M.D., Professor of Administrative Medicine, Columbia University, and Executive Director, New York Labor-Management Council of Health and Welfare Plans, New York City

■ PRIVATE HEALTH INSURANCE: PROGRESS AND PROBLEMS 187

Herman M. Somers, Professor of Politics and Public Affairs, Woodrow Wilson School of Public and International Affairs, Princeton University

■ THE SOCIAL SECURITY SYSTEM AND MEDICAL CARE 201

Charles I. Schottland, Dean, The Florence Heller Graduate School for Advanced Studies in Social Welfare, Brandeis University; formerly Commissioner of Social Security, Washington, D.C.

■ MEDICAL EDUCATION IN THE HOSPITAL 221

Edward D. Churchill, M.D., John Homans Professor of Surgery, Emeritus, Harvard Medical School; member of the Board of Consultation, Massachusetts General Hospital

■ THE HOSPITAL AND THE CONTINUING EDUCATION OF THE PHYSICIAN 237

Russell A. Nelson, M.D., President of The Johns Hopkins Hospital, Baltimore, Maryland

■ MEDICAL EDUCATION AND MEDICAL CARE: AN EXAMINATION OF TRADITIONAL CONCEPTS AND SUGGESTIONS FOR CHANGE 254

Thomas McKeown, M.D., Professor of Social Medicine, University of Birmingham School of Medicine, Birmingham, England

■ THE HEALTH NEEDS OF COMMUNITIES 271

Erich Lindemann, M.D., Chief of Psychiatric Service, Massachusetts General Hospital; Professor of Psychiatry, Harvard Medical School

■ AT THE TURN OF THE NEXT CENTURY 293

David D. Rutstein, M.D., Professor and Head of the Department of Preventive Medicine, Harvard Medical School

■ NOTES 321

■ INDEX 335

# Hospitals, Doctors, and
# The Public Interest

# THE TEACHING HOSPITAL:
## HISTORICAL PERSPECTIVE AND
## A CONTEMPORARY VIEW

John H. Knowles, M.D.


THE emergence of the hospital as a health center has been occasioned by the successes of medical science. The doctor has seen himself change from an intuitive, independent artist far removed from the hospital as a House of Despair to a scientific social worker, heavily dependent on what is now the House of Hope with its centralization of specialists and expensive machinery. As Titmuss has said . . . "progress in medical science, in psychological theories and in the specialized division of medical skill has converted medicine from an individual intuitive enterprise into a social service." [1]

The steadily mounting benefits of scientific medicine have created the social problem of rising expectations in a rapidly expanding, longer-lived population progressively less able individually to afford the inexorably rising cost of medical care. As expectations are relentlessly fulfilled by the advance of medical science, the frustrations of a parallel rise in costs coupled with the discontinuity and depersonalization of care resulting from specialization has led doctor, patient, and politician into the public arena for a series of continuing debates. The cacophony has been joined by the drug houses, commercial insurance companies and the Blue Cross, organized labor, and by the experts of other disciplines, such as economists and sociologists.

The problems of medicine and hospitals today demand a more effective social technology for their solution. In the case of the hospital, social action by the total institution becomes mandatory if effective solution of some of the social, political, and economic problems of medicine is to be found. The public looks with rising expectations to the medical profession and to those in politics, and the hospital finds itself squarely in the middle providing the center stage where all the forces and vested interests meet. Better understanding of the hospital is necessary if the medical profession wishes to play the main role in shaping its future. The consuming public needs understanding also, or the hospital will begin to reflect something undesirable and distorted. For the present form of the hospital has been molded and shaped by the wants and needs of society as well as its beliefs, values, and attitudes. As such it mirrors society and reflects not only its culture, but its economy, and it has never pretended to be better or worse than the times and the environment in which it finds itself.

Historical perspective is necessary as we view the evolution of the hospital to its present central position in the provision of health services and its unique role as a social instrument.

## HISTORICAL PERSPECTIVE

The earliest hospitals were the healing temples of ancient Egypt, the public hospitals of Buddhist India and the Mohammedan East, and the sick houses (Beth Holem) of Israel. The earliest physicians were both priest and magician. Disease was thought to represent the work of evil spirits and could be induced by infractions of religious codes. In Greek mythology, Aesculapius, the pupil of the centaur, Chiron, became the son of Apollo and the god of medicine. The cult of Aesculapius was centered at the Temple of Epidaurus where the priest-physicians received the sick with their votive offerings and practiced their magic, mainly using ritual and hypnotic suggestion. The temple at Kos was one of the most famous sanctuaries of Aesculapius; it was here that Hippocrates was born about 460 B.C. Elsewhere, the ancient Oriental custom of hospitality for guests and travelers pervaded the Levant and houses were built where weary travelers and strangers could stop for food and lodging, and if sick, nursing care. Indeed the very derivation of the word hospital shows what an important part these travelers and their hosts played in the evolution of the hospital. Hospital comes from the Latin, *hospes*, meaning "host" or "guest." The English word "hospital" comes from the Old French *hospitale* as do the words "hostel" and "hotel" and all were originally derived from the Latin. These three words, hospital, hostel, and hotel, although of different meaning today, were at one time used interchangeably.

The evolution of the modern hospital is usually associated with the advent of Christianity. The Christian ethic of faith, humanitarianism, and charity resulted in the creation of a vast hospital system. At the Council of Nicaea in A.D. 325, the bishops were instructed to establish hospitals in every cathedral city. Emperor Constantine, the first of the Roman emperors to embrace Christianity, ordered the closing of all pagan temples of healing in A.D. 335. The practices of Greco-Roman medicine were discarded and the authority of the church in medical practice was complete.

The great Crusades between 1096 and 1291 established numerous hostels for the sick which dotted the way to the Holy Land. In England, St. Bartholomew's and St. Thomas' hospitals were founded by monks in 1123 and 1215. Medicine was practiced by monks and priests in the hostels adjacent to or in designated areas of the monasteries. Peripatetic apothecaries and blood-letting surgeons plied their trade in the houses of their patients and only the destitute, the weary traveler, and those with diseases regarded as hopeless found their way to the hospitals. Special hospitals were founded during this period for the halt, the blind, the aged infirm, lepers, and orphans.

With the arrival of the Renaissance in the late 1200's and the Reformation in the 1500's, the Middle Ages, which had seen the great development of the Christian hospital system, came to a close and the age of individualism and humanism began. The fetters of religious dogma and scholasticism were loosed; new medical curricula were established from the experience at Salerno, Bologna, Montpellier, and Oxford; and the practice of medicine became an important way to make one's living as an individual, intuitive enterprise.

The Reformation Parliament of Henry VIII dissolved the monastery system of England between 1536 and 1539 and the hospital system disappeared with it. Thousands of impoverished and homeless people along with the halt, the blind, the aged infirm, and lepers were cast adrift to roam the countryside. Out of this chaotic and bleak situation arose the voluntary private, nonprofit hospital system of England, the direct forebear of the major part of our American hospital system. First, however, the Royal hospital system came into being when Henry VIII refounded by Royal Charter St. Bartholomew's in 1546 and St. Thomas' in 1552, on a secular basis, the latter named, "The King's Hospital in Southwark."

These two hospitals cared for the entire sick population of London for the next 170 years. Whereas the monastery system had cared for incurables, the sick poor, and those with specific disabilities, the enormous burden shared by these two hospitals forced them to limit their work to the *curable* sick, and in 1700 it is recorded in the orders, "No incurables are to be received"[2] at St. Thomas'. This was an important turning point in the functional evolution of the hospital, which was to lead to its present-day limitations as an acute, curative institution. Simultaneously, it accelerated the development of *separate* institutions for others in need, such as the workhouse for the able-bodied ne'er-do-well and the almshouse for the care of incurables.

With the growth of mercantilism, urbanization, and the Industrial Revolution, individuals were able to amass large fortunes. A social conscience matured and was to find its expression in private philanthropic work. Sir Thomas Guy, a wealthy London merchant, began the construction of a hospital for incurables in 1722, which received its first patients in 1725, one year after his death. Because of ambiguity in his will, it ultimately housed both curable and incurable patients. Guy's Hospital was one of the first voluntary, privately endowed hospitals of modern times, passing to the control of the state, under the National Health Service in 1948, two hundred and twenty-four years after its founding.

The new age saw further development of the medical profession into three main guilds, the Physicians, Barber-Surgeons, and Apothecaries. There were rules for apprenticeship training and licensing, designed to set standards and protect the members from outside domination and unfair competition. The apprentice system of training held sway and the honorary physicians and surgeons of the London hospitals were paid by the apprentice for their training. No longer peripatetic merchants, the physicians gave freely of their time to the care of the sick poor and, imbued with enquiring minds, added to the knowledge of clinical medicine. To provide free medicine for the impoverished, which the Apothecaries had refused to give, the College of Physicians of London founded the first dispensary in 1696.

The eighteenth and particularly the nineteenth centuries in England saw the founding of *special hospitals* because of the social, financial, and medical restrictions for admission to the "general" hospitals; the necessity for segregation of lunatics and patients with infectious diseases; and the desire of the profession to group patients with similar diseases for observation and study. Thus smallpox and venereal disease hospitals in 1746, obstetrical in 1750, and mental in 1751 were followed by fever (1802) and eye (1804) specialty hospitals in London, frequently situated on Harley Street, hence the term, "Harley Street specialist."

It is important to emphasize that during the eighteenth century most of the care given in hospitals was nursing and the hospital remained an institution for the sick poor. The Hôtel Dieu, founded in A.D. 651 by the Bishop of Paris and the oldest hospital in existence today, contained some 2000 beds. In 1788 the death rate amongst patients was nearly 25 per cent and frequently two and sometimes eight patients occupied one bed. Attendants living in the hospital were noted to have an increased death rate of 6 to 12 per cent per year. It wasn't until 1793 that the Convention of the French Revolution ruled that there should be only one patient to a bed and the beds should be separated by at least three feet.[3]

## Origins of the American Hospital

It was the prototype of the British voluntary teaching hospitals of London that ultimately arose in America, but only after more than a century following the first settlements in colonial America. As Shyrock has noted, "In Spanish and French colonies the church set up such institutions more promptly. But the Anglican and non-conformist English churches had given up the hospital tradition, and state or 'voluntary' agencies acted only under the cumulative pressures of public need, secular humanitarianism, and professional initiative." [4]

I shall confine my comments to the Massachusetts Bay Colony and Boston in the evolution of the institutions that housed the sick. I am also primarily concerned here with the development of the university-affiliated teaching hospital and shall therefore finally focus on the Massachusetts General Hospital. Of the roughly 7000 hospitals that exist in the United States today, there are 140 with university affiliation, 1000 accredited as teaching institutions, and over 5000 which are not classified or accredited as teaching institutions. It should also be noted that we are a nation of small hospitals (under 200 beds) and not large ones.

The most powerful stimulus to the founding of the American hospital was the process of urbanization, and indeed the history of the city is the history of social progress (or social decline I might add) in any civilization. Urbanization concentrated the need for care in a small area and provided the tools for the solution of the problems. Public health measures for the segregation of infectious disease in quarantine hospitals very early fell under the jurisdiction of the General Court of Massachusetts, establishing the state's responsibility in these matters. Intellectual activity abounded and flourished in the city. Educational institutions were founded, and finally, schools of medicine which needed institutions where they could teach and learn from first-hand experience.

### Urbanization

The progressive urbanization of Boston was slow initially and gained rapidly only with the arrival of the nineteenth century. The population grew from 4,500 in 1680 to 11,000 in 1720[5] and to 32,896 in 1810.[6] As late as 1845 "Boston remained . . . a town of small traders, of petty artisans and handicraftsmen, and of great merchant princes who built fortunes out of their 'enterprise, intelligence, and frugality.' "[7] The merchant princes amassed their fortunes from entrepreneurial triangular traffic between Boston, Oregon, and Canton; Southern ports and Liverpool; and the West Indies and Russia. The town did not have a fertile back country, had no large source of labor, and lacked the power of a good water supply. Entrepreneurial activity was the only answer. The resultant wealth was wisely invested and Boston became a great center of finance and banking, supplying the money for the first railroads in this country and gaining a firm hold on the development of the textile and shoe industries in Massachusetts. The home of the merchant prince and the petty artisan contained favorable social conditions and in 1790 it was said that poverty and pauperism were declining relative to the total population,[8] and well they might for "Boston offered few opportunities to those who lacked the twin advantages of birth and capital." [9] Most immigrants until the Irish hegira of the 1840's, passed through Boston on their way West or went directly to Philadelphia or New York.

*Institutions for the Care of the Sick*

What of the state of the public's health during this time and the institutions for the care of the sick? The original colonial practice of "outdoor relief" whereby local citizens were paid to take the sick into their homes was soon outmoded as the burden increased and infectious diseases became the main public health problem.

Smallpox was the chief public health problem of the seventeenth and eighteenth centuries. Major epidemics hit Boston at least four times between 1644 and 1689 and seven times in the eighteenth century beginning in 1721 with the last great epidemic in 1792. The General Court had taken measures in 1699 and 1700 to provide for the isolation of townsfolk and quarantine of ships crews known to have "the plague, small pox, pestilential or malignant feaver, or other contagious sickness, the infection whereof may probably be communicated to others." [10] The earlier pesthouse was replaced by the quarantine hospital built on Spectacle Island by the order of the General Court in 1717. This was abandoned later and was replaced by one on Rainsford Island in 1737 which was managed by the Town Selectmen.

Some idea of the seriousness and magnitude of the smallpox epidemic can be gained from the figures in 1721, when the disease was introduced by the infected crew of a British ship newly arrived from the West Indies. With a total population of 10,700 in the town, 5,759 contracted the disease and 842 died, nearly 8 per cent of the total population. It was during this epidemic that Cotton Mather had written to Dr. Zabdiel Boylston, urging him to try the inoculation method developed by Timoni of Constantinople. Subsequently, he inoculated 242 persons in nearby towns with only 6 deaths. After much prolonged controversy, inoculation hospitals for the practice of inoculation and segregation of infected patients were approved and set up by the General Court as well as private physicians between 1764 and 1790. The "Grand Inoculation Hospital" was Dr. William Aspinwall's and it had 150 beds. Games, music, and parades were arranged for the inmates.

The inoculation hospital disappeared with the introduction of Jenner's vaccination by Professor Benjamin Waterhouse of the Harvard Medical School in 1800.

The first almshouse in Boston opened its doors in 1665. It was consumed by fire and a new one was built in 1686, which by 1790 had 300 occupants.[11] A bridewell for the disorderly and the insane in the early 1700's and a workhouse for the able-bodied ne'er-do-wells built in 1735 were immediately adjacent. It was stated that ". . . the earlier almshouses of Massachusetts were indicative of all that is evil in the eyes of social service. They admitted of slight if any separation of the sexes. They afforded no classification according to age. They housed little children with the prostitute, the vagrant, the drunkard, the idiot and the maniac . . . they were schools for crime — breeders of immorality and chronic pauperism," [12] and, I might add, they facilitated the transmission of infectious disease among the impoverished sick.

In 1800, a new almshouse, designed by Charles Bulfinch, was built on the north side of Leverett Street in the West End of Boston, which was to stand until 1825. The Reverend John Bartlett was its Chaplain, a fortunate assignment as will be shown.

Meanwhile another institution, the forerunner of the present-day ambulatory medical clinic, was established through the efforts of the Massachusetts Humane Society, which had been founded in 1780. This was the Boston Dispensary, which was founded in 1796 for two reasons: so that the sick could be cared for in their own houses and so that they could be assisted at less expense to the public than in a hospital or the almshouse.[13] Although described as a drug store with a physician for ambulatory patients,[14] it served both the humanitarian and the economical reason for its existence.

A final institution for the care of the sick was established at the turn of the nineteenth century. The Boston Marine Society had agitated for the construction of a hospital at their meeting in October 1790. Its purpose was to care for merchant mariners, frequently far from home, where most medical care was being given for those fortunate enough to avoid the pesthouses. A congressional bill entitled, "An Act for the Relief of Sick and Disabled Seamen" was signed by President John Adams on July 16, 1798, and established a form of governmental compulsory sickness and accident insurance to provide medical care and hospitalization for seamen by the collection of *20¢ per month* per mariner on every American merchant ship coming from a foreign port.[15] In 1803 a Marine hospital was completed in Charlestown for the port of Boston, and in 1804 the one that had been located in the barracks buildings at Fort Independence on Castle Island since 1799 moved to the new quarters. The new institution housed an average of 30 patients.

Thus, progressing from outdoor relief to pesthouse, quarantine and inoculation hospitals, to the dispensary, the almshouse, and finally, the Marine hospital, there remained no single institution adequate to care humanely or safely for the impoverished sick of Boston, who could not be cared for in their homes.

### The Medical Profession and Medical Education

The medical profession and the founding of the Harvard Medical School in 1782 must now be considered, as they played a crucial role ultimately in the founding of the Massachusetts General Hospital. Colonial America, whether for praise or blame, was traditionally English. The middle classes emigrated to America and the first physicians were "ships surgeons" or apprentices from London hospitals, and not English physicians who enjoyed high social prestige and good incomes in London. Most of the early practitioners were nomadic surgeon-apothecaries, and commonly, ministers doubling as physicians. Medical education consisted of the indentured apprentice system. On the eve of the Revolution, only 5 per cent of the 3,500 established medical practitioners held degrees, and scarcely 10 per cent had had any formal training.[16]

Harvard College had been founded in 1636 on a strongly puritanical and theological basis and its first two presidents, in keeping with the times, were minister-physicians. Its second and third presidents were graduates in medicine of Cambridge, England. By 1700, there were said to be 26 graduates of Harvard College who had practiced medicine in New England, although none had a medical degree.[17] The indentured apprentice system remained the main form of medical education.

In 1772 Dr. Ezekiel Hersey of Hingham left 1000 pounds to Harvard College to support a resident professor of anatomy and surgery. Edward Augustus Holyoke of Salem, a graduate of Harvard College in 1746, had amongst his many apprentices, John

Warren. On September 19, 1782, the Harvard Corporation adopted some 22 articles, probably written by John Warren, which established the Harvard Medical School. John Warren in Anatomy and Surgery, Benjamin Waterhouse, a Quaker, M.D. Leiden, 1780, in Physic, and Aaron Dexter in Chemistry and Materia Medica were appointed the first three professors. The first lectures were given in the basement of Harvard Hall in the fall of 1784 and thence the quarters were shifted to Harvard's Holden Chapel.

This new method of teaching which was in direct competition with the individual indentured apprentice system was not universally applauded, as is shown by the several public clashes of the Massachusetts Medical Society with the new medical school in Cambridge. The Society, founded in 1781, demanded the right to examine and license all physicians,[18] prevented the faculty from using the Boston Almshouse for the teaching of medical students in 1784, and defeated a proposal by the Harvard Corporation to the General Court for the establishment of a "public infirmary" in Cambridge for the care of the sick and the teaching of medical students.[19] The Boston Medical Society (founded in 1780 and the forerunner of the Massachusetts Medical Society) wrote that "the scheme of annexing a Medical Establishment in this Town to the College in Cambridge is not only impractical, but nugatory." [20] Fortunately for the democratic concepts of our young nation, it was not discovered until later how wrong this "majority vote" would prove to be.

In 1782 John Warren was appointed to care for the sick in the almshouse (on Park Street) and, although he took his apprentices there, it was not until 1810 that Harvard medical students were allowed to enter the new almshouse on Leverett Street for clinical training. At this time the almshouse had approximately 350 occupants of which about 50 were sick and infirm. Medical education at Harvard consisted of two winters of lectures and a third year as apprentice to a practitioner before the student could qualify for his degree in medicine. Benjamin Waterhouse urged the use of the new Boston Marine Hospital for teaching medical students and was Chief Physician there in 1807. Professor Waterhouse was to be succeeded by James Jackson on September 15, 1812, at the Harvard Medical School. In 1810 the medical school had moved from Cambridge to Boston in rooms over W. B. White's apothecary shop (the present location of Filene's Department Store). In 1816 it was to move to Mason Street and thence to the head of North Grove Street adjacent to the Massachusetts General Hospital in 1847. Thirty-six years later it was to make another move to larger quarters in the newly developed Back Bay almost equidistant between the Massachusetts General Hospital and the rapidly growing Boston City Hospital in the South End. The Boston City Hospital had opened its doors in 1864 to meet the growing needs of a rapidly expanding immigrant population, drawn from Ireland during the great potato famines.

## The Founding of the Massachusetts General Hospital

We have attempted to describe the various factors that were to result in the founding of the Massachusetts General Hospital in 1811 — the advent of Christianity with its humanitarian spirit; the age of individualism with its development of the merchant prince with a social conscience, indulging in benevolent philanthropic work; the process of urbanization with its resultant concentration of misery and social need, as well as with its concentration of energy, intellect, and resource which could provide for social needs; the relative inadequacy of the existing institutions for the care of the sick; and finally, the rise of the enquiring medical mind, scientific thought, and the new concern for an improvement in medical education requiring that a hospital be available for teaching.

The well-to-do were cared for in their homes, a situation which was to prevail until the turn of the twentieth century. Philadelphia and New York had already established their hospitals under almost identical but better developed circumstances and the Boston philanthropists and doctors were equally anxious to have such a humanitarian institution grace their city.

The stage was set and the sequence of events seems totally rational. All the factors and forces for the creation of such an institution were present and in person. A minister, the Rev. John Bartlett, the Chaplain of the Boston Almshouse, called the meeting spurred on by the Christian ethic and the inhumane conditions in the almshouse. James Jackson and John Collins Warren were present representing the medical profession and the needs for medical education. The merchant princes were represented by John Phillips and Peter Brooks.[21] The letter that Warren and Jackson were to compose to the wealthy and influential citizens of Boston and the subsequent report of the legislative committee recommending the state's approval of the hospital's charter summarize beautifully the social need for such an institution and the responsibility with which it would be charged.

The legislative report stated: "The Hospital, thus established, is intended to be a receptacle for patients from all parts of the Commonwealth, afflicted with diseases of a peculiar nature, requiring the most skilful treatment, and presenting cases for instruction in the study and practice of surgery and physic. Among the unfortunate objects of this charitable project, particular provision is to be made for such as the wisdom of Providence may have seen fit to visit with the most terrible of all human maladies — a deprivation of reason . . ." [22]

On February 25, 1811, the General Court granted a charter for the incorporation of the Massachusetts General Hospital to James Bowdoin and 55 other prominent Bostonians. Active interest and participation by the State in the conduct and maintenance of the hospital was assured from the outset, not only through repeated financial aid, but by the practice which continues to this day of the governor's appointment of 4 of the 12 trustees.

The War of 1812 interfered with the raising of funds, but by 1817 enough private money was available so that final aid from the state in the form of prison labor and granite allowed the construction to begin. Charles Bulfinch was the architect. James Jackson was appointed Physician and John C. Warren, Surgeon to the Massachusetts General Hospital. On September 3, 1821, the first patient was admitted, and no other application was made until September 20th.[23] The first "Annual Report," printed in March 1822, contained what today would be regarded as direct advertising. It began, "We entreat all those into whose hands this address may fall, to reflect well upon the advantages which this Institution offers . . ." and then listed the comforts and advantages of hospital care.[24] The public was slow to forget their experiences in the pesthouse and almshouse and as late as 1849 the hospital was yet to be completely filled.[25]

By 1823, the west wing of the Bulfinch building was completed and there was a total of 93 beds. In 1824 the trustees ordered that medical students and doctors attending operations should be admitted free of charge, rather than be charged by the staff.

In the early years (as well as today), the most pressing problem was the discrepancy between the expense of running the hospital and the income from patients, friends, and endowment. The free bed subscription idea was instituted by the Massachusetts Humane Society in 1824, when it gave the hospital enough money to support 6 free beds for 5 years. Subsequent annual drives were conducted for gifts for the support of free beds and in 1826 "23 beds were occupied . . . at an everage expense of $3.52 per week for an average stay of 5½ weeks." [26]

## Three Contributions of the Hospital as a Social Instrument

I would like now to narrow our historical view to three examples of one hospital's role as a social instrument — that combined or total institutional effort which enabled the hospital to contribute solutions to the social problems of the times. These are the founding and development of the McLean Hospital, Medical Social Service, and the Baker Memorial Plan. There are others, but these represent examples of the social conscience of the hospital and a total institutional effort to fulfill the needs of the community. The contributions were unique and represent a pioneering effort by the Massachusetts General Hospital.

### McLean Hospital

We have reviewed some of the conditions which resulted in the state's charter of the hospital designating the humane treatment of the mentally ill as one of its prime functions. The shackling of lunatics in the almshouse, the extreme financial and emotional expense of caring for such patients, and the necessity for their segregation from the community as well as the other occupants of the almshouse were the main considerations. In England, the inhuman treatment of the insane was slowly being rectified through the efforts of John Howard and William Tuke, both Quakers. In 1792, the York Retreat was founded by Tuke — stressing kindness; no restraints; and a favorable environment as regarded food, lodging, occupational work, fresh air, and exercise. In the same year Philippe Pinel, the great advocate of "moral treatment," was placed in charge of the large Paris institution, the Bicêtre, for insane men. His success in "striking off the chains" of the insane here and later at the Salpêtrière Hospital for women was perhaps the turning point in the humane and moral treatment of the insane.[27] Prior to that time the insane had been social outcasts. The public paid an admission fee to watch the bizarre activity at St. Mary of Bethlehem in England, more popularly known as "Bedlam."

The trustees of the Massachusetts General Hospital proceeded with dispatch and by 1818 the first patient was admitted to what was then called the Asylum in Charlestown, a mansion redesigned by Bulfinch. The name was changed to the McLean Asylum for the Insane in 1826 and was known as such until 1892, when it became the McLean Hospital. In 1833, Dr. Rufus Wyman, the first superintendent, wrote, "chains or strait jackets have never been used or provided in this asylum."[28] Dr. Luther Bell, appointed in 1836, gave considerable support to the efforts of Dorothea Dix, by his professional statements on the treatment of the mentally ill, and therefore at least indirectly aided Miss Dix's efforts to correct the squalor, crowding, and heartless indifference that she found in the state asylums.[29] By 1847, in contrast with the General Hospital, the Asylum was full, with 173 patients, and only two-thirds of all who applied could be admitted.

In 1882 the new superintendent, Dr. Edward Cowles, established a training school for psychiatric nurses and this was the first such school to be established in a mental hospital in America. At the turn of the century he also established the importance of biological research in mental illness with the addition of Otto Folin and Philip Schaeffer to the staff.

More recently (1962), the new McLean Rehabilitation Center has been opened with its day care, educational and vocational units, civic center, and music therapy room. With the introduction of newer methods of treatment in psychiatry, particularly the use of drugs ("tranquilizers," if you will), and the tendency for society and the community to reintegrate the mentally ill into their own care, this effort should facilitate the ambulatory and day care of patients who can now be cared for in their homes. This should help to reduce the cost and obviate the necessity of prolonged and expensive in-hospital care for an ever-increasing segment of the population that wants and needs psychiatric help.

*Medical Social Service*

The second example of an institutional social conscience arose in 1905, after Dr. Richard Cabot had been appointed physician to the Out-Patient Department in the new out-patient building. As Washburn stated,

From its very earliest days the General Hospital has shown an interest in its patients' problems and a humane attempt to lighten their burdens. When the Hospital was a small affair, the Trustees themselves visited the patients regularly. In many instances they saw to it that relief over and above medical care was provided. As doctors and patients and Hospital officers were a small family, the troubles of the patients, the underlying causes of their disease, their disposition upon discharge were considered, and often remedied and alleviated . . . the Resident Physician (Director) or his assistant took great pains to see to it that discharged patients were properly escorted to their homes, that patients left on the doorstep were suitably placed, and that allied administrative problems were handled as humanely and efficiently as the means and facilities at their disposal would permit. The problems were not so difficult when New England had a homogeneous, uncrowded population, with a good standard of living.

With the tremendous unrestricted immigration of the latter part of the 19th and the early part of the 20th century, the difficulties became greater and more complex.[30]

It was Dr. Richard Cabot who recognized the necessity for a more coordinated and formalized program of social help when he employed two full-time workers in 1905, whose sole function was service for problems relating to the care of the patient. Their report in 1906 listed their work which included hygiene teaching, infant feeding and care, "vacations and country outings" where it seemed a necessary part of treatment, help in finding jobs or changing jobs according to the medical need, provision for patients "dumped" at the hospital, and "assistance to patients needing treatment after discharge from the hospital wards." The report of 1918 added utilization of "all the sanataria, convalescent homes, vacation funds, employment agencies and charitable agencies that may . . . help the patient or his family to pay for the medicine, apparatus, or vacation that may assure recovery."

In 1914 the trustees appointed Miss Ida Cannon Chief of Hospital Social Service. The service developed rapidly, demonstrated its usefulness, and in 1919 was made a department of the hospital. In 1930 the service was extended to McLean Hospital as well as the newly opened Baker Memorial, where Miss Cannon appointed Miss Josephine Barbour the head. This was important because it established the fact that Social Service is needed at all economic levels.

By 1935, Dr. Washburn could write, "No hospital in the United States, of any size worthy of the name, is without such a department, and in many other countries the example has been followed." [31]

Expensive? Yes — very much so. In 1918 the expenses of the department were roughly $25,000. In 1961 the expenses exceeded $250,000. The value of the contributions cannot be priced however, and under Miss Barbour's guidance now, it continues as a vital example of the social conscience of the hospital and its determination to fulfill optimally its primary function, the care of the sick.

### The Baker Memorial Hospital and Fee Plan of 1930

In 1917 the Phillips House was opened and for the first time provided completely private rooms for the well-to-do, a milestone of great significance as will be shown later. This left a large segment of the population unable to afford completely private care and unable to qualify for admission to the General Hospital and its wards. As Washburn said in 1914, "This group in the community must often be ill in their homes, dependent upon physicians who cannot provide the necessary laboratory tests and scientific examinations which are readily available in a general hospital." [32]

Sixteen years later on February 27, 1930, the Baker Memorial Hospital for patients of moderate means was opened, the patients being admitted if they fell within certain income limits. The average income of the patients admitted during the first year of operation was $2,101.74. Hospital charges were $6.50 per day for a single room and $4.50 for a four-bedded room. The staff had agreed to a set of fees regulated by the hospital, with a maximum of $150 no matter how long the patient stayed or how complicated the condition. As Dr. Washburn wrote: "The Massachusetts General Hospital is blessed with a medical and surgical staff which is public spirited and desires to co-operate with the Hospital in any progressive movement for the good of the community. Of its own volition the staff has agreed to accept at the Baker Memorial a small regulated fee for its professional services." [33]

In this first year, the average all-inclusive charge was $158.94. The average length of stay was 13 days. Fifteen per cent of the patients needed special nursing care with an average additional charge of $121.40, demonstrating vividly how important and costly special nursing care was even in those days.

The experiment was a success and the patient of moderate means was indeed protected from excessive hospital costs and professional fees. Here stands a fine example of a cooperative institutional effort to solve a pressing social and economic problem of medicine — doctors, administration, and trustees working together to utilize the maximum potential of the hospital as a social instrument.

## THE PAST TO THE PRESENT

Turning back once more in an attempt to summarize the critical events which were to determine the place of today's hospital in contemporary life, we note that in 1850, the beds of the Bulfinch building were yet to be completely filled and roughly 10 per cent of admissions died in hospital.[34] Hospital care consisted of food, shelter, and the comforting ministrations of a nurse. Individuals with means avoided the hospital and were treated at home or in the doctor's office. The life-threatening dangers of cross-infection in surgical wounds, known as "hospitalism," were yet to come under some semblance of control.

Meanwhile, medicine as a social science was gaining momentum. In Germany in 1848 Neumann and Virchow were advocating that the state concern itself with health; that there be established a critical interrelationship of health to social, economic, and political conditions; and finally, that social action be taken to maintain health and combat disease. In England, John Simon, serving as Central Medical Officer from 1855 to 1876, was to establish the obligatory relationship of health to social progress and the necessary intervention of the State in matters of the public health. Following the work of Pasteur and Koch, public health and preventive medicine was splintered off from clinical medicine and concerned itself mainly with sanitary reform and the control of communicable disease, a situation which persists to this day.

The hospital began to assume shape and form as an acute, curative, health-restoring institution following the discovery at Massachusetts General Hospital in 1846 that ether could be used as an anesthetic agent. This has been called justifiably the most important single contribution of American medicine during the nineteenth century. The surgical experience gained during the Civil War enabled the surgeon to deal more effectively with disease and the work of Lister in the 1860's, following Pasteur's discoveries, led to the development of the carbolic acid spray which was to result in better control of cross-infection of surgical wounds in the hospital. The pioneer work of Florence Nightingale at Scutari, in the Crimean War, between 1854 and 1856, was to establish the importance of nursing in reducing the morbidity and mortality of disease and result in the founding of nursing schools in hospitals.

Meanwhile, the introduction of science and the scientific method, which had its origins with Bacon, Descartes, and Galileo in the sixteenth and seventeenth centuries began to affect medicine and hospitals. The nineteenth century was notable for the development of clinical medicine, physiology, and pathology and the description of clinico-pathological entities. Guy's Hospital flowered with such giants as Bright, Addison, and Hodgkin. In this country, such men as O. W. Holmes, Marion Sims, Daniel Drake, and Reginald Fitz took the lead. Clinical investigation flowered locally when Fitz described the clinical and pathological condition of appendicitis in 1886. Meanwhile President Eliot of Harvard had succeeded in extending the course of instruction in the medical school to three years with formal lectures and laboratories and mandatory attendance.[35]

The new developments in pathology and bacteriology were recognized, and in 1896 a laboratory for pathology, clinical chemistry, and bacteriology was established at the Massachusetts General Hospital with James Homer Wright (of the Wright stain) at its head. Both service to patients and research were established immediately. As if these developments were not enough to contend with, Roentgen announced the discovery of x-rays in 1895.

By 1901, Walter Dodd, apothecary and photographer to the Massachusetts General Hospital, built an x-ray machine for the hospital, an historic event presaging what is today a massive and expensive technology in the fields of x-ray diagnosis and treatment.

It was David Linn Edsall who established clinical investigation and the full-time support of teacher-investigators at the Massachusetts General Hospital. From 1912, when he came as Chief of the East Medical Service, to 1924, when he became Dean of the Harvard Medical School, he created and maintained a good environment for the enquiring mind and displayed unusual ability in picking the right men, such as James Howard Means, George Minot, and Paul Dudley White.

With the development of the clinical chemistry laboratory, the institution of x-ray machinery for diagnosis and treatment, the examination of pathological tissues at the time of operation by the technique of frozen section, the establishment of full-time heads of the Departments of Medicine and Surgery in 1912, all added to the use of anesthesia, the better control of hospitalism, and the professionalization of nursing, the "peripatetic home surgeon" (and much later the medical man) now found it best to do his work in the hospital and society agreed — it was safer and the technical equipment as well as the experts were there. The opening of the Phillips House in 1917 as a division of the Massachusetts General Hospital for the well-to-do stands as a milestone in this change of attitude which was to result in the development of the hospital as a health center. People who could afford to avoid the hospital now came to it with what was to become increasing hope, instead of fear.

The first three decades of the twentieth century saw the establishment of mass immunization procedures and an expanding role for departments of public health, the discovery of insulin, liver diet in pernicious anemia, as well as other advances in the field of nutrition, cholecystography, blood grouping and successful blood transfusion, and antibiotics, to say nothing of the increasing triumphs of surgery.

The great depression of 1929 brought the social and economic problems of medicine into sharp relief and the 1930's saw the establishment of the Blue Cross system of health insurance, the Social

Security Act, and on the local scene the building of the Baker Memorial.

By 1935 the Baker Memorial and the Baker Plan initiated for patients of moderate means were successfully filling the gap between the Phillips House and the General Hospital. Medical education had expanded to four years of rigorous undergraduate work followed by anywhere from one to five years of hospital-based postgraduate (house staff) training. Research support was listed at $51,639.[36] There were 728 beds. The daily rate was under $4 in the General Hospital to a top of $12 in the Phillips House. There were nearly 15,000 patients admitted and 300,000 visits to the Outpatient Department.

Dr. Nathaniel Faxon, Director of the Massachusetts General Hospital from 1935 to 1949, played a major role in organizing Massachusetts Blue Cross and signed the hospital's first contract in 1937. Hospitals agree to provide hospitalization and stipulated services by contract, regardless of cost of these services to the hospital. As of December 1962, over 141 million people (76 per cent of the population) had some form of health insurance and nearly one-half of these had Blue Cross.[37] Major medical expense coverage (initial deductible clause and payment of 75 to 80 per cent of remaining bills up to 5, 10, or $15,000) has enjoyed remarkable growth to the point where over 38 million people enjoyed this protection, an increase of 4½ million people over 1961.[38]

The past twenty years have seen the development of tranquilizers and reintegration of mental patients into the community; the steady expansion of medical research through federal support and the establishment of a separate Department of Health, Education and Welfare; advances in cardiovascular surgery; transplantation of organs and reimplantation of severed extremities; and the steady accumulation of social and economic problems attendant upon the successes of medicine. Today's problems concern a rapidly expanding aged population with chronic disease and the fact that over 50 per cent of our hospital beds in this country are filled with patients with mental disease. Rising costs and rising expectations; the increasing short supply of doctors, nurses, and technical help; and the problems of financing care and the necessary facilities occupy the center stage.

## CONCLUSION

This brief review has traced the historical foundations of the American teaching hospital. It has stressed the role of the hospital as a social instrument and new departures have been suggested. The hospital has now emerged as the "health center" and provides the platform on which the profession meets the public. Its tremendous responsibility is matched by an equally great opportunity as an organized, coordinated social instrument for the study and solution of the social and economic problems which beset medicine and the community today. Medical schools and the staffs of many hospitals have not turned their faces readily to these problems. Health has now become a birthright and the benefits of medical science must be available to all. The public looks with rising expectations to the medical profession and its political representation, and the hospital finds itself squarely in the middle, providing the center stage where all the forces meet.

The Lowell Lectures have been established to bring a number of experts here to comment upon the social and economic problems of medicine and hospitals today. Hopefully, their perturbations and peregrinations will enlighten both community and hospital as regards their mutual problems and stimulate their possible solutions.

# THE BALANCED BIOLOGY
# OF THE TEACHING HOSPITAL

## John H. Knowles, M.D.

THE time-honored functions of the teaching hospital are the indivisible and interdependent triad of patient care, teaching, and research. The present conventional wisdom states that the medical school's launching pad rests on an immovable and indisputably appropriate foundation of basic, biologic science for the first two years, followed by two more years of clinical training in the subdivisions of medicine. This, in turn, is followed by two to six years of postgraduate training in an accredited teaching hospital with one or two years' additional time in a "research laboratory." Armed with M.D. and "boards," the physician can now practice medicine, do research, and teach, or attempt varying combinations of all three, depending on the predominance of the influences and attitudes that have prevailed upon him at home, in school, and finally in the world at large. With the present massive technical facilities of medicine, he must locate his office as a practicing physician in or as near as possible to the hospital and spend increasing amounts of time there, utilizing all the machines, health personnel, fellow specialists, and available agencies that can be brought to bear on the patient's problems, all the while ministering directly to the needs of his patient. Suddenly, the social, economic, and political realities of medical practice and hospital life are thrust upon him, literally overnight.

His bedfellows in the teaching hospital are a curious and motley crew: the administrator in the dark suit, whose name he doesn't know and who is concerned mainly with "money"; the research worker with frayed coat, carrying an ice bucket and preoccupied with thoughts of DNA and RNA, whose lectures he cannot under-

This material was presented in part as one of the annual Alpha Omega Lectures at Boston University, and it is reprinted from the *New England Journal of Medicine*, 269:401–406, 450–455 (August 22 and 29, 1963).

stand; the harassed nurse, obliged to give everything it seems but personal care at the bedside; the social worker, arranging for the nursing home; the bevy of technicians and the clinical and research fellows, who multiply exponentially each year; the maintenance man, who seems eternally preoccupied with elevators and light bulbs; and a variety of other people, who might be accountants, housekeepers, or visitors, the last looking dazed, worried, and usually asking for directions. Finally, at regular intervals on a certain day of the week, a procession of distinguished-looking "businessmen" hurry in as the great oak door near the front entrance of the hospital swings shut, to indulge in a continuing series of rather mysterious deliberations with the hospital's director.

All told, roughly 10,000 people daily pass through the doors of the urban teaching hospital with 1000 beds. Of this 10,000 people, over 4000 work there, 2000 are sick and seeking help, 2000 are accompanying or visiting the sick, and the rest are "doing business" with the people who work there. It is this frenetic microcosm with which the individual physician is concerned, in which the major part of his professional life is spent, and that he is inadequately prepared to understand. It is this microcosm of individuals, groups, skills, and machines, and the balance of all their activities, that collectively describes the function and direction of the teaching hospital.

## THE INDIVIDUALS

The hospital remains highly individualistic in its function as a complex organization because of the intensely personal and critical nature of its work. The individual patient and his care remains the elemental reason for the existence of the hospital. The individual doctor enjoys a necessary degree of autonomy and authority in the hospital that serves the best interests of his patient. These two individuals form the primary human equation around which the hospital is structured so far as its buildings, its people, and its machines are concerned. That a hospital is only as good as its staff is a time-honored verity. The hospital's influence and its place in society, however, are determined by its community of patients. They, and only they, can judge the end result.

The tremendous expansion of science in the past half-century has led to an enormous increase in medical knowledge and medical technology, which in turn has necessitated the development of specialization. Therefore, the doctor has become increasingly dependent on the hospital and on other health personnel. The patient has endured more encounters with more people and more machines leading to discontinuity, less personal care, and increasing costs. Both doctor and patient remain highly individualistic in their hospital needs, but now, other people and other things are necessary for the best care of the patient. With the increasing subdivision of labor in all areas of the health profession, medicine has changed from an individual, intuitive, and intensely personal enterprise into a highly complex, interdependent, and increasingly impersonal social service. The individual patient and his own individual doctor should always form the most crucial and enduring relation in medical care. Both are concerned about the increasing discontinuity of care attendant upon specialization, which is reducing the ability of both patient and doctor to maintain this basic relation. A detailed look at some of the individuals and their problems is necessary here.

## The Patient

The individual who ultimately becomes the subject of the teaching hospital's efforts is, in most cases, a highly selected person. It has been estimated that in a period of one month, in an adult population of 1000, subjective illness or injury will be experienced by 750 people, and 250 of these will seek the advice of a physician. In turn, 9 of them will be hospitalized, 5 will be referred to another physician, and 1, and only 1, will find himself, by referral in a teaching (university-affiliated) hospital! [1] Before the patient reaches the doctor, and depending on his own cultural beliefs and other attitudes, he will have indulged for varying periods in a definite sequence of events involving, first, self-diagnosis, followed by consultation with family, friends, the corner druggist, or even a "casual" exploration of the local doctor at cocktails. Finally, in the nonemergency situation, a trial of procrastination and self-treatment ensues. If the patient is a doctor or a nurse the time involved in this ritual is usually extended considerably before final "surrender" to medical authority.[2]

In the emergency or complicated situation, he will be referred to the emergency ward of the urban teaching hospital by himself, his friends, or his doctor, or he will be transferred from the scene by the police or from another hospital. Transfer from community hospitals may occur because of any one or a combination of the following: the patient or his family requests it; the community doctor feels the need for specialist consultation; there is a need for special techniques available only in the teaching hospital; and, rarely, because the patient is unable to pay the local bills. The emergency ward of the urban hospital has become the doctor for the aged and medically indigent, particularly on weekends and at night. There are many reasons for its ever-increasing use, including convenience for both patient and doctor and the fact that the public has accepted the hospital as a medical center and looks to the institution and its technical facilities for its medical care.[3]

The ward services of teaching hospitals today contain a highly selected patient population of the medically indigent. If there is no selective and exclusive admitting procedure the average patient is elderly and has been admitted through the emergency ward with one of the degenerative diseases or cancer. The signs of his disease and the results of special tests are more important to the diagnosis than the history. House staff and medical students are taught and learn here.

Over the past fifteen years, with the enormous growth of Blue Cross and other third-party payers, the patient who was formerly admitted to the ward service now finds himself on the semiprivate service, as his means are judged by his health insurance and, to a now lesser extent, his income. Health insurance has become an important "fringe benefit," and roughly three-quarters of health insurance is provided by employers. Therefore, the active, wage-earning population (the great middle class of America) now has the right to a semiprivate bed and a private doctor. Consequently, the semiprivate service cares for the man power of the nation and generally represents a better cross-section of the "active" community's health needs and wants. There is much organic disease in this group, as well as more patients with mental illness, than one finds on the ward service. The care and rehabilitation of this group is crucial to their heavily dependent, growing families and is equally vital to the economy of the country.

As one moves on to the private service, one again finds an aged population with cancer and degenerative disease, and an older, actively working executive group with cardiovascular and psychosomatic disease. In contradistinction to the ward service there are more patients with alcoholism and psychoneurosis, as well as more diseases in their subtle, incipient stages. Here, the history is more important to the diagnosis than the signs of disease. The patients are more articulate in their demands as well as in giving their histories. More preventive medicine is practiced here. The least teaching of house staff and medical students is done here, a peculiar paradox.

To turn from the objective to the subjective patient, as he enters the hospital acutely ill, he assumes the sick role of selfishness, egocentricity, and passive dependency.[4] There is a marked constriction of interests and a heightening of sensory acuity. He accepts with faith the technical competence of the institution and wants primarily personal care and a steady atmosphere of caring about himself. With his hypersensitivity and hyperacuity, he is able to judge this critically and is a hard taskmaster. Frequent tests and encounters with a steady succession of medical students, house officers, and consultants produce an ambivalent state of mind. He yearns for personal and continuous care but feels depersonalized as he is stripped of his clothes and has no clock or calendar on his wall to tell him who or where or "when" he is. He feels like a guinea pig and thinks he is being "used" for the benefit of the scientist and the student of medicine. People are learning and benefiting from his being there, and he wonders how much his bill is being run up because of it. At the opposite end of the pole he believes that many people are helping him to get well, and he is the center of attraction.

At the time of discharge from the hospital he is presented with his bill, which, for an average stay of ten days, may amount to $500, without the doctor's fee. If he is over sixty-five he has stayed an average of fifteen days at a cost nearer $750, which for a little over 50 per cent of the entire aged population represents three quarters of annual income.[5] After the initial shock a number of questions enter his mind, and he is unable to find answers from friends and, just as frequently, from his doctor. The day rate is incredible as he compares it with the only comparison available to him, the hotel. Nobody has told him that the 1000-bed hotel has 1000 employees whereas the comparable hospital has nearly 4000 employees. Nobody has explained the "room service" of the hospital and reminded him of the costs of room service in the hotel. Little does he know that only 30 per cent of his total bill represents the hotel function of the hospital and that 70 per cent is what he cannot get in a hotel and is controlled by his doctor. The costs of nursing and dietary service do not come readily to mind, as well as many other special facets of the hospital. He wonders about teaching and research and how much they contribute to the bill. This, in short, has been one of medicine's failures, to explain adequately why costs *are* so high in teaching hospitals and why they will continue to rise. The costs remain unjustified in large segments of the public mind through a combination of ignorance and frustrated inability to afford them. Health has become a basic inalienable birthright, and its procurement, the public believes, should not interfere with other rights such as housing, food, the enjoyment of leisure, and credit.

The patient on the private service respects and admires his doctor. The poor and impoverished of the United States, which may number some 40,000,000, or one quarter of the total population (family income less than $4,000, and single person's income less than $2,000 per year — thus including the house staffs of most teaching hospitals!) and have been termed "our invisible poor," [6] are more likely to share the attitudes expressed by Friedson: they "will continue to get along but will present the evasive, resentful but desperately demanding face to the medical world that all people present when confronted by forces they cannot control, which they know are sometimes indifferent to them, but which they cannot do without." [7]

## The Doctor

Turning to the doctor, when and why did he decide to become one? Was it a deep-felt need for love and adulation, individuality and independence, power over people and money, emulation of his father, or just plain interest in man, and more recently, an interest in biological science? Whatever the reason, being a doctor remains one of the most honorable and biologically unassailable ways of earning one's living and spending one's life, and the physician remains, as R. L. Stevenson said, "the flower . . . of our civilization." By what course did he finally reach his position in the teaching hospital?

First of all, one should turn one's attention to the premedical student. Once he has declared himself, two forces are set in motion, neither of which is entirely desirable. The first is acceleration of the curriculum, and the second is an "overwhelming obsession for science," [8] so that his interests are constricted and restricted and the liberal arts are not given the full measure of attention. What emerges from college may thus be an incomplete product, politically and socially naïve, and not optimally prepared to be, as Lionel Trilling[9] has said, "at home in and in control of the modern world, . . . the true purpose of all study." President Pusey,[10] of Harvard, has said, "The humanities have a very special place in a university, especially perhaps because of the pleasure they give, but also because of the heightened effects which experience of them can produce in individuals in terms of enlivened imagination, increased responsiveness, broadened interest, clarified purpose and in the end also, quickened ethical sense."

The medical school curriculum accelerates the constricting effect of his premedical education by its complete emphasis on a foundation of basic science in the first two years of medical school. The opportunity still exists to introduce the liberal arts, humanities, and social sciences of *medicine* but is not seized. The history of medicine, its people, its institutions, and its social setting is neglected, as are the politics and the economics of medicine. The student is relentlessly forced to focus on the individual doctor-patient relation as an object, and his own subjective self-understanding and his understanding of the world around him flags.

At the end of his four years he is a highly individualistic person, trained to take immediate action with the individual patient and to expect immediate rewards, with his knowledge firmly grounded in science. The primary purpose of medical education — that is, to understand disease and to be able to manage sick people — *has* been fulfilled, but the broader issue of the physician's place and problems in the world at large has been neglected. The world of the health profession and its institutions has been left undescribed and unstudied.

During his medical school days the student's acculturation takes a number of interesting tacks. As his intellect grows, he simultaneously acquires the values, attitudes, habits, and expectations of his profession through didactic teaching sessions, as well as, and more importantly, through constant, informal association with the faculty and "the others" who habitate the hospital. His understanding of these people is acquired informally and intuitively. It has to be, because his curriculum does not include a study of the sociology of these groups or the complex institution known as the hospital. His knowledge of the nurse and the nursing profession is acquired informally outside working hours. He begins to assign various specialists and specialties to his own system of values. He views the internist as a thinker and the surgeon as the doer, cavalier, forceful and occupying the central stage of the theater. The pediatrician is short, frequently plump, quiet and gentle natured, endomorphic and motherly. The radiologist, the dermatologist, and the eye, ear, nose, and throat man are associated with good hours and large income. The neurologist is thought to be an extremely profound, careful thinker with infinite patience. The neurosurgeon is marveled at for his emotional strength in the face of such high mortality in his patients. The hospital administrator is usually never seen or known but is generally viewed as a low-order businessman hired to keep the place clean. If he is a doctor he was "unable to make it" in the practice of medicine and wanted "better hours."

Having acquired knowledge of disease and the "subculture" of medicine, he begins his long stint on the house staff and rapidly acquires the technical competence of his particular specialty. He enjoys for the first time "real responsibility." The patients are his own, and the internship is judged by just how complete his responsibility is.

Up to this time, he has been taught and trained and has grasped for knowledge and understanding. He has been the receiver and the obtainer or "taker" in the intensely competitive environment of medicine. If he is a good student and his acquisitive powers are strong he will receive the best internship. At the time of graduation, his degree is awarded and he recites the Hippocratic oath, in which he now swears to *give* to his patients and to *give* his knowledge by teaching those who follow him. His willingness to give and his ability to give must now develop, and the conflicting demands of giving and taking lead, as they do in all men, to discomfort and continuing attempts to reconcile the two.

As he leaves the house staff and follows the usual course into the laboratory to do "some research," he once again becomes the acquirer, and his acquisition of research techniques and scientific knowledge is limited by time. The degree of success in the self-acquisition process determines his final starting position on the academic ladder in the medical school's teaching hospital. Now he is expected both to give and to take to succeed. He gives of his time, his emotion, and his intellect as a teacher (and also his income if he becomes a practicing physician). The best teacher is not always the best researcher, as judged by both his peers and the medical students. He now finds himself squarely on the horns of a dilemma of conflicting and antagonistic demands. If too much time is taken up with teaching and seeing patients, he is unable to devote sufficient time to his research. The same thing is true of the "administrative chores" that he is asked to assume. The balance of his time is tipped toward research if his satisfactions are richest here in terms of his own intellect and the approval of his peers. If the balance is tipped toward teaching, patient care, and administration (giving to patients, students and the department, the hospital and the medical school), he fears he may not be promoted to the tenure position, he may not obtain financial support from the federal government, and he may be pushed off the academic ladder. He notes with dismay that "teaching and research" has become an academic cliché, and believes that research and its reporting is the final determinant of his advancement.

Every individual strikes his own best balance in the hospital, and if the sum total tips the balance to the giving side, so the balance of the hospital's activities will be centered on giving — and the most dependent member of the institution, the patient, will believe that the primary function of the (teaching) hospital is the care of the sick today because that *will* be the environment of the hospital. He will also realize that teaching and research will benefit tomorrow's patient, and will appreciate their valuable place in the function and economy of the hospital, even though *he* may not be tomorrow's and assuredly not the next generation's patient.

Progressively frustrated by wanting to excel at teaching and research, but seeing that his research in medicine is being removed farther and farther from the bedside and into the constant-temperature bath, he finds it increasingly difficult to teach clinical medicine as his research is no longer clinical research. Furthermore, he notes that there is little federal support and even less approval or admiration by his colleagues for clinical research. And, finally, the best experience for teaching clinical medicine, the actual direct care of patients and of the *whole* patient, takes him too far away and for too long a time from his research.

At this point he may "go away" for more training in basic research, he may continue to struggle and ultimately, he hopes, to reach his own best balance, or he may finally devote more and more time to the practice of medicine. A few of his colleagues will excel in all three areas, but they are becoming increasingly scarce as the expansion of medical and scientific knowledge continues its inexorable march. In his research he has become increasingly dependent on the nonclinical investigators representing the basic biological and biophysical sciences, and he finds their numbers increasing in the hospital.

A few of his colleagues will study the social scene and contribute solutions to the present dilemma for themselves and others, but most will be swept with the tide and may never "be at home and in control of the modern world," except as others around them have defined it. In this event his "outer-directedness" harnesses him, and he is locked in by the conventional wisdom and the status quo. He continues to feel uncomfortable.

The man who finds himself practicing his specialty in the teaching hospital has a different set of problems. A slow process of isolation occurs in some cases, imposed from both within and without. He enjoys less teaching responsibility, and his assignments are more in the out-patient department and less on the wards. He finds it progressively more difficult to understand "grand rounds," which used to be clinical exercises and are now an excuse for launching into the biochemical mechanisms of disease. He doesn't understand the organizational and policy-making structure of the hospital and is vaguely aware that "somebody else" is making the decisions that may determine his fate. Attempts to coordinate staff opinion and present a united front to the decision-makers seem fruitless, as his colleagues all seem hell-bent on their own particular bias and "nobody knows the facts" and "nobody tells us what's going on."

Fifteen per cent of his colleagues do know what's going on and participate in the decision-making; 15 per cent "never know what's going on," believe that communication is nonexistent, and are automatically against change; the other 70 per cent (whom the hospital director never sees) are happy in their work and believe the hospital is doing well. All are frustrated with their increasing interdependence and the multiple administrative decisions that they are forced to make regarding the use of tests and other consultants. A steadily increasing amount of their time is spent on making arrangements for their patients and interacting with the number of people in the hospital, constantly multiplying, whose skills and techniques must be brought to bear on their patients' problems. They think the pendulum may have swung too far toward science, and firmly believe that the primary function of the teaching hospital is the care of the patient.

## The Nurse

As Nietzsche said, "God created woman. And boredom did indeed cease from that moment . . ." As the American nurse looks back on the short history of her profession and interrelates it with the changing social position of women generally, she finds much of interest, tinctured with turmoil and struggle. Florence Nightingale's astounding success at Scutari in caring for the British soldiers and reducing their morbidity and mortality allowed her to obtain endowment for the first school of nursing when she returned to London in 1856. Subsequently, two major events were to change the history of the nursing profession, one an accident, and the other an inexorable and not-to-be-denied human development. The accident concerned the school.[11] Miss Nightingale's was founded as an endowed institution, totally separate from the hospital, its budget, and its administrator. Subsequent copies of the original school, however, were brought in under the hospital, which expected a return from the school in the form of apprenticeship. The indentured-apprentice system of medical education was to disappear but not that of nursing. With no separate endowment the schools lost their autonomy, and their function and direction were dictated and governed by the stringencies and exigencies of the hospital's budget. Education costs money and gives no immediate return. Nursing education, just as any other form of education, and its length and depth facilitates and achieves full professionalization by developing and passing on a special body of knowledge not available to all. Education provides for upward mobility in the social scale, and the person thus professionalized enjoys higher status *and* higher pay. Today, the nurse still has not achieved full professional status (in her own eyes or in the eyes of the doctor) by virtue of an inability to expand her educational process. The pay is too low, flexibility is constricted, and a return on the apprentice is still expected by the hospital.

The human development was the expansion of scientific thought and its application to the problems of human suffering and disease. Florence Nightingale's revolution was to be carried on by a steadily enlarging group of women devoted to the advancement of the nursing profession. But the very triumphs of medical science that were steadily enlarging their life's horizon now created the dilemma in their profession that exists today. Nursing, which had consisted of comforting ministration and personal caring while the doctor's orders were carried out, has now become a highly technical, specialized, and demanding skill. The nurse today has assumed many of the functions of last generation's doctors and is expected to be an expert technician, therapeutician, administrator, and social worker, and still to give highly personal care. Yet full professionalization has not been achieved, and the educational and economic advantages not realized. As Miss Russell [12] has said, "Hospital authorities, government officials and the senior profession of medicine — all these have been transferring new responsibilities to nursing in steadily increasing quantity ever since the opening of the First World War, but these same groups have not done enough to support the development of nursing education in corresponding measure." In 1948 the statement was made in a detailed study of the profession, "Successful reorganization of the nursing profession will depend largely on the soundness of its educational structure." [13] This same statement can be made today.

The nurse, just as the doctor and the patient, has been caught in the constantly accelerating advance of science and technology, leaving her with more specialized functions and the necessity for assuming somewhat incompatible, or at least hard-to-rationalize, roles. For nursing there are two basic functional roles, which

Schulman[14] has termed "mother surrogate and healer." The mother surrogate gives the personal care in an affective role, and the healer is all business and efficiency, allowing little flexibility of emotion and no room for "idle" behavior. The mother surrogate enjoys high emotional rewards but little pay whereas the healer role demands more skill, more technical competence, and therefore more education. With more education, there is more professionalization, higher status, and higher pay. Nursing education today does not provide adequately for this flexible pattern of roles, particularly that of the healer, and recruitment is therefore difficult in an age when more and more nurses are needed.

The nurse has become the central figure on any floor in the hospital devoted to patient care. The operating room, the recovery room, and the intensive-care unit all revolve about the strength and ability of this person, who at the present time has to be all things to all people in the hospital. Her frustrations are understandable. Increasing educational opportunities and increased pay will solve some of her problems as well as the emergent problem of recruitment. Adequate time for personal care will remain a problem but may ultimately be subdivided amongst nurse, doctor, practical nurse, orderly, and the patient's family. Meanwhile, there will be an increasing overlap of activities between medicine and nursing, and more specialization will be demanded as new responsibilities are shifted from the doctor to the nurse.

### The Administrator

Somewhere in the midst of doctor, patient, and nurse stands the administrator, whose job it is to set the stage and implement all the activities of the teaching hospital. The name administrator has become a less objectionable word in hospitals in recent times as specialization has made administrators of everyone. The paradoxical arrangements of physician authority and administrator responsibility still remain, however — a situation that has fascinated the medical sociologist. The informal hierarchical structure of such a complex institution along with the responsibility of the administrator unmatched by commensurate authority makes the "outsider" wonder "how anything ever gets done." The prima donnas of the hospital are the doctor and the patient, and well they should be.

The relatively loose organizational structure allows flexibility and freedom of action and thought, the best atmosphere for patient care and for teaching and research. Only a few usurp this freedom in their own interests.

The administrator occupies an exceedingly complex position, the prime function of which is planning. He spends much of his time arbitrating conflicting interests while he attempts to direct the energies of the institution toward certain goals. His ability to tolerate ambiguity is vital to the success of his plans. As A. Lawrence Lowell [15] said, "one cannot both do things and get the credit for them . . . It tends to arouse opposition, and . . . to distract the administrator's own mind from the single object he is trying to pursue." The administrator's job is to create the intellectual and emotional atmosphere by setting the stage for others to do and get the credit for doing. If this consideration is coupled with the necessary central position of the doctor and patient in the hospital perhaps the invisible nature of the hospital director is explained.

There are other considerations, however. For years the administrator was responsible for the financial structure and the hotel-service function of the hospital. As such he was, and still is, primarily a lay business manager, who had no experience with the subculture of medicine by virtue of the experience of medical school and subsequent patient care, teaching, and research activities. He was a nonexpert in the most vital function of the hospital, the care of the patient, and therefore progressively less able in this era of expanding knowledge to educate and advise his trustees. The trustees consequently looked to the staff directly for their advice, frequently easily obtained as a patient of the staff man or at social gatherings. This more often than not led to difficulties because of a lack of unanimity of opinion among the highly individualistic physicians and surgeons. More important, the staff doctor's advice was inadequate because of a lack of knowledge of the complexity of the institution and of its socioeconomic structure. The staff too often viewed the administrator as a bottleneck to professional advances, choked with financial considerations.

Most teaching hospitals have had the doctor administrators who have had formal training in schools of medical administration and public health or who have left the practice of medicine or medical research to enter the field. Assistant directors as well as assistant

deans have been said to be mice training to be rats! Regardless of
their formal or informal training, I agree with those who say that
books on (hospital) administration are about as convincing as books
on the art of making love.[16] It has also been said that being an administrator is more of a strain on the character than on the intellect,
and in keeping with this, that the dean or hospital director as an
intellectual man of action can only rarely combine the talents of,
or remain, a scholar.

As the teaching hospital has increased in complexity and in the
pace of its advances in research and patient care, the position of the
administrator has become more difficult and potentially more important and crucial to the life of the institution. He must be an
expert in business management, in social welfare and public health,
and he must understand intimately the teaching, research, and patient-care functions of the hospital. He is sociologist, psychologist,
politician, and statesman, or should be. He functions best, however,
by knowing how to use the minds of others, a technique that Eric
Ashby[17] has likened to the use of an electronic computer. He must
know how to program his information and questions and whom to
ask for help on different problems. He must then know how to
code his questions so as to be able to retrieve relevant information
to answer his questions. Once the information and advice is obtained, he must be able to decide what is capable of being turned
into action (his political sense) as well as what must be done (his
statesmanship sense) for the benefit of the community and society
at large.

> The bad administrator may fail for any of three reasons: because he
> cannot elicit appropriate replies from experts (because he does not know
> how to "program" his questions to them); because, having secured the in-
> formation, he cannot create a simple and persuasive decision out of it (be-
> cause his own "integration mechanism" is at fault); or because his decisions
> underestimate the political component (they may be excellent in theory but
> they are not viable; they overlook the adage that politics is the art of the
> possible).[18]

Finally, it is true that neither the expert doctor nor the expert
hospital director should have the ultimate authority to determine
policy, any more than the Secretary of Defense should be a general.
This is the function of the hospital's trustees. Harold Laski[19] expressed this as follows:

. . . expertise . . . sacrifices the insight of common sense to intensity of experience . . . Intensity of vision destroys the sense of proportion . . . the knowledge of what can be done with the results obtained in special disciplines seems to require a type of coordinating mind to which the expert as such is simply irrelevant . . . it is only the juxtaposition of the statesman between the expert and the public which makes specialist conclusions capable of application . . . that indeed is the statesman's basic task. He represents at his best supreme common sense in relation to expertise.

The hospital trustee must occupy the statesman's position. If the hospital director is a layman and therefore a "nonexpert" he will seldom find it possible to obtain authority in the hospital commensurate with his responsibility. Therefore, it is difficult for him to qualify as a statesman although he can make politically viable decisions. If he is a doctor administrator he is disqualified because of his expert status. Simultaneously, however, he is given more authority by the hospital staff. Small wonder that hospital trusteeship is so important and also such a difficult job and subject to so many different pressures. It is the trustee's job to articulate the expertise of the institution with the wants and nedes of the community. The magnitude of his job is such that in recent times some hospital directors have been made trustees *ex officio*. In his best capacity the director combines expertise regarding what the profession wants and needs with nonexpertise (or nonprofessionalism), and in that capacity, he will reflect the wants and needs of the community.

## THE BALANCE OF FUNCTIONS

The three functions of the teaching hospital are patient care, teaching, and research, and their sum total defines the place of the hospital in society and its effectiveness as a social instrument. The direction of the contemporary teaching hospital and the success of its operation are determined by the degree of fulfillment of both its community function — that is, the care of the sick — and its university function, which is teaching and research. The goals of both hospital and university are the same, but they are separated to a certain extent by the element of time: the hospital cares for today's patient and provides for the contemporary health wants and needs of the community; and the university provides for tomorrow's patient by teaching medicine, training practitioners, and conducting research. The orientation, or the balance of activities, may be primarily toward the community or toward the university. A heavy imbalance in either direction is not desirable. The best patient care can be provided most easily in the environment of the university, and the best university function can exist only on a demonstrated foundation of hospital service to the community.

It is my contention that the primary function of the hospital, any hospital, is the care of the patient and that the environment or the attitude of the hospital must be one of giving to the patient today. If the hospital places teaching and research as its primary function, and budget, space, and admitting policies are all geared selectively to this end, tomorrow's patient may well benefit, but today's atmosphere is one of obtaining knowledge and using the patient to this end.

### The Care of the Patient

If the care of the patient is indeed the primary function of the hospital there are several material ways of proving it. Is there an active, well equipped and well staffed emergency ward operating twenty-four hours a day? Does the hospital admit any patient who needs hospitalization, regardless of his disease, its relative rarity, or its interest? If the admitting policies are selective and predicated on research and teaching needs, the accent is here for the benefit of the academicians and "tomorrow's patient" and not on the community for the benefit primarily of today's patient.

Are the staff of practicing physicians given appropriate academic and hospital titles, and do they share the ward teaching duties with the full-time members of the department, or are they given the jobs in the clinic, which unfortunately, in most teaching hospitals, remains an undesirable place to work in?

Is the chief of the nursing service a full member of the medical-policy board, participating actively in the medical-care problems of the hospital?

Are new departures in medical care initiated because of community and patient wants and needs, or are they set up for teaching and research uses? In the latter event, I think that they have a lesser chance of succeeding, believing that patient-care programs of demonstrated worth are the best foundation on which to conduct research and teaching, which then, in turn, serve to expand and improve the demonstrated service.

Is there an active medical social-service department, and is it fully supported in terms of space and budget?

Finally, is there an active program of medical-care research, studying the organizational arrangements for the provision of health services, the quality of medical care, the gigantic social and economic problems and, generally, the ways of best bringing the steadily increasing benefits of medical science to an expanding population with rising expectations and increasing wants and needs?

## *Teaching*

Medical education shares the aims of all education, which, from its Latin derivation, means the process of leading forth. A. N. Whitehead defined it as "the acquisition of the art of the utilization of knowledge." John Dewey said, "All education proceeds by the participation of the individual in the social consciousness of the race" and "Education is the fundamental method of social progress and reform."

I shall assume that the aim of medical education are to develop the intellectual capacity to its fullest extent; to pass on the culture and the ethics of medicine, its attitudes, values, expectations, and beliefs; and, finally, shading into the area of postgraduate education, to provide for training in the techniques of the profession, so that one may earn one's living — the vocational aspect of one's education. The final object of the medical student's study is, once again, to "be at home in and in control of the modern world," in this case, the world of medicine. I shall assume that the aim of the medical school is to provide those who will take care of the sick, teach, and advance the knowledge of medicine through research.

I have already spoken of the undergraduate acceleration and the constricting effects of the premedical course with its preoccupation with science. This is reinforced and accentuated in medical school, to which unquestioned faith in the technology or machinery of medicine is added in the hospital. Fully "expert" and ultimately specialized, the young physician finds himself, not independent, which was very probably one of the reasons he entered medicine, but quite dependent on the people and the machines around him in the hospital. He also finds that more and more people have something to say about what he is doing, and several outside agents, such as the Blue Shield and the Blue Cross, as well as state and federal welfare plans, are playing an increasing part in determining just what he can or cannot do with his patient. His medical education, while developing his scientific intellect, did not provide him with the tools with which to understand the people and institutions around him, the historical forces that molded his profession to what it is today, or the numerous and increasingly powerful social, economic, and political forces that are sure to shape his future. This is the world he is *not* in control of, and the substance of which is being determined by someone else.

I agree with the statement that "The independence of education from social pressures must be defended not merely for the sake of education but primarily for the sake of society. Education is almost the only force *within* society that is capable, in some measure, of altering society." [20] That is true, but there will be no alteration of society regarding its view of medicine and hospitals by the product of the medical school unless there is some relevancy, some content of the curriculum devoted to the social problems of medicine today. In their blind insistence on the ultimate veracity and benefit of science, both for the public and for the primacy that it has assumed in the development of the student's intellect, educators have neglected the twin sister (or the afterbirth) of the science struggle, the social and economic problems of medicine.

The Flexner report accentuated, crystallized, and established the place of science in medicine and medical education,[21] and no one would question the necessity, the value, or the benefit of this establishment. Now, however, the role of healer is being overwhelmed by the mass exodus of young physicians from the bedside and into the laboratories of medicine and the acquisition of new scientific knowledge. As the pace of science accelerates in all walks of life, who will be the medical statesmen and medical politicians who can solve some of the resultant problems so that the benefits are more readily available to society? Will medicine do this, or will the voter, with his "desperately demanding face," [22] determine the future of doctors and hospitals by turning to central authority, with all its bureaucracy and political expediency?

There can be little doubt that the training and experience gained in the teaching hospital are out of touch with reality and do not provide the student of medicine with a complete set of Betz cells with which to face the world of medicine. The deficiencies are real and occur for several key reasons: the patient population, stated above, is highly selective, representing on the teaching service a gathering of the aged and medically indigent with acute, advanced, complicated, and frequently rare somatic disease; there is little emphasis on the social and economic factors of disease and hospitalization except for a brief recording of the type of health insurance and the occupational and family history; there has been inadequate integration of the semiprivate and private patient into a meaningful teaching situation; because of the restrictions of the traditional, acute, curative function of the teaching hospital,[23] preventive medicine and public health play almost no part in the teaching process, and there is no extension of the student and house officer's interest or knowledge into the community so far as existing facilities for the aftercare of the chronically ill are concerned; and there remains little or no knowledge of the hospital as one of society's major institutions, its history, its organizational structure, its contemporary social and economic problems, its various people, and its machines.

The restrictions and inadequacies in the education and training of the house officer are a result of both the medical curriculum and the traditional function of the teaching hospital. In the former, little or no attention is given to the social history of medicine and hospitals, the broader field of social welfare, and the socioeconomic problems of patients, doctors, and hospitals. In the latter, the teaching hospital has restricted itself to the acute curative function at a time when it has emerged as the community health center and finds itself with no active preventive-medicine, public-health and socioeconomic or "medical-care" departments. Medical social service and hospital administration are as close as they get, and in many hospitals these areas are secondary interests and are effectively excluded from the mainstream of the teaching function.

### Research

The incredible growth of science and the benefits that have accrued to mankind are well known to all. Derek Price[24] analyzed this growth as follows:

All other things in population, economics, non-scientific culture, are growing so as to double in roughly every human generation of say thirty to fifty years. Science in America is growing so as to double in only ten years, it multiplies by eight in each successive doubling of all non-scientific things in our civilization. If you care to regard it this way, the density of science in our culture is quadrupling during each generation.

The benefits are well known, but the resultant social and economic problems are dimly perceived. The scientist is of little help in this regard. He has sacrificed (and necessarily so) "the insight of common sense to intensity of experience." He decides what *could* be done. Someone else (namely, the politician or the statesman) has to decide what is applicable and *should* be done by and for society in terms of the allocation of man power and economic resources to the applied technology of science.

While science advances, the social and economic problems pile up. The atomic bomb, overpopulation, mass transportation, and the cost of medical care are but a few. Attempts to solve this type of problem are reflected by the increasing importance of the nonexpert in society, the politician, the increasing numbers of civil servants, expanding bureaucratization, and the tendency of a highly expectant public to look to central authority for the provision of its needs and a full share in the fruits of medical science. Increasing emphasis on the social sciences and their expansion culminated in the report of the President's Science Advisory Committee,[25] which stressed the importance and potential contributions of the social sciences to public affairs and the multiple social and economic problems of a scientific society.

When this view is narrowed to the teaching hospital the experience of one institution is of interest. In 1935 at the Massachusetts General Hospital, a little over $50,000 was spent on medical research, largely clinical and financed totally by private means. Dr. Paul D. White is a good example of the person involved. The budget for patient-care activities in that year was $2,300,000. This year, nearly $7,000,000 will be spent on research, of which the greatest portion represents federal money. The budget for patient care is nearly $22,000,000. The balance of research activity is heavily weighted toward the biological sciences, most of the work is done *in vitro*, and the two cultures of medical practice and medical science find it increasingly difficult to communicate and understand each other's problems. A new type of Renaissance man has emerged, however, who maintains excellent research while he teaches and applies his knowledge at the bedside of the patient. It is apparently still possible in certain extraordinary men to reconcile and effect a rapprochement of the two cultures of the present teaching hospital, represented by the extremes of the practicing physician and the "basic," biologically oriented scientist.

Still, with the increasing federal support of scientific research, the direction of many an individual and many an institution has been determined by the path of least resistance to financial security and status as determined by an outside agent with much money to give. The outside agent is subject to pressures too, as witnessed by the recent change in policy adopted by the United States Public Health Service and its National Institutes of Health brought on by the activities of the Fountain Committee, which presumably reflects the "public interest."

## THE BALANCE OF ACTIVITIES

How can one assess objectively the balance of activities in the teaching hospital and determine whether its goals and its primary mission are being realized? I have spoken of the primary function as the care of the patient and the vital importance of an over-all institutional attitude, which is geared to giving to today's patient. I have also recognized the obligatory relation of teaching and research if the best care of the patient is to be achieved and if contributions to tomorrow's community are to be realized. There are certain material measures that can be made such as budgetary and space allocations, the uses of new construction, the distribution of man power, the hours spent in various pursuits, and finally the patient-care activities. "Facts" help but do not reflect the "personality" or traditions or the "feeling" of the hospital that are passed from one generation of workers to the next.

Allowing a certain degree of provincialism, I should like to review the years 1950 and 1960 regarding these material measures at the Massachusetts General Hospital. My provincialism may be excused by necessity, for it has been difficult to obtain comparable studies from other university-affiliated, teaching hospitals. I have summarized these measures in Tables 1 to 4, which are self-explana-

TABLE 1. CHANGES IN EXPENDITURES AND AREA

| Item | 1950 | 1960 |
|------|------|------|
| Expense | | |
| Patient care (dollars) | 7,800,000 | 17,200,000 |
| Research (dollars) | 1,400,000 | 5,200,000 |
| Per cent of total for research | 15.2 | 23.2 |
| New construction (dollars)[a] | | |
| Patient care | | 4,600,000 |
| Teaching and housing | | 2,000,000 |
| Research | | 6,200,000 |
| Area of hospital | | |
| Research (sq ft) | 30,075 | 96,262 |
| Total hospital (sq ft) | 607,616 | 642,995 |
| Per cent of total for research | 4.9 | 15.1 |

[a] Over 10-yr period.

tory. The trend is unmistakable and represents one institution's heavy participation in the expansion of scientific research in medi-

TABLE 2. CHANGES IN THE STAFF

| Category | 1950 | 1960 |
|----------|------|------|
| Practicing staff (practitioners) | 216 | 211 |
| Full-time Harvard system | 52 | 61 |
| Physician-Scientists | 17 | 27 |
| Nonclinical investigators | 7 | 38 |
| House staff | 105 | 136 |
| Clinical and research fellows | 84 | 161 |

cine. The Trustees' Scientific Advisory Committee of the Hospital stated, "The recent expansion of the Hospital's research program

TABLE 3. CHANGES IN CLINICAL AREAS

| Item | 1950 | 1960 |
|------|------|------|
| Patients admitted | 16,939 | 24,610 |
| Operations | 11,777 | 13,861 |
| Patients examined and treated in | | |
| Radiology Department | 61,841 | 127,363 |
| Total out-patient visits | 195,849 | 225,456 |
| Patients treated in emergency | 15,335 | 38,258 |
| Number of beds used | 851[a] | 1,012[b] |

[a] 1952.
[b] 1963.

has stimulated a significant improvement in the standards of patient care and teaching." I share that conclusion. The patient still comes

TABLE 4. PERSONNEL HOURS

| Personnel classification | Number of hours | |
|---|---|---|
| | 1952 | 1960 |
| Administrative and general functions | 408,464 | 650,914 |
| Nursing service | 1,144,506 | 1,456,411 |
| Radiology | 144,311 | 258,153 |
| Clinical services[a] | 305,398 | 397,256 |
| Research | 462,558 | 986,590 |

[a] Includes house staff, ward secretaries, etc., and chiefs of all clinical services.

first and has not been lost while the institution has taught tomorrow's doctors and health personnel and contributed new knowledge through scientific research to the problems of life and disease.

## THE FUTURE

The past and present are established. The next Flexner report will deal with the social and economic aspects of medicine. New departments will be created, and changes in medical curricula and the function of the teaching hospital will result. Medical research in the biological and behavioral sciences will continue to expand and contribute heavily to the advancement of knowledge and the attainment of health. Medical-care research will increase, and medical administration will assume a more important and central issue in the complex life of the teaching hospital, which will allow a clearer translation and a more rapid articulation of the work of the institution with the wants and needs of the public.

The next generation's medical student will have better understanding of himself and of those people and institutions around him. He will find that he can once again achieve a feeling of independence by virtue of a deeper and broader understanding and a new ability to "be at home in and control of the modern world." This will be accomplished by courses designed to present and study the social history of medicine and hospitals, the social and economic problems confronting the public, their universities and their teaching hospitals, and a strengthening of the humanities, liberal arts, and social sciences in premedical education. The student will become a better medical ambassador to the public.

In an age in which specialization is making people strangers to each other, an individual may develop who can continue to combine the best of two worlds and be an intellectual man of action at the bedside while continuing his scholarly work in the biology laboratory or even the medical-care field.

Medical-care research concerns itself with the assessment of medical needs, the provision of health services, their quality and quantity, the broader field of social welfare, the economics of medicine, medical administration, and the implementation of preventive medicine and public-health measures. Perhaps a new breed of practicing physician will arise who maintains his clinical skills and who will conduct medical care research. Surely, these two disciplines are relevant to and complement each other. The opportunity to contribute to mankind is great in this area, and the problems are even more difficult of solution than those concerned with the mechanisms of disease or the size of the moon rocket's booster.

Every generation thinks its problems are the greatest, and its time the most important and the most exciting, and I am no exception. The present generation is faced with solving the accumulated problems of its heritage of science and applied technology over the past five hundred and particularly the last fifty years. It is desirable not to leave all this to someone else. It would be nice to develop in one's medical life what Max Weber called the three cardinal qualities of the successful politician: "passion, a feeling of responsibility, and a sense of proportion." "Proportion" and "responsibility" can be achieved through study of those neglected and excluded areas that have pertinency to the social and economic problems of medicine. Passion — the totality of giving and feeling and sacrificing — is something that the doctor acquires when he finds his own best role in medicine. It is still possible for physicians, individually and collectively, to shape their own futures and to "be at home in and in control of the modern world" of medicine.

# THE TEACHING HOSPITAL
# AND THE COMMUNITY

Ellsworth T. Neumann, M.D.

Each of us has a personal philosophy which guides us in our personal conduct and everyday life. It is our mental compass — our distillate of wisdom — our feelings about human nature, about morality, about life, about reality. Some of these feelings were taught us in childhood, and some we developed ourselves. With some we are vague and inarticulate, but with others definite in the way we show them in discussions and in decisions. So too, the teaching hospital has a guiding philosophy which expresses its distinctive personality and nature. It is shown in the conduct and everyday life of the hospital, but it is seldom discussed because it is a deceptively simple philosophy based solely on the spirit and act of giving.

When the concept of total commitment to giving is recognized, it provides clearer meaning to the work, the conduct, and the individual natures of those involved in patient care, teaching, and research. Furthermore, it can be used intellectually in determining organizational decisions and plans, the selection of leaders, the pattern of organizational hierarchy, the intellectual climate, and the relative priority of goals. But is this philosophical concept in keeping with our changing culture? Will it and its subsidiary principles push a teaching hospital forward to keep pace with the future needs of a changing community? In discussing the philosophy and nature of the hospital and community, I will try to use only my observations of those everyday situations in the home or hospital which are familiar through participation in one way or another.

Looking back over the sixty-odd years of this century should produce the necessary reference points from which to chart our course. This period has been one of continuous change in our national society. All of us have either seen the changes for ourselves or have heard the changes discussed by our parents. I would like to examine only three of the many changes which affect the hospital and its future course.

## THREE CHANGES

### Social Responsibility

The first of these is the change in our understanding of social responsibility. At the turn of the century, it was a generally accepted view that everyone was his brother's keeper, but its meaning was something different from what it is today. It meant that if there was a sudden catastrophe such as fire, neighbors would house, feed, and clothe the dispossessed on a temporary basis. Community giving was more intimate, local, and temporary. Now one needs only to look to his taxes to understand the change in meaning. In the local community, we provide, through our government, a livelihood for the older person or invalid who cannot work or for perhaps the deserted wife whose children we feed, clothe, and educate until maturity. We do this across the nation; and each year we increase the number of those whom we feel worthy of our support. And after the Second World War we set new standards of national giving by not looting our defeated enemies but giving generously to them. To almost every nation in need we have been giving not only capital, food, and tools, but also knowledge through the Point 4 Program. All of us may not agree with this; but our legislators here and in congress represent fairly well the social understanding of the majority. They give as we wish them to give. And the trend toward assuming greater responsibility as shown over the past half century indicates no sign of slowing or changing direction.

This major change provides both reference points and guide lines for the teaching hospital. There are obvious implications of the method and degree of giving to be assumed by the community (government) in medical care. There are also less obvious implications of the impact to be felt by the teaching services of the hospital. One should remember the possibilities that teaching services and charity care may no longer be synonymous; and that the open ward with its current social connotations may become an anachronism in tomorrow's society. However, we know that society will demand well educated doctors and nurses from the teaching hospital; and this, therefore, means that the teaching hospital must look carefully to its traditional concept that teaching is possible only in conjunction with the gift of "free" medical care by the hospital and hospital medical staff.

### The Family Structure and the Nursing Service

The second change which affects the course of the teaching hospital is the most important because it implies so much in organizational patterns and in the personal conduct, attitudes, and relationships of all of us who contribute in one way or another to the total functioning of the hospital. It is the revolutionary change in the basic organizational structure upon which our entire society rests, the family. We cannot help but be familiar with the American family's many changing aspects if we read any of the popular magazines. Articles entitled "What Has Happened to the American Wife?" or "What Has Happened to the American Man?" or "Why Our Children Go Wrong?" are on the continuous bill of fare and are primarily devoted to the problems created by this change in family relationships and conduct. None of the articles is calculated to make us more tranquil!

Sensational as these articles may be, they nevertheless do serve a useful purpose. We are all in the position of being unable to see the individual trees around us because we are so deep in the woods. And these articles often focus our attention on the singular aspects of this cultural revolution. Some of these changing aspects also affect the organizational structure and conduct of the hospital.

A hospital, like a nation, is an organization created of people, by people, and for people. This is its greatest protection because the hospital is only an instrument of our society; and its growth, its usefulness, and its life must depend on how well it fits our society and its needs. Fortunately, society provides new patients and new participating members to test this. If they are uncomfortable, they express it in words or actions. If those who make up the organization are sensitive enough and flexible enough, the necessary changes in relationships and atmosphere occur. The basic organizational unit of society, the family, is, of course, the training ground for the new participating members and patients of the hospital. It is here that they develop most of their abilities for relating with other humans and their individualized preferences and concepts. And it is to the changing nature of these relationships in the American family and the consequential changing relationships in the hospital that I would like to address myself.

The American family at the turn of the century had a structure easily understood by all. There was no question that the father was the head of the family. In a subsidiary position was his wife who had promised in their marriage ceremony to love, honor, and obey him — and in that era very likely meant every word of it. In the most subsidiary position came the children. The aphorism of that day, "Children are better seen than heard," provides the best clue to assessing their situation. Orders went down this structure to the children. Any discussion of these orders by the children was apt to be considered "back-talk" requiring a "summary court martial" on the spot. Articulate, imaginative children in those days were considered undisciplined and probably brought more shame than praise to their parents. And, furthermore, the children of the average American family completed their schooling in the fourth grade. From that point on, whether in the city or rural area, the children worked in some way and contributed to the welfare of the family. How this contribution was to be utilized by the family was largely determined by the father. With this as the structure of the basic organizational unit in society, it shouldn't come as a surprise to find the structure of other organizations in the same society bearing a marked resemblance.

### The Nursing Service Yesterday

In the hospital of that era, as in the hospital of today, the nursing service provided the most readily identifiable hierarchy of the hospital. Its easily observable authority structure also provided strength, cohesiveness, and a communications system from top to bottom. For these reasons, I would like to use it to represent the more complex and less easily understood total hospital structure.

Like all women executives of her day, the director of nursing service and school naïvely assumed that success and strength in her position lay in her absolute imitation of male executives. She played the role of "Captain of the Ship" both in and out of the hospital. Any friendliness or intimacy with her subordinates was forbidden in this role because it might lead to disrespect and contempt and she designed her speech and action so as to create awe.

She also distrusted information coming from her subordinates and, therefore, devoted much of her time to detailed inspection of her ship. Everything had to be in exact order. And this included the posture and appearance of patients as well as nurses and students. There was no excuse for individual variations partly because individuality was frowned upon and partly because an excuse had to be verbalized and this was tantamount to "back-talk." Her communication system, in short, went only from top to bottom and then only in writing so that subordinates who did their own thinking and speaking could be spotted and terminated. Her resemblance to the classical "father" of the era is easily seen. And her immediate subordinates, teachers and supervisors, gave her honor and obedience, if not love. In turn, they were vigorous and demanding in their approach to their subordinates.

The head nurses, more likely third-year students, thought and acted like all students of the era. They learned and repeated again and again in word and action exactly what they had been told by the teacher or supervisor. Individual or imaginative thinking was the exclusive prerogative of age and position. Any student who might be inclined toward a research pattern of thinking was rigorously reoriented. And the student went to work quickly and contributed maximally to the welfare of the organization.

The patients were the subordinates of all subordinates. No matter how dignified by age, they were usually called by their first names. So little was required in conversation from the patient that a complete foreign language barrier presented few problems. Textbooks of nursing care were devoted primarily to the patient's physical care which could be well regularized. Little effort was wasted by the authors on the care of the patient's emotional problems other than by their solution through the use of physical restraints. The apocryphal story of the little old non-English speaking man who accompanied a friend to an out-patient department and was finally returned to his grieving family three weeks later after surgery speaks volumes, whether or not it actually happened.

*Today's Family Structure*

Next I would like to discuss the family structure which is evolving in our society today and which is affecting the hospital in many ways.

According to the "scare" articles in the popular magazines the father has abrogated his traditional authority by his venturing into diaper-changing and dishwashing; his role in the eyes of his sons is so neutral as to produce young men with no interest in young women; or he is a corporate executive, living on an expense account and giving so little emotional support to his children that they become the delinquents of the suburbs and exurbs. Obviously this corporate executive of today has replaced the minister or psychiatrist of yesteryear in his ability to produce delinquent sons.

The articles about today's mothers are still more deprecating. She is out of her home and working; and that's bad. Or she is at home wasting her intelligence and education; and that's bad. Or when she isn't buying ready-to-bake cakes or using an automatic dishwasher, she is busily inventing new ways to destroy her husband's ego, all of which is worse.

The children are treated more sympathetically in these articles. Although most of them would appear to be delinquents, their faults are happily blamed entirely on their badly motivated parents, their modern teachers, or those violent Western morality plays on television. With modern teaching, which requires articulate and responsive students, and television, which does not encourage conversational development, it is only natural that many of these articles resolve the conflict by recommending the junkheap for one or both. Fortunately, fathers and mothers are still considered useful.

But amid all this terrifying cacophony there is one melodic phrase which appears again and again: the primary responsibility of parents is to give their children understanding and love. No longer is there much discussion of providing for the physical needs of the children. This is a rich country. Other than giving vitamins for unobservable and indeed nonexistent vitamin deficiencies, the parents must only worry about their lack of restraint in giving too many calories and too many convertibles to their teen-age children. Furthermore, in a society which prefers thinking about Freud and psychiatry to thinking about Einstein and the atom bomb, parents are becoming relatively sophisticated about the giving of love and understanding to their children. They can easily differentiate firmness and consistency of policy and emotion from the physical disciplining of bygone generations. Finally, they usually do understand the ideal of equal and mutual support by both mates. Analysis of contemporary marriage often indicates that one mate gives most of the emotional support in the family to the other mate as well as to the children.

And the mate who has a need or tendency to give more than to take may be either the husband or wife. Strangely enough, he or she may not be the "boss" who makes most of the family's important decisions. This person is the one, however, who "carries the family"; and it is to this person that troubled members of the family first turn for emotional support and decisions. The growing climate for the children probably also depends on the emotional reservoir and understanding of this person.

### Today's Nursing Service

If the family is involved in so radical a reorientation, what is happening in our society's less important organizations such as the hospitals? Certainly the doctors, nurses, employees, executives, students and patients are affected by their family lives consciously or unconsciously. Their thinking, their behavior, their expectations must have some perceptible effects on the direction taken by the hospital whether it be personnel policy, organization, medical care, teaching, research, or whatever. Nursing service may well be developing an upside-down organization in which the patients are at the top and the nursing director is at the bottom with assistant directors, supervisors, head nurses, graduate nurses, practical nurses, floor secretaries, aides, ward-helpers, and the student nurse arranged properly inside a massive organization.

In her position at the bottom of this inverted pyramid representing the total nursing service, it is obvious that the present director of the service must be a much stronger woman and executive than was her counterpart at the turn of the century. Nothing so foolish as imitating male executives ever enters her head, for she knows full well that the equality of men and women resembles the equality of apples and pears, both equally valuable but totally different. In her supportive role she works mostly with four or five immediate lieutenants, each of whom, in turn, does the same. This seems to follow throughout the organization with the bedside nurse on the day shift ideally caring for four or five patients. This pattern of support resembles that of the family, in which one person supports a mate and the current average of three or four children, bringing the total to four or five.

In addition, the director at the bottom of the heap must be a good "applied social scientist." She must know how to build and maintain a fast and accurate two-way communications system within her organization. The information coming now through her lieutenants must provide her with the necessary clues to the most minor fluctuations in individual or group attitudes and efforts. She must also be sophisticated enough to analyze the information properly and redirect or strengthen these attitudes and efforts without jarring her organization. In doing so, she must always remember that each person with whom she works must be considered an end in herself and not a means to an end. This implies a step ladder methodology whereby each level in her hierarchy will support those for whom they are responsible in the same manner as the patients are supported by those who are at the bedside. This, of course, provides a supportive giving hierarchy rather than a manipulative hierarchy, and in turn enhances the possibility that each person will receive the attention and encouragement which she deserves as an individual working in this hierarchy.

Like the good parent, the Nursing Director is responsible for providing a growing climate for the nurses and nursing students for whom she is responsible. Although she must recognize and act quickly in times of crises to provide the firm autocratic posture needed by those who are less secure emotionally, in ordinary times and circumstances she must act in the restrained role of the leader, guiding rather than directing. Her use of dialogue, her mental flexibility, and her encouragement should help her provide an intellectual and emotional atmosphere which promotes the production of new ideas and encourages experimental improvements. Her respect for other individuals and disciplines around her and consequently her giving of greater freedom of action and thought to these other individuals and disciplines will also be reflected in a more respectful, considerate, free and creative atmosphere in which patients, nurses, and doctors inevitably benefit. This description of the Nursing Director must also, with slight modification, describe any executive in the hospital who has the responsibility of guiding others and uses this philosophy in carrying out this responsibility.

### The Patient

Let us next consider the patients. The quite important and mature corporate executive who comes in for surgery may reveal something. Why is it that before the operation he will look to a young graduate or student nurse for reassurance when he is so accustomed to calling only for the professional services of others equal in importance to himself, such as the surgeon who is to operate on him shortly? Why is he so upset when he hears the nurses or doctors joking among themselves as they go about their work? Why is it that, although he is going nowhere for the next ten days he must ask the time of the nurse and then get upset if she isn't definite about it? And why does he call for the nurse in the middle of the night although he has no evident need?

We, of course, know the answers to these questions. He is doing what all "good" patients do. He becomes as dependent as a child and manifests the same characteristics. He unconsciously places doctors and nurses of all ages in the role of parents. Naturally, like any child he is upset that such important people may be joking among themselves and laughing at each other. And, moreover, he expects such individuals to be definite about everything including the time. He calls for the nurse in the middle of the night, of course, for the same reason that a child calls his mother for a glass of water, simply to be sure that she is there.

After the operation all this will gradually change as he pursues an upward road from dependency to maturity. His demanding ways will diminish. He will start to see the doctors and nurses as men and women rather than fathers and mothers. And, consequently, he will start joking with the nurses. Unfortunately, we still tend to evaluate physical condition rather than emotional condition and we will, therefore, probably discharge him before he has regained his former maturity and ability to give his family and subordinate executives their customary support. We must upset and disorganize a lot of families and commercial corporations in this way.

This man represented well the "good" patient who immediately falls into a "taking" posture when admitted. We also know of the patient who refuses to take and who through true courage or foolhardiness is determined to brazen out the entire preoperative and postoperative periods. For some reason he tends to a rocky postoperative period with more chance of physical and emotional complications and a longer stay in the hospital. "The best givers," be they doctor, nurse, or hospital executive all seem to fall into the category of bad patients. Perhaps they are so used to their own "giving" roles in this same environment that they have difficulty assuming the necessarily dependent and "taking" role of the good patient.

We might now discuss those who give the care to the patients by first scrutinizing the statement heard so often from patients, "I had such an understanding nurse." Certainly none of us would assume that these patients considered their nurses to be psychoanalysts well trained to understand the emotional conflicts and problems of the patients. They simply meant that their nurses "stood under" them and supported them emotionally during their crisis. The equal distribution of praise for the understanding of both nurses and doctors bodes well for both professions and their future social images.

What I have done so far is point out that the nursing service organization can be a magnificent method for providing emotional support and care from one end of it to the other. It is not perfect, however, because the head nurse position is almost untenable in this new turnabout. She alone of all the executives in the hospital is expected to support an unlimited number of others. She should be working with a few doctors and teamleaders. But in actuality, dozens of doctors, nurses, patients, relatives, and individuals from other departments approach her directly at the tested rate of more than thirty an hour. If she is also in an emotionally trying situation in her private life, it is inevitable that her emotional reservoir will be drained. As she becomes less able to give, her ability to make decisions diminishes and her absenteeism increases. When this happens, everyone around starts to shield her by giving to her. During this period of breakdown, which may be lengthy, the organization devoted to giving is short-circuited at her level. At this point both patients and doctors note the change of atmosphere and lack of care at the bedside. Fortunately, there is often a supervisor, floor secretary, or physician who heads off this eventuality by a quiet, unostentatious daily ministration of support to the head nurse. The physician's help is worth noting because it represents the most natural and most easily given support, that between the two sexes. This natural support, so taken for granted, may be basic to some of our successes and failures and may possibly explain the occasional impasse in relationship which occurs between physician and nurse.

Why are we so successful in gaining the appreciation of male patients of all ages? Or why is it that we fail so often in giving sufficient personal care to please the elderly woman? I once pondered the possibilities that either younger women were intolerant of older women or that younger women were unsuccessful in maintaining a mother role with older women. But my detailed questioning of both patients and nurses revealed that the women patients received as much or more care than did the men patients. Could it simply be that a few minutes of support of one sex by the other sex is equivalent to an hour's support of one sex by the same sex? This is probably so; and particularly so in the case of the elderly woman who has so many unfulfilled emotional needs. With so many more women than men supplying care, she has much less chance of being satisfied.

*Doctors and Nurses*

The occasional impasse between doctor and nurse may often be based on a similar situation in reverse. The situation may be familiar to us. It appears to start when a physician in or near a nursing station complains that the nursing profession has reached a sorry state of affairs, that nurses have become cold and interested only in paper work and that the schools of nursing are turning out chemists rather than nurses. The response is inevitable. A verbal defense may not be forthcoming but the action is surely forthcoming. He is given the "deep-freeze" treatment. Frigid cooperation — just one step above no cooperation at all — only serves to aggravate him more and apparently prove his point. Rapid communication insures the same treatment for him on other floors until he is pushed to the point of retreating to his own office or going to the office of either the hospital administrator or nursing director to denounce the nursing profession. Questioning of the original nurses involved brings forth the following defense: the doctor was a boor who insulted the nursing profession without provocation, and was guilty himself of overordering tests, medications, and repetitive checking of his patients, all of which is responsible for excessive paper work.

Investigation of this familiar situation makes me believe that the complaints of both physician and nurses leading to this impasse were incorrect. I would like to suggest instead that something far simpler occurred in the following manner. First, let me say that almost all doctors and nurses are "giving people" who frequently go beyond their endurance not only in the hospitals but in their homes as well. The demands of their mates and children compete with the demands of their patients. It is natural that they occasionally forget that they must each give support to the other when it's needed, just as must the two parents in the "typical family."

In this instance, it is quite possible that the physician, after having been up late caring for a patient, was vigorously reminded by his wife that she and the children needed more of his time and attention. It is understandable that he arrived at the hospital with a headache and feelings of oppression and depression. It is possible that he entered a nursing station and wandered about disconsolately before he was interrupted with the question: "Would you like to give some orders, Doctor?" This may have been a perfectly business-like courteous question which befitted the environment; but it was not fitted to his mood. He was in no mood to give anything, including orders. His answer and perhaps his facial expression should have provided a clue to the nurse that he was in as much need of solicitude as any patient under care. Apparently, however, she failed to respond. Perhaps because she and his wife, as women, failed in giving, and because the members of the nursing profession are mostly women, he arrived on the next floor with his commentary on the nursing profession. Had the first nurse offered only a few minutes to his care, perhaps the whole impasse would have been averted. Had she asked him whether he had a headache and then offered sympathy or two aspirin tablets, she might have given the necessary support.

## Expansion of Knowledge

The last of the changes affecting the teaching hospital's course is the rapidity with which the new knowledge has been discovered and spread. All of us are familiar with the claim that the knowledge accumulated by man before this century has been doubled already in this century and, furthermore, that it may well be redoubled in the next twenty years or so. The impact of this can be felt best by the simple expedient of talking to any reasonably intelligent 10-year-old child. The comparison of that child's conceptual and factual knowledge with your own at that age should provide both understanding and shock.

The increase in knowledge has also led to a better spread of knowledge. Teachers have obviously exploited the research work of the social scientists and put it to good use. Although the invention and exploitation of television as a mass communication medium has not made our young people more articulate, it has certainly contributed to this astonishing spread of conceptual and factual knowledge. Keeping this in mind, these inferential statements can be understood: (1) Those who are in teaching and executive work must continuously learn, accept, and use new social and scientific concepts and facts in order to avoid the intellectual scrapheap to which young people are so prone to assign their elders. (2) Each new generation of students and workers has a more sophisticated set of concepts than had the previous generation. Because a hospital should be thought of as a group of persons rather than a group of buildings, it is the responsibility of the existing group not only to orient the new members to the concepts of those already there but also to orient themselves to the concepts of those who join now and those who join in the future. This implies a guiding principle: Any teaching hospital which hopes to remain a pioneering organization must anticipate the concepts and reality of the future community far enough in advance to provide the time necessary for the changes to take place and to be in readiness. (3) In the complicated organizational patterns of a hospital with its many hazards for the inexperienced, it is naturally difficult for the older established person to give the younger unestablished person an opportunity to experiment with unsolved problems, particularly those located at the interface of multiple disciplines. You often hear the sentiment: "The brash youngster succeeds only because he doesn't know that the problem can't be solved." Perhaps this is true to a point but it is also possible that he knows more than does his elder of the contributions made by the social scientists in the areas of group dynamics and communications. (4) We should be wary of harsh criticism of the occasional student nurse or student physician who appears in some way to be unaware of the patient's needs or who appears to show irresponsible apathy by failure to match the dedication of the group primarily responsible for the patient's care. Perhaps we and the vast increase of knowledge are equally at fault. The amount of factual material a student must absorb in a limited time increases annually. A student's security and rewards depend on his absorption powers, that is, his ability to take. Certainly, we shouldn't assume that a person's "giving" propensities must automatically match his "taking" propensities. At present we can only select students whose taking abilities are shown by their previous grades and hope that all the candidates for selection have the intuitive judgment to have selected themselves for these giving professions because of their own need to give.

## THE PHILOSOPHY OF GIVING

The discussion so far has been devoted to the changing forces affecting the teaching hospital in the past and the present. It has also included some examples of the ways in which giving plays a role and gives meaning to the work, the conduct, and the individual natures of those involved in patient care.

What about those working in the fields of teaching and research? Does giving also play a role there? It will not be necessary to go into the detail given to patient care because most people feel that the good teacher's relationship to the student is the same as that borne by the parent to the child or the physician or nurse to the patient. As mentioned before, this relationship has changed in our culture gradually from an authoritarian and demanding one to an understanding and encouraging one. Perhaps the metamorphosis of the schoolmaster in the famous novel "Goodbye, Mr. Chips" best exemplifies this change in role.

At the turn of the century, the student of unusual sensitivity and imaginative thinking ability rapidly developed the habit of repressing his aberrant thinking to avoid personal destruction, a sorry pattern for the development of sensitive and imaginative physicians and nurses. Those students made of sterner material often suffered the consequences of rebellion and were forced to finish their education under their own tutelage. Fortunately, most students survived this jungle, and had enough originality and sensitivity left to become the great researchers, teachers, doctors, and nurses of the past half century. How many students were "stifled" or totally lost can only be surmised.

In the medical world where completion of a formal education has been a basic requirement and rebels have been irretrievably lost, the profession has been particularly fortunate in having a select group of individuals who were naturally equipped to provide the understanding or supportive teaching that has only recently been given in the nonmedical disciplines. The Flexner report earlier in the century also did much by eliminating those medical schools which gave too little to their students. Our present accreditation standards for hospital residencies and schools of nursing lead to excellency in teaching by setting a constantly rising minimum standard for this giving. If I am not overly optimistic about the improved teaching in the teaching hospital, there should be an ever-increasing number of young individuals whose trained minds retain conceptual originality and thereby qualify them for careers in research. The increasing flow of such young candidates indicates some grounds for my optimism. Their dedication to providing a gift of knowledge to us all puts them in a special category of giving.

We have been talking primarily about those who are directly involved in the patient care, teaching, and research of the teaching hospital. We must also touch briefly on those whose responsibility and privilege it is to provide the proper "growing climate" and environment for those who are so directly involved. This responsibility belongs to the individual in any position of leadership whether it be that of a trustee, a department of service chief, a hospital administrator, or someone serving on a committee. This leadership must provide an environment which fosters the creativity and change so necessary to the pioneering function of the teaching hospital as well as its three primary functions. Such an environment is one in which a new idea is capable of exciting individuals and groups throughout the organization. It is one in which the leadership, in a risk-taking spirit, stretches the organization to the limit of its capacities to effect the implementation of an idea.

The environment is one in which the individual's right to think and act in an unorthodox fashion is defended and encouraged whenever possible; in which rules are flexible, not restrictive; in which errors of commission are not considered in the same light as errors of omission. It is one in which the relationships among all professions, skills, and ranks are fluid, respectful, and easily maintained; and ideas are quickly communicated back and forth formally and informally so as to make cross-pollination of thinking a matter of casual routine. It is one in which the tradition most respected is that of constant change and improvement. It is the type that cannot be ordered into being but must be nurtured by an understanding and spirited leadership.

Leadership of this type can be successful over a long period of time only if it is aware of the teaching hospital's total commitment to giving. If it accepts the primacy of giving in the work, the conduct and the individual natures of those involved in patient care, teaching, and research, this leadership may well use certain principles subsidiary to the central giving concept in guiding the hospital forward in keeping with the future needs of the community. Of the many possible subsidiary ideas, I would like to suggest only four: (1) The striving for excellence in every area, no matter how minor, is essential to the idea of giving to the utmost. (2) Patient care should have or should appear to have priority over teaching and research in order to maintain the sanctity of the individual patient to whom so much must be given now and for whose future care so much education and research must be provided. Assigning priority to teaching activities or research activities suggests that the patient of the future is more important than the patient of today — a suggestion that the patient of today naturally finds unreasonable even though he may be the patient of the future. As long as he and his care are more important than the learning going on about him, he is comfortable in his proper role. With any reversal of that role,

he may appear to be the giver and those around him the takers —
a possible distortion of care and of teaching discernible to both the
patient and the student. (3) The self-sacrificial nature of greatness
in man or institution poses a constant threat of overextension and
self-destruction for the man or institution aspiring to maximal contribution. However, the mediocrity that comes from moderate effort is a quality which the teaching hospital can ill afford to show
in policy, in action, or in goals. (4) As greater insight into man
and his illnesses is gained, this insight must be put to use for the
benefit of not only the patients but those who care for the patients
as well. This means when put into practice that an understanding
leadership by its very nature comes to constantly greater understanding and gives more and more to those who give.

These four principles with the others mentioned earlier may
also serve the teaching hospital as guide lines in meeting the changing needs of our society, a society whose direction of evolutionary
change in some ways may be predicted from analysis of its recent
past. The nature of the teaching hospital in its present development
provides reason for believing that these needs will be well met.

# HOSPITALS, MEDICINE, AND THE
## BEHAVIORAL SCIENCES

George G. Reader, M.D.

THE behavioral science with which I have had the most experience is sociology, and the realm of application most familiar to me is the illumination of problems encountered in the care of ambulatory patients. Accordingly, this paper will focus on certain results and implications of several interrelated studies which were carried out collaboratively with sociologists in the Out-patient Department of The New York Hospital-Cornell Medical Center over the past ten years. The studies encompass demonstration and evaluation of the teaching of medical students, appraisal of patient attitudes, in part as an attempt to determine quality of care, and observations on administrative organization. Although the locus of these studies was an out-patient clinic, they have obvious implications for the understanding of other areas of hospital function. And although the approach was mainly sociological, I shall try to indicate a possible role for other behavioral sciences in studies of the hospital.

A large and growing field of behavioral science research in medicine has developed in the past decade, but this report will restrict itself to studies carried out at The New York Hospital-Cornell Medical Center in relation to the Comprehensive Care and Teaching Program (CC & TP). Some of these have been published previously and will be mentioned in summary form; others as yet unpublished will be presented more fully.

Before coming to the results of this research, however, it is appropriate to give some reasons for focusing on ambulatory patients and to explain the significant role of the Out-patient Department within the hospital.

Research reported here was supported by grants from the Commonwealth Fund of New York and by United States Public Health Service grant GN 5687 (C3S1).

## THE OUT-PATIENT DEPARTMENT
## IN PERSPECTIVE

The Out-patient Department plays an essential part in fulfilling the hospital's responsibility to its community. It is a major point of contact with the people of the community as many more patients visit the OPD per year than enter the hospital for bed care, the ratio at the New York Hospital in 1961, for example, being almost two to one. A hospital without out-patient clinics is limited in the service, research, and teaching it can provide. Follow-up of patients to determine outcome of therapy cannot be done effectively without an ambulatory service. The future of medical care, moreover, seems definitely to be in the direction of greater emphasis on ambulatory service, both for reasons of cost as well as convenience. With the technological evolution of medicine requiring a locus for the complex machinery of diagnosis and treatment, the hospital is bound to assume even greater importance as the central point in the medical care network of the community. The hospital's ambulatory service will inevitably grow with the hospital. If the hospital is to develop as a responsible community agency, the presence of a strong out-patient clinic as a base for extension of its activities into the community is essential. Organized home care, for instance, represents the projection of hospital standards of patient care into the homes of patients. It flourishes when part of an excellent, hospital-based, ambulatory service.

With the prolongation of life and the consequent increasing prevalence of chronic disease, hospitalization becomes but one of many episodes in the course of an illness. Between periods of being homebound and of being hospitalized for acute exacerbations of a disease process, the patient is the responsibility of the physician who sees him as an ambulatory patient. The maintenance of health and the long-range prevention of disability lie in the physician's hands. As a result, the out-patient clinic physician today is becoming more and more a manager, and together with the nurse, social worker, dietitian, and other specialists, the manipulator of the therapeutic environment. He must know how community agencies may be brought into play in the patient's behalf, how the home situation may be improved, and what facilities are available for rehabilitation and for reinforcement of recommended therapeutic modalities.

As the out-patient service increases in prominence, the difficulties inherent in providing proper service to patients in that setting become more evident. Without planning and special precautions, patient care tends to become fragmented and discontinuous. The large number of patients passing through the clinic doors can lead to emphasis on symptomatic treatment rather than careful evaluation of patient needs as the basis for therapy. Providing patient care of high quality is much more difficult than on the in-patient service. This is not to imply, as is sometimes done, that ambulatory medical care cannot approach the level of care on a university-hospital ward. The out-patient clinic is in many ways unique, and in-patient and out-patient medicine are not directly comparable; they require different techniques and somewhat different criteria for judging their success.

Because the out-patient clinic of the hospital presents distinctive problems in organization and because the patients' environmental relationships and relative autonomy are important considerations, the need for behavioral science concepts and methods is particularly acute in this setting. In order to understand and control the process of providing care for ambulatory patients, one must learn something of the administrative principles at work, the possible ways of evaluating patient attitudes and expectations, and the methods of measuring environmental influences. In addition, if young physicians are to be taught the art of providing care for ambulatory patients, the process must be dissected to the point where at least some features of it can be readily communicated didactically rather than merely by precept and example. The Comprehensive Care and Teaching Program applied sociological principles to the attainment of these ends both in patient care and teaching. A brief description of the program is necessary to an understanding of what was attempted, and to an appreciation of the teaching-learning environment provided.

## CONTEXT OF THE STUDIES

### *The Cornell Comprehensive Care and Teaching Program*

The Comprehensive Care and Teaching Program at Cornell was conceived as an experiment in medical education and patient care; it was to be a demonstration with evaluation of its effects. The demonstration encompassed a reorganization of the fourth-year medical school curriculum, introduction of full-time staff into OPD teaching, and improvement of service to ambulatory patients. Details have been published elsewhere;[1] suffice it to say that in the Comprehensive Medicine course, medical students at Cornell spend 22½ weeks, or half of their fourth year, in an integrated program of study in the Departments of Medicine, Pediatrics, Psychiatry, and Public Health. They serve as physicians to ambulatory patients under the supervision of senior staff members. The General Medical and General Pediatrics Clinics of The New York Hospital are the main sites of operation and full-time faculty members provide over-all supervision of the teaching and patient care. A consultation system permits relatively complete diagnostic study of patients within the two clinics; internists and pediatricians see to it that patients receive coordinated and continuous care.

The evaluation of the effects of the Comprehensive Care and Teaching Program on student learning and on patient care has been a large-scale effort, and only a few selected findings will be described here. First, however, the aims of the research and the methods employed deserve brief attention.

It was assumed that the integrated experience with patients provided to Cornell students by the revised curriculum would not result in a large increment in factual knowledge, either in comparison with previous classes or between the third and fourth years. On the other hand, the added emphasis on social and psychological attributes of patients was expected to result in no diminution in the high level of achievement on objective tests of medical information, and this has indeed been true. The primary increment anticipated was in the development of student attitudes toward medicine and patient care appropriate to mature physicians, along with an increase in the students' ability to solve patient problems, while improving their clinical judgment.

The process of medical education consists of learning facts and technical skills and acquiring the role-attributes of the physician. In the first two years of most medical schools the emphasis is on facts and technical skills; in the third and fourth years it shifts gradually to include learning the values and attitudes of physicians as well. Learning the social role, such as that of the physician, is called socialization by sociologists; generally speaking, it is the process by which individuals acquire the social attributes appropriate to the statuses they occupy in society.[2] In the CC & TP, socialization with respect to the professional role of the physician might be expected to be the dominant process, and sociologists, therefore, seemed the appropriate investigators to analyze it. Professor Merton, Dr. Patricia Kendall, and their colleagues at the Bureau of Applied Social Research (BASR) at Columbia University had already developed an interest in professional socialization and had acquired a formidable experience in the methodology of attitude research. In a happy convergence of interests a collaborative enterprise was therefore established to evaluate the effects of the CC & TP on medical student learning, with Professor Merton and his colleagues providing some of the information on which medical educators might later base their judgment of success or failure.[3]

Since the Cornell medical students spend half of their fourth year in the Course in Comprehensive Medicine and the other half in a more traditional experience in Surgery, Obstetrics, and Gynecology, and full-time elective work, appraisal of student attitudes and values prior to the fourth year, at the middle, and at the end would permit a comparison of the differential effect of the Course in Comprehensive Medicine with more traditional teaching. The whole medical school experience is a significant social context for student learning and for this reason it was determined that observations would be carried out on all four classes over a period of years; in this way development of attitudes and values and their relationship to a variety of learning situations might be traced.

*Methods*

The investigators used a number of research methods in the study of medical student learning as well as in the other studies to be reported here, and it may be helpful to describe some of them briefly. Participant observation was one technique where the sociologist would, for example, attend classes with students or clinics with patients and interview them informally about their reactions to the situation they were both experiencing. In addition the investigators analyzed the salient social factors in the clinic setting as well as those emerging from conversations with staff, students, and patients. They also carried out formal interviews with structured interview guides. From these data they constructed questionnaires which could be administered to all the students or to a sample of patients or faculty members. Based on further observations the questionnaires were constantly subject to modification, although core questions were retained so that responses to the same stimuli could be measured over time. Some students were asked to keep diaries and were interviewed at regular intervals to indicate to them the appropriate material to record. In this way the sociologists multiplied their observation posts and obtained special insights into the student culture. Other techniques included use of reports of contact with patients, analysis of patient charts, and factual quizzes. The investigators had access to all the usual sources of information about the hospital and medical school as well, such as annual reports, attendance statistics, and student grades, and all were used in one way or another to characterize the social structure and interaction of the hospital-medical school community.

## RESULTS OF STUDIES

### Teaching and Learning

Preliminary findings from the research into medical student learning have been reported previously;[4,5,6] some of the findings from three studies, two of faculty attitudes and one of the effects of the Course in Comprehensive Medicine on student attitudes, will be presented and discussed.

#### Faculty Attitudes

In 1954, while determining points of view on student teaching of the various clinical departments in order to gauge their effect on the learning environment, members of the BASR staff interviewed 89 members of the clinical faculty.[7] Faculty members were asked to indicate how they perform two of their most important roles — teacher and physician. They were also asked about their expectations of the good fourth-year student as well as what kind of abilities were demanded by the practice of medicine. The 89 faculty members were distributed throughout the clinical departments about equally. Full-time and part-time physicians were included, and junior as well as senior staff members. From the analysis of the responses it was possible to characterize the points of view of the various clinical departments and make some distinctions among them that have bearing on how medical students are taught and how these departments tend to function in the care of patients.

There appeared to be a dichotomy of views regarding what performance should be expected of students in the clinical years, which the sociologists labeled "social-interactional" and "technical-medical." The social-interactional approach represents an emphasis on knowledge of social and psychological factors in illness and the ability to develop and maintain an optimal relationship with patients. A technical-medical outlook implies that the instructor believes a definite body of factual knowledge and skills must be communicated to students, even to the exclusion of developing ability in the interactional sphere. Nearly all instructors placed some value on both points of view but there were some who appeared to be oriented most of the time toward the technical-medical; others, toward the social-interactional; and still others who gave about equal emphasis to both. In general, instructors seemed to feel that a good student would value highest the instructor's own orientation toward what was most important in patient care, a projection of their attitudes onto students. Another way of describing these views of instructors is to say that some thought it important to place formal emphasis on teaching social-interactional skills because students would naturally learn the necessary technical facts in the ordinary course of their medical education; others thought it important to concentrate on facts because students would readily learn how to deal with patients during their medical careers, and some thought both interactional skills and medical facts needed explicit attention.

In all departments there were some faculty members of one

persuasion or another, but there seemed to be a particular point of view that predominated in each department even though the numbers of respondents were too few to make a definitive statement in this regard. Surgery and Obstetrics and Gynecology, for example, appeared to place the greatest emphasis on the medical-technical outlook; Psychiatry and Pediatrics tended to be oriented interactionally, while the Department of Medicine placed equal emphasis on both. This is shown in Table 1.

TABLE 1. THE RELATION OF DEPARTMENT AFFILIATION TO INSTRUCTORS' MEDICAL ORIENTATION

| Instructors' medical orientations | Departmental affiliation (per cent) | | | | |
|---|---|---|---|---|---|
| | Surgery | Obstetrics and gynecology | Medicine | Pediatric | Psychiatry |
| Primarily technical | 70 | 83 | 23 | — | — |
| Technical and interactional | 20 | 37 | 73 | 23 | — |
| Primarily interactional | 10 | — | 4 | 77 | 100 |
| Total | 100 | 100 | 100 | 100 | 100 |
| Total number of instructors | 20 | 8 | 26 | 13 | 14 |

Source: Modified from Gene N. Levine, Natalie Rogoff, and David Caplovitz, "Diversities in Role Conceptions," Bureau of Applied Social Research, Columbia University, 1955 (mimeographed, 65pp), p. 28.

Taking all faculty members interviewed and relating their basic orientations, departmental affiliations aside, to preferences for types of patients and opinions about appropriate experiences for students produced some other provocative associations. When asked, "What kinds of patients do you find uninteresting?," about one-third of the instructors denied that any patient was not of interest to them. Moreover, no instructor felt that a patient was uninteresting whose problem was both complex and organic in origin. Nine out of ten of the technically oriented, however, felt that some patients are less interesting than others whereas only 7 out of 10 of those with the other orientations felt this was so, as is indicated in Table 2.

In addition, 8 out of 10 of the technically oriented prefer to refer out-patients with social or psychiatric problems, that is, they do not wish to accept personal responsibility for such problems, while only half of the others would refer them out of their care.

TABLE 2. THE RELATION OF INSTRUCTORS' MEDICAL ORIENTATION
TO THEIR JUDGMENT OF INTERESTING PATIENTS

| | Medical orientation (per cent) | | |
|---|---|---|---|
| Instructors' judgment of patients | Primarily technical | Technical and interactional | Primarily interactional |
| All patients interesting | 13 | 28 | 33 |
| Some less interesting | 87 | 72 | 67 |
| Total | 100 | 100 | 100 |
| Total number of instructors | 24 | 29 | 27 |

Source: Modified from Gene N. Levine, Natalie Rogoff, and David Caplovitz, "Diversities in Role Conception," Bureau of Applied Social Research, Columbia University, 1955 (mimeographed, 65pp), p. 37.

In terms of student experience, two out of three of those who put some emphasis on the social-interactional orientation believe a medical student should have some personal, supervised responsibility for patients because this will enhance attitudinal learning, but only half of the technically oriented group would permit students an autonomous role.

This diversity of opinion has suggestive implications for student learning, for the success in acceptance of one type of teaching program over another, and for the type of environments provided for patients. First and most important is the probable effect of a lack of faculty consensus on formation of consistent student attitudes and values. It is not surprising that students develop a variety of attitudes about patient care when such a variety exists among their teachers. On the other hand, it would be antithetical to the university ideal to expect complete conformity with one set of values or another from the faculty. Moreover, the technically oriented and the interactionally oriented teacher each plays an essential part in fostering the growth of knowledge, and the medical school has need of both.

The constellation of attitudes represented by lack of interest in some patients, desire to refer out-patients with social and psychiatric problems, and doubt that students gain anything from working with patients on their own, suggests that a number of faculty members may be disinclined to favor a teaching program like the CC & TP, which emphasizes interest in all patients, responsibility for social and psychological problems, and some student autonomy. A service characterized by this set of attitudes too might be expected to be somewhat more authoritarian, bureaucratic in the sociological sense, and impersonal toward patients than the one where social-interactional attitudes are dominant. It should be noted, however, that conditions treated on the two services may be expected to be dealt with most efficiently and effectively in the environment suitable to them; there can be little question, for example, that surgical conditions are handled best where there is a premium on technical skill, and children flourish most satisfactorily in an atmosphere of technical competence tempered by large amounts of tender loving care.

The data on this relatively small sample of 89 faculty members prompted further exploration of faculty attitudes through a questionnaire mailed to all members of the clinical faculty in 1956.[8] By comparing the student questionnaire responses with the faculty responses it was hoped that we would be able to determine which faculty values and attitudes were communicated to the students in the course of their medical school years and to what extent. A chief finding was that both students and faculty gave more emphasis to acquisition of technical knowledge and skill than to value learning. Even those faculty members who were interactionally oriented tended to believe that technical knowledge and skill is of the greatest importance. This finding is not really surprising, for the medical profession necessarily recognizes that medical knowledge and technical skill define the professional role. The physician who knows nothing of modern medicine or who cannot distinguish an evident heart murmur is not a physician at all, but social-interactional attributes must be added to the technical for the physician to fulfill his social role completely.

It was also discovered that students are aware of the social-interaction values held by some of their teachers but do not necessarily accept them. As students, they feel that it is more appropriate for them to concentrate on the technical aspects of medicine, and that later as practitioners these other attributes will be more appropriate. Compared with their elders on the faculty, younger faculty members, too, tended to eschew the social-interactional values. From these data, one might conclude that it may take many years of maturation or of socialization to the medical culture for a patient-orientation to develop in some physicians, and a few, of course, may never develop it. Since house-staff training was not found to enhance concern for patients, the question may be asked what influences *do* result in adding an appreciation of patients' total needs to the young physician's understanding of disease mechanisms and the techniques of treatment. Caplovitz suggests a concept of delayed learning, whereby once having been exposed to certain values and attitudes, students respond to them later in life when they appear more applicable to the professional role and status then occupied.

If the function of the teaching hospital is to meet the needs of patients and communicate these skills to young physicians, how can this be done most effectively in the light of the findings just cited? One way may be to attempt more intensive teaching programs for undergraduates, and the next section will give some indication of the success to be expected in that area. Another way is to recognize that physicians' learning about patients' social and psychological needs may be infinitely delayed and to provide for a division of labor. An enlarged role for the social worker and nurse may help to fill the gap in the hospital and allow those physicians with a purely technical orientation to proceed with their work, unencumbered by a feeling of responsibility for patients' social and psychological needs. This will require a nurse or social worker to have routine access to all patients, and training that will permit her to identify and act on the problems presented.

### Student Attitudes

Professor Merton and his colleagues arranged to administer the questionnaire, which they designed to obtain information about student attitudes and values, to all four classes of students in Cornell University Medical College from 1952 through 1956. The questionnaire was given in May to all classes, but the fourth-year class had an additional opportunity to express their opinions in December just after completing the first semester and before starting the second. Group A represented the half of the fourth-year class taking the Course in Comprehensive Medicine in the fall semester and Group B, the half taking it in the spring semester. This is a so-called "panel design" which provides repeated observations on the same individual using the same criteria, or may be looked upon as administering the same stimulus a number of times and observing changes in the response. Data were collected in this way on about 300 students.

Patricia Kendall, James A. Jones, and Candace Rogers of the BASR staff carried out the analysis of these data.[9] Two sets of their findings are of particular interest in this context: student attitudes toward patient contact and student response to time pressures in their work.

Students were asked: "Do you look upon your contact with patients while in medical school primarily as an opportunity to learn medicine? primarily as an opportunity to help patients? as presenting equal opportunities to learn medicine and to help patients?" Table 3 shows the distribution of their responses.

TABLE 3. STUDENTS' CLASS IN MEDICAL SCHOOL AND THEIR ATTITUDES REGARDING PATIENT CONTACT

| | Medical school (per cent) | | |
|---|---|---|---|
| Attitudes regarding patient contact | 1st year | 2nd year | 3rd year |
| Opportunity both to learn medicine and help patient | 75 | 50 | 57 |
| Opportunity only to learn medicine⎫<br>Opportunity only to help patients ⎭ | 25 | 50 | 43 |
| Total | 100 | 100 | 100 |
| Total number of students | 325 | 324 | 336 |

Source: Modified from Patricia L. Kendall, James A. Jones, and Candace Rogers, "The Effects of the Cornell Comprehensive Care and Teaching Program on the Attitudes and Values of Fourth Year Medical Students," Bureau of Applied Social Research, Columbia University, 1960 (mimeographed, 203pp), Confidential Report, p. 45.

The proportion of students who looked upon patients as an opportunity both to learn and to help rather than just learn dropped steadily from the first through the third year, from 75 per cent to 57 per cent. In the fourth year, however, at the end of the first semester, those who had completed the course in Comprehensive Medicine, when compared with those who had not, showed a jump to 79 per cent viewing patient contacts as an opportunity both to learn and to help patients, as may be seen in Table 4. Moreover, this orientation tended to persist up to graduation. Students beginning the course in Comprehensive Medicine in December, Group B, also demonstrated a gratifying increase in viewing patient con-

TABLE 4. THE IMPACT OF EXPOSURE TO CC & TP ON CHANGE
IN ATTITUDES REGARDING PATIENT CONTACT
AMONG TWO GROUPS OF STUDENTS

| | *Point of time in medical school (per cent)* | | | | | |
| | *Group A* | | | *Group B* | | |
| *Attitudes regarding patient contact* | *End of 3rd year* | *Middle of 4th year* | *End of 4th year* | *End of 3rd year* | *Middle of 4th year* | *End of 4th year* |
|---|---|---|---|---|---|---|
| Opportunity both to learn medicine and help patient | 59 | 79 | 64 | 52 | 53 | 72 |
| Opportunity only to help patient<br>Opportunity only to learn medicine | 41 | 21 | 36 | 48 | 47 | 28 |
| Total | 100 | 100 | 100 | 100 | 100 | 100 |

Source: Modified from Patricia L. Kendall, James A. Jones, and Candace Rogers,
"The Effects of the Cornell Comprehensive Care and Teaching Program on the Attitudes
and Values of Fourth Year Medical Students," Bureau of Applied Social Research,
Columbia University, 1960 (mimeographed, 203pp), Confidential Report, p. 46.

tacts as an opportunity to help as well as learn, indicating that the
CC & TP was successful in providing an environment where patients could be perceived as needing help from students as well as
illustrating instances of disease.

Turning next to student preferences for types of patients, there
is a distinct trend found of increasing preference for patients with
physical illness from the first to the third year, as Table 5 shows.

TABLE 5. STUDENTS' CLASS IN MEDICAL SCHOOL AND
THEIR PREFERENCE FOR PATIENT TYPES

| | *Medical school class (per cent)* | | |
| *Patient type preferred* | *1st year* | *2nd year* | *3rd year* |
|---|---|---|---|
| No preference | 66 | 58 | 52 |
| Patient with physical illness | 27 | 39 | 45 |
| Patient with emotional illness | 7 | 3 | 3 |
| Total | 100 | 100 | 100 |
| Total number of students | 245 | 241 | 253 |

Source: Modified from Patricia L. Kendall, James A. Jones, and Candace Rogers,
"The Effects of the Cornell Comprehensive Care and Teaching Program on the Attitudes
and Values of Fourth Year Medical Students," Bureau of Applied Social Research,
Columbia University, 1960 (mimeographed, 203pp), Confidential Report, p. 56.

Again the effect of the Course in Comprehensive Medicine was in the direction of slowing down this trend as we see in Table 6. The

TABLE 6. THE IMPACT OF EXPOSURE TO CC & TP ON CHANGE
IN PREFERENCE FOR TYPES OF PATIENTS
AMONG TWO GROUPS OF STUDENTS

| | Point of time in medical school (per cent) | | | | | |
| | Group A | | | Group B | | |
| Patient type preferred | End of 3rd year | Middle of 4th year | End of 4th year | End of 3rd year | Middle of 4th year | End of 4th year |
|---|---|---|---|---|---|---|
| Patient with physical illness | 47 | 46 | 54 | 46 | 57 | 58 |
| Patient with emotional illness No preferences | 53 | 54 | 46 | 54 | 43 | 42 |
| Total | 100 | 100 | 100 | 100 | 100 | 100 |

Source: Modified from Patricia L. Kendall, James A. Jones, and Candace Rogers, "The Effects of the Cornell Comprehensive Care and Teaching Program on the Attitudes and Values of Fourth Year Medical Students," Bureau of Applied Social Research, Columbia University, 1960 (mimeographed, 203pp), Confidential Report, p. 57.

program had a limited success in halting the trend toward preferring physically ill patients, however, because it was not able to reverse it. Once students developed this preference, the Course in Comprehensive Medicine did not succeed in modifying their position.

The second set of findings of interest here related to the effect of time pressures on students. Students were asked: "About how often have you felt rushed during Comprehensive Care Clinic sessions?" They could answer, frequently, once in a while, or practically never. When their responses about pressure of time are analyzed in relation to patient preference, the data show that those students not experiencing particularly serious time pressures in the General Medical Clinic were less likely to shift to a preference for physically ill patients. As Kendall says,

This relationship between time pressures and a preference for a patient with a physical illness is readily understandable. A patient with a clearly-defined illness is generally not as time-consuming as a patient with vague symptoms which must be systematically checked.[10]

Also, feeling rushed in the General Medical Clinic seemed related to a loss of interest in the social-emotional problems of patients. Kendall writes,

When students feel rushed during a clinic session, they are likely to become impatient with what they may consider the non-medical aspects of a case. They want to get on with the establishment of a diagnosis and a plan for treatment and not be side-tracked by other time-consuming problems.[11]

Time pressures seemed to have a deleterious effect not only on sympathy for patients but also on development of clinical judgment. In discussing the interpretation of her data on that score, Kendall says,

A student who experiences heavy demands on his time, and feels himself under pressure, is probably more likely to develop a set of standardized reactions to situations which he faces recurrently . . . Only when he has time to think and weigh the consequences of alternative lines of action is the student likely to develop discrimination.[12]

One other finding from this study that should be mentioned is the effect of continuity of patient care on the student's conception of a physician's responsibility for patients' social and emotional problems. Over 80 per cent of students who did not endorse the belief initially that it is the physician's responsibility to investigate the patient's background did so if they averaged 2.5 or more contacts with their clinic patients. Repeated visits with patients over time cause the student to become involved in their problems, and he tends to acknowledge the relevance of the patient's background to his illness and its treatment.

Implication from these findings for hospital function are clear but at the same time they pose a dilemma. If students are to develop optimally in terms of their sense of responsibility for total patient care, they must not feel rushed and they must have an opportunity for observation of ambulatory patients over time, averaging at least 2.5 visits per patient. Presumably even mature physicians will function more comprehensively under such circumstances than when they are rushed or where patient care is fragmented. But this means that only a relatively small number of patients may be seen; the large numbers who seek admission to a hospital out-patient service must be turned away or dealt with in some other fashion. At the New York Hospital-Cornell Medical Center this problem has been partially solved by providing an appointment system in the Medical and Pediatric Clinics and in addition, organizing special clinics to take care of patients with the most pressing complaints. A patient who comes to the hospital, for example, with a cough and fever must be evaluated at once to determine whether a serious respiratory infection is present. A large number of such patients would quickly disrupt an appointment system and lead to the kind of rushed atmosphere in the clinic that would inhibit physicians from practicing in a comprehensive fashion. On the other hand, such patients are not regularly candidates for admission to the bed service and do not belong in the Emergency Room, which should be reserved for true emergencies. Instead they are better served in a clinic, such as the one that has been established at The New York Hospital, where treatment may be begun after a quick evaluation is completed, and the patient referred for later follow-up and further study in the General Clinic.

## Clinic Administration

Although the development of the Stat Clinic represented an empirical response to the perceived problem of time pressures in the clinic, a more systematic review of the administrative procedures and the ways in which they related to clinic functioning was obviously called for. Dr. Mary Goss carried out such a study, beginning first with an analysis of the role of the full-time staff physicians in the clinic.[13] Her sources of information included several years of participant observation, the content of formal interviews with full-time staff members, and various CC & TP documents. Her survey of day-to-day activities of full-time staff indicated that each full-time person to a greater or lesser extent takes a direct part in educating students, serving patients, investigating aspects of the teaching or patient care process, and administering the clinic as well as the CC & TP as a whole. The Assistant Director for Medicine, for example, when serving as the administrative officer of the Medical Clinic, regularly reviews charts in order to maintain standards of patient care both in terms of professional ideals and CC & TP organizational goals and teaches and sees patients as well, filling in the part-time instructors absent that day.

Another most important aspect of the administrative role she identifies as "innovation" or the constant re-evaluation of organizational functions to determine new and more optimal ways of achieving goals. This is explored further in another paper.[14] It is also manifested in the research orientation of the CC & TP staff which has resulted in a number of studies, some of which will be reported here. Innovation is the result of creative activity and is greatly impaired by time pressures and the distraction of multiple responsibilities such as practice affords. A certain amount of contemplation is essential to the development of new ideas, and the introduction of full-time personnel into clinic work provides time for contemplation of clinic problems and for consequent innovation.

In continuing her investigations into the administrative structure of the Medical Clinic, Dr. Goss turned her attention to the supervisory relations within the medical hierarchy and found that physicians were able to retain the autonomy required by professionals in their work despite the clinic's administrative arrangements.[15] Physicians accepted supervision if it came from other physicians whom they respected and it was viewed as advice, that is, as a formal advisory or consultative relationship. This system worked, in her view, because of the long process of socialization to which physicians are exposed in their student and house-staff training, whereby they learn to accept the advice and supervision of respected professional superiors. These findings identify a problem for lay administrators for, as she points out, "If the non-physician is unfamiliar with professional norms and values, or unwilling to accept them as guides for his conduct with physicians, he may experience considerable frustration in attempting to exercise control, even in administrative matters." [16]

Most physicians view administration as a nonprofessional activity, and Goss next turned to a study of attitudes of clinical faculty members toward the administrative role.[17] Data were obtained from a questionnaire survey as well as from participant observation. She found that physicians openly viewed administration as a relatively nonprofessional and unappealing type of activity in comparison with patient care, teaching, or research, yet most of the full-time faculty respondents reported spending at least some time in administration. Full-time men, moreover, expressed a greater personal interest in administration than did the part-time staff. Younger instructors tended to have more interest in administration than senior faculty members, who were perhaps surfeited with their administrative responsibilities.

These findings suggest the need in hospital staffing for clinician-administrators who will accept responsibility for organizing and supervising patient care services as well as lay administrators who will supervise important housekeeping services. Lay administrators or those physician-administrators who have allowed their professional skills to atrophy may, however, have to tread warily in their relations with medical staff and may, therefore, be less effective in some areas of administration than their professionally respected colleagues. Fortunately, a number of people are available in full-time academic posts who are interested in administration and would welcome the opportunity to participate in it. The hospital must be structured to make optimal use of their talents without threatening their technical competence or their role as innovators through the pressure of routine duties. Proper support by adequate secretarial help and the assistance of junior lay executives to whom nonprofessional tasks could be delegated would free them for important decisions about patient care. As hospitals enlarge their responsibility for medical care through development of group practices, enlarged ambulatory services, and prepaid insurance programs, the need will be ever greater for clinician-administrators to maintain quality and create new patterns of service.

## Patients and Patient Care

Patients are the reason hospitals exist; they are also the substance of medical teaching and the subjects of research. In understanding the hospital's functions in service, teaching, and research, therefore, knowledge of the patient population served is essential. Over the past ten years at The New York Hospital-Cornell Medical Center a number of studies have been done of the ambulatory patients served by the Comprehensive Care and Teaching Program.

### Statistical Data on Clinic Population

The patient population has been analyzed in terms of numbers and kinds of people, their needs, their behavior, and their expectations of the kind of help the hospital has to offer. The arrangements provided by the hospital for care have also been examined to see whether continuity and coordination of care is possible, how the doctor-patient relationship functions optimally and what kind of changes are required to fulfill organizational goals.

To determine, among other things, the social and economic characteristics of patients and their range of diagnoses, Margaret Olendzki, of the CC & TP staff, analyzed in 1955 a 50 per cent random sample of patients attending or having appointments to the General Medical Clinic for the month of April.[18] This study indicated that more women than men attended the clinic, but that otherwise the clinic population was fairly representative of the aging lower middle class group in New York City with somewhat fewer Negroes than might have been expected. The diagnoses are what one might expect to find in such a group of older patients, where the General Medical Clinic functions as a diagnostic service for the whole Medical Out-patient Department.

A longitudinal view of patients' attendance in the clinic is even more useful than the cross-section just described, and Olendzki went on to examine appointment-keeping behavior and statistical trends over time. Over a three-year period the crude rate of missed appointments in the Medical Clinic varied from 15 to 25 per cent in any given month.[19] During the year of careful and intensive study from April 1955 to March 1956 it averaged 21 per cent. Further investigation of the appointment-breakers showed that appointment-breaking is widespread; more than half of the patients would break at least one appointment in the course of the year. Thus, contrary to a belief common among hospital personnel, a considerable proportion of broken appointments are made by patients who do not make a habit of it.

Good appointment-keepers were more likely to be over than under 60 years of age, and more likely to be women than men. The typical good appointment-keeper at The New York Hospital is a woman over 70, foreign-born, of East European non-Jewish origin, living near the hospital, with a low income, and multiple ailments. Surprisingly, there was little evidence that appointment-breaking represented a poor doctor-patient relationship or could be related to poor continuity of care. These findings are interesting but clearly indicate the need for further investigation to provide a basis for prediction that may be useful in clinic management. Although the broken appointment rate runs at a relatively constant level, it is apparent that a large number of factors contribute to it, few if any of which are readily controllable at the present time.

Olendzki examined other trends in the statistics of the General

Medical Clinic as well as those relating to broken appointments.[20] She summarizes the trends from 1950 to 1955, as follows: (the CC & TP was established in 1952 in the middle of that period). There was an increase of 65 per cent in the total number of patient visits per year after institution of the CC & TP; an increase in the number of patients served per year of 22 per cent; an increase in average yearly number of visits per patient from 2.4 to 3.5; and a decrease in the yearly rate of patient turnover of 15 per cent. As she says, "The pattern presented by these interrelated trends rather clearly reflects the interest of the CC & TP in encouraging comprehensive, continuing patient care. The total number of visits per year increased more than did the number of patients; thus the average yearly number of visits per patient also increased. The greater number of visits per patient had its price, however, in the form of a trend toward reaching fewer patients yearly who were entirely new to the General Medical Clinic." [21] This conclusion again reflects the dilemma of wanting to admit as many new patients as possible to serve the community better and provide students with a diversity of experience and, at the same time, of wishing to follow as many old patients as possible who require continuing care and who provide students with experience in long-term patient management. As the aging population brings more and more chronic illness and multiple ailments to physicians and hospitals, the problem of accepting sufficient numbers of new patients while following the old ones will become more and more acute. Revisit patients continually increase in numbers, and the attrition through therapeutic success or failure, or because the patient moves away, is less than the number of new patients applying. Accordingly, new means must be developed for dealing efficiently with large numbers of chronically ill, older people without losing consideration for their personal dignity and proper care.

*Further Studies of Patients*

CC & TP research staff members made various attempts to assess the quality of patient care in the out-patient clinics; the study of statistical trends just described was one such effort. It had been expected that those trying to give and teach a more comprehensive kind of care would make some measurable impact that would be discernible in review of patient records as well as in the attendance statistics. A medical audit of charts yielded little comparative information about patient care before and after initiation of the CC & TP. Charts were generally complete; diagnoses were accurate; and follow-up of patients was satisfactory. The investigators' attention, therefore, turned to dimensions of patient care other than those usually recorded in patients' charts, such as patient satisfaction. The approach used was not merely that of asking patients whether or not they were pleased with their treatment. A great deal of thought was devoted to finding out the kind of expectations patients have of medical care. Special efforts were made to ascertain what actually happened to them and how this met or failed to meet their expectations.

Lois Pratt, a sociologist on the CC & TP staff, began this study by randomly selecting 50 patients admitted to the Medical Clinic.[22] Each was interviewed on admission and before and after their visits with a physician. Another social scientist sat in the room with the physician and patient and recorded the interaction. Patients were followed as long as they continued to see a clinic physician, ranging up to 34 visits over an 18-month period. Pratt found that a large majority of the patients initially defined their problems as a serious illness. The dominant goal of two-thirds of the patients was to find out if they had a serious disease; the other one third either wanted a thorough study and diagnosis, or were primarily concerned with treatment. Almost three quarters of the patients wanted some kind of treatment or symptomatic relief. Patients exhibited a remarkable uncertainty about what would happen to them; they lacked hope that they would really be cured, but expected mainly symptomatic help and reassurance. After seeing a physician for weeks or months two thirds had a fairly firm and accurate notion of their diagnosis, but one third failed to learn their diagnosis at all; and most of this group had symptoms of emotional origin. Patients' concepts of a good doctor showed an almost even split between attributes related to medical competence and those that related to skill in interpersonal relations. It may be noted that patients emphasized the social-interactional orientation as much as the technical-medical. Thus, if their criteria of high quality care are to be recognized, the proper preparation of physicians to deal with social and emotional problems of patients, either themselves or with the help of nurses and social workers, is essential.

Further investigations of the level of knowledge of 214 clinic patients as determined by a factual quiz about ten common diseases demonstrated that patients knew only about 55 per cent correct answers on etiology, prognosis, and treatment.[23] Information tended to improve with educational level, but patients with particular diseases were no better informed about their own illness than the rest of the group. In a companion study, physicians in the Medical Clinic were asked their views on information appropriate for patients and the amount they believed patients had.[24] The physicians considered it best for patients to know most of the information asked for on the quiz, but consistently underestimated the amount the patients did know. Those physicians who seriously underestimated patients' knowledge were unlikely to discuss the patient's illness with him. Furthermore, observation of patient-physician interaction indicated that the clinic patients tend to be unaggressive about obtaining information even though they have a desire to know more than they are told. Physicians, too, make little effort to communicate to patients even though they believe it best for the patient to be well-informed. An explanation of this phenomenon offered by Pratt is that "the doctor perceives the patient as rather poorly informed; he considers the tremendous difficulties of translating his knowledge into language the patient can understand along with the dangers of frightening the patient; and therefore, avoids involving himself in an elaborate discussion with the patient; the patient in turn reacts duly to this limited information, either asking uninspired questions or refraining from questioning the doctor at all, thus reinforcing the doctor's view that the patient is ill-equipped to comprehend his problem, and further reinforcing his tendency to skirt discussions of it." [25] The opposite kind of circular process can be set off if the doctor takes the initiative and is gratified by the patient's response, so that he continues to communicate as the patient continues to respond.

Pratt's findings indicate that greater effort is needed to inform patients about their illnesses. She has suggested that facts about common diseases should be introduced in elementary school since people may learn more readily then. Later, when they are ill, they tend to block their own understanding when they identify the information supplied as relating to their own symptomatology. She has further suggested that people be given training in appropriate patient behavior when they first come to see a physician. They might well be taught, she believes, to take the initiative in requesting information from physicians and nurses. It is clear from her studies, though, that the clinic patients she observed are a passive and fearful lot, and that it must be incumbent upon the hospital to receive them with warmth and understanding and send them forth with support, symptomatic relief at least, and a better comprehension of their state of health and the means of maintaining or improving it. This may well require increased staffing to permit a better educational job on the part of the nurse as well as the physician.

In a somewhat different, but related vein, two other studies are worthy of mention: One concerns medical social work referrals by Alice Ullmann, a social worker, and Gene Kassebaum, a sociologist; the other is a study by Doris Schwartz, a public health nurse, and Barbara Henley, a social worker (with the advice and help of physicians and sociologists), of the nursing and psychosocial needs of chronically ill ambulatory patients. Ullmann and Kassebaum studied the social work referrals at The New York Hospital over a six-month period in medicine, pediatrics, and surgery.[26] They found social workers giving casework services more frequently than any other kind of help. In the younger age groups the work was mostly geared to improving family relationships; while for older patients, caseworkers were more likely to use community social agencies in planning for chronic and terminal care, with intensive but short-term casework. In pediatrics there was the greatest convergence between reasons for referrals and services actually given, and in surgery the least. Ward patients received the most intensive casework help. Terminal-care arrangements stand out as the major problem on the surgical service, while casework constitutes the major service on the medical and pediatric wards. There are relatively few referrals from private and semiprivate services and referrals from the out-patient department tend to be superficial. This suggests that extension of formal social service rounds to the private service and the OPD might result in greater and more appropiate use of social workers. The social worker evidently has an important place in the hospital, and on her own casework terms, rather than merely as an aide to the physician. She may become even more valuable as physicians and nurses learn of her special skills and call on her more frequently to use them. Also, as the need for understanding of patients' social and psychological problems grows, she may find her role enlarging to free the physician for fuller exercise of his technical competence.

The study of nursing care was of a 10 per cent random sample of 220 elderly, ambulant patients attending the General Medical Clinic. The complete findings will be reported in a volume to be published in 1966,[27] but a part of the study, already published relating to medication errors is of particular interest to this discussion.[28] The investigators found a majority of the patients to be making one or more errors in their medications; 26 per cent were making serious errors. The type of error that occurred most frequently was omission of medication; next, inaccurate knowledge, followed by errors in self-medication, incorrect dosage, and lastly improper timing or sequence. As Schwartz says, "Initially it was hoped that the error-prone patient could be recognized by some simple means and protected from the consequences of his error-making by delegating responsibility to a relative, neighbor, or to a community agency, such as the Visiting Nurse Service. The evidence accumulated in this study would lead us to consider this a nearly hopeless task at present unless each individual patient is carefully interviewed about what he is doing or plans to do, regarding medications. . . . In determining how much responsibility can be delegated to a particular person for carrying on a self-administered drug treatment program, therefore, individual assessment of what a patient is doing or plans to do, and what he knows or feels he knows about the drugs he is taking, appears to be essential." [29] The implications for hospital function are clear: if medication regimens for ambulatory patients are to be effective, time must be provided for interviewing patients periodically about their drug usage, and staffing must be planned with this in mind.

## THE ROLE OF RESEARCH IN PATIENT CARE

The behavioral sciences have now reached a stage of development where they are beginning to be applied with considerable success to the elucidation of the elements that comprise high-quality medical care. The nature of the medical care process makes the use of methods from the behavioral sciences particularly appropriate to analysis of the best application of a rapidly evolving medical technology to the community. One of the most exciting features of the introduction of the behavioral sciences into the work of the hospital and medical school is that much of what has formerly been thought of as the art of medicine can be studied objectively and scientifically. The art will always remain, of course, because it represents the personal style of the practitioner in applying medical facts and techniques to problems patients present, but the factors that inhibit or promote communication between doctors and patients, or among health personnel, or the best type of organization for effective service, are now amenable to study.

If a patient care research group is to be developed in the hospital, what should its composition be and where is it best located? Behavioral Science encompasses a number of disciplines, the most relevant of which are sociology and psychology, the combined discipline of social psychology, and cultural anthropology.

Sociologists are essential for an investigation of the organizational structure of the hospital and for examining the social system, comprising doctors, nurses, social workers, and patients. They are also necessary for properly surveying attitudes of patients and others in the community at large. Psychologists, on the other hand, may be expected to make their greatest contribution in studying the individual differences of patients which are relevant to their medical care and in delineating their personality structure and the idiosyncrasies related to personality development. Cultural anthropologists have been most helpful thus far in examining the therapeutic milieu of the mental hospital and in cross-cultural studies of medical care. Their talents lie particularly in identifying cultural norms and values. Where there is ethnic variety in a patient population or where health personnel differ markedly from patients in cultural background, they may be indispensable in bridging barriers to understanding.

Physicians, nurses, social workers, and other health personnel should plan to work collaboratively with the social scientists, if the problems most relevant to health care are to be explored and the findings most applicable to improving service discovered. By working together, too, physicians and others may be expected to learn from their behavioral science colleagues to the point that they are contributing more than ideas and critique, and are, indeed, full working partners in the research.[30]

Depending on the situation in a particular hospital, the research group may be located within hospital administration or in one of the clinical departments. It may even stem from a division or department of behavioral science that is coequal with other sections of the hospital organization. Eventually every hospital may be expected to make use of its operating statistics to maintain a continuous review of its function, as many in fact do now. A group of sophisticated investigators may be able to add much to the interpretation of the routine statistics by building in specific questions to be asked of these data or by adding special *ad hoc* studies to the on-going data collection. One or another of the clinical departments may set up investigations of its own services or of the community at large in terms of special interests, such as epidemiological studies or follow-up of special patient groups. In a university hospital, the Dean's office may have a particular concern with evaluation of student learning behavior and ultimate performance. A behavioral science division in a teaching hospital may well provide research services to the entire institution as well as carrying out investigations basic to its own discipline.

Some of the kinds of research that may be carried out have been indicated in this paper. A more systematic listing of possible research topics is provided by Dr. Mary Goss:

## SOME CATEGORIES AND QUESTIONS INVOLVED IN GENERATING PAST, PRESENT, AND PERHAPS FUTURE RESEARCH IN PATIENT CARE

I. *Who receives care: characteristics of the patient population*
   A. Background characteristics
   B. Diagnoses
   C. Functional capacity
   D. Attitudes, values, opinions, expectations, information relevant to health, disease, health personnel, and medical care
   E. Behavior of relevance to medical care, health, and disease
   F. Needs for particular types of care — expressed and inferred

II. *Who gives care: characteristics of the staff and students*
   A. Background characteristics and technical qualifications

B. Attitudes, values, opinions, expectations, information relevant to health, disease, medical care, and patients
C. Behavior of relevance to medical care

III. *Nature of Medical Care*
   A. As a social process
   Interaction processes: among personnel as a team; between health personnel and patients, patients' relatives
   B. As a technical process
      1. Volume: patients, visit/year
      2. Services rendered
      3. Continuity and centralization
      4. Standard routines: general and for particular types of disease entities, cases
      5. Quality of care: indices

IV. *Organizational Context of Care*
   A. Coordination and control structure
   B. Division of work responsibilities among staff
   C. Aims, values, and principles underlying organization
   D. Communication, social cohesion, staff morale, and consensus
   E. Organizational continuity and change
   F. Relation to larger structure (medical center) and community

V. *Situational Context of Care*
   A. Clinic
   B. Home
   C. In-service of hospital
   D. Private office
   E. Other

VI. *Cost of care*
   A. To patient
   B. To hospital and/or other organization providing it

SUMMARY AND CONCLUSIONS

These studies at The New York Hospital-Cornell Medical Center carried out collaboratively by physicians, nurses, social workers, and social scientists have indicated some of the diverse functions of research in defining the relationship of the hospital to its community. Although focused on the out-patient service, they have ranged widely from evaluation of medical teaching and physician attitudes to appraisal of patient needs. The findings have had implications for many areas of hospital activity, for hospital-community relationships, and for the place of behavioral science research itself in the hospital structure.

More specifically, evaluation of the Course in Comprehensive Medicine revealed a range of student and faculty attitudes relevant to patient care. The sociologists found three orientations toward student learning: a technical-medical emphasis, a social-interactional emphasis, and among some faculty members, an equal emphasis on both. Students and faculty were both found to place more importance on the technical-medical and the acquisition of factual knowledge than on the social-interactional and the learning of values and attitudes. The Course in Comprehensive Medicine was found to slow down the tendency to disregard the social-interactional orientation, without interfering with the acquisition of technical knowledge and skill. Reducing time and work pressures and providing for patient follow-up over time appeared to be central to success in inculcating consideration for patient needs.

A sociologist's observations of the administrative arrangements in the medical out-patient clinic led her to conclude tentatively that the long process of socialization to which physicians are exposed during their training conditions them to accept structured ways of relating to supervisors. The supervising physician to be successful must be respected professionally. His direction in medical matters is then accepted as consultative advice rather than as an order. Physicians thus retain essential professional autonomy while submitting to the strictures of an administrative framework necessary to effective clinic function. These findings suggest that clinician administrators must be developed within the hospital structure to supervise maintenance of standards in quality of care in addition to the lay administrators who concern themselves with housekeeping functions.

Collaborative studies by sociologists, physicians, nurses, and social workers of patients' attitudes, knowledge, and needs indicated that many clinic patients considered themselves to be seriously ill, and although lacking hope or cure, expected symptomatic help and reassurance. Patients emphasized the social-interactional orientation in their physicians as much as technical skill, indicating the importance of these attributes of the physicians' role for patient satisfaction and for high-quality care. Patient's knowledge of disease was found to be a salient factor in communication between doctors and patients, and the physician's responsibility for taking the initiative in the interaction was found to be crucial in increasing patient's understanding. The implications for hospital function of all these findings relate to staffing patterns, organization of services, and the place of on-going research in patient care as a means of steadily improving the ways in which patient needs — medical, social, and psychological — may best be met.

The behavioral sciences appear to have made a place for themselves within the hospital and will have an increasingly important role in the future as medical care becomes technologically and organizationally more complex. The hospital of the future with a well-founded patient care research division may be compared to a highly-developed organism, its research staff acting like organs of perception to evaluate internal function and to probe areas of community need. As the perceptions are integrated and acted upon, the hospital can then homeostatically adjust itself in ever more satisfactory fashion to its internal and external environment. It may then become a more and more active and effective part of the community to which it belongs.

# THE HOSPITAL AS A SOCIAL INSTRUMENT: RECENT EXPERIENCES AT MONTEFIORE HOSPITAL

Martin Cherkasky, M.D.

ALL hospitals are social instruments. The hospitals of our country, however, vary widely in their assumption of social responsibility. At one end of a hypothetical spectrum is the hospital which has a narrow categorical function for a particular kind of in-patient and for whom the hospital is prepared to provide a very limited kind of service. Moving along the spectrum, the functions of the hospital broaden continually both in the kinds of care they are able to provide for in-patients and in the development of ambulatory services along with teaching and research programs. At the other end of the spectrum are the country's major teaching hospitals. Here society has an instrument of extraordinary complexity with a bewildering array of facilities and services and with great numbers of highly specialized personnel successfully carrying out functions that were undreamed of a generation ago.

Despite the fact that these great hospitals are hard put to manage and finance the tasks they have already assumed, I believe that their mission must be expanded. New areas of service need to be explored because of changes in the medical care needs and expectations of society. The nature of the illnesses with which we deal has been altered. We are beginning to think about health as well as disease. Finally, advances not only in the physical and biological sciences but also in the social sciences inevitably must lead the large teaching hospitals to redefine and extend their role as social instruments within the community. It is quite clear that many have already done this and numerous instances come to mind which demonstrate the ingenuity, interest, and broad sense of social responsibility of the more forward-looking hospitals of the country.

The purpose of this paper is to describe the program of one such institution, Montefiore Hospital in New York City, and how it has seen fit to expand its communal responsibilities. These programs were undertaken because we believe that there are medical care problems which face society for which we at the hospital can help provide constructive solutions.

## MONTEFIORE HOSPITAL

When the first President of the Montefiore Home for Chronic Invalids (as it was then called) made his initial annual report in 1885, he noted that the home had been created to care for those incurables for whom none of the existing hospitals were willing to provide. He rightly noted that this was philanthropy of the highest order. Almost eighty years ago the founding fathers of the hospital committed it to the care of the chronically sick at a time when such care was not of great interest to most physicians and certainly not to hospitals.

It was Montefiore's preoccupation with these people and their long obdurate illnesses, and with the social and emotional problems arising from such illnesses, that inevitably turned the institution more toward the family and community than was the case with those hospitals which cared for the acutely ill. Lest this seem obscure, it has seemed to us that the acutely ill patient, whose sickness usually occupies only a brief interlude, comes to the hospital as a stranger, and is the focus of intense activity which usually results in a satisfactory and definitive conclusion. He then slips back to the usual life in the community. His problems can often be dealt with effectively without any probing into the social situation or the family from which the patient came and to which he will return. Chronic illness represents the other side of the coin: here the course is long and the result of treatment is often unsatisfactory and unclear. Handicap and disability are most common.

When Montefiore first became involved with the chronically sick, the available tools with which to deal definitively with the illness were meager indeed. Despite extraordinary advances in our ability to treat some of the chronic illnesses, our scientific weapons are still inadequate to the needs of those so afflicted. The inability to cure, coupled with the long-term nature of the illness and frequent disability, place enormous strains upon the emotional as well as the fiscal resources of the family. Inevitably, we were led to the realization that in attempting to help the patient we would have to concern ourselves with more than just the pathology and physiology of his disease. We would have to deal with the social pathology and some of the emotional and social aberrations which accompany every long-term illness. It was these considerations that led us to understand that the family and the patient's relationship to it could be both a source of "dis-ease," as well as a source of support and comfort.

Through all the years of Montefiore's existence, both as a home for chronic invalids and as a hospital for the last fifty years, the attitude of the governing board, as reflected in its administration and staff, has been that we must provide, in the words of our first Chief of Medicine, Dr. Simon Baruch, "medical, hygienic and moral assistance" to these patients hoping to obtain recovery or improvement. A parallel objective was the utilization of the hospital and its patients for education and research in chronic diseases. By 1947, Montefiore Hospital had a well established program of high-quality patient care, education, and research. In fact, the needs of the very complex and difficult patient problems led us by 1930 to introduce a program of full-time chiefs of divisions well before most of the voluntary hospitals in our area. By 1947 all the major divisions were directed by full-time, academically trained and oriented physicians who devoted all their efforts to the goals of the institution.

While I plan to review those programs and developments at Montefiore Hospital which express a somewhat unique view of the hospital's social responsibility, I wish to state unequivocally that such new responsibilities are in addition to, not in lieu of, the generally accepted purposes of a major patient care, teaching, and research institution. A hospital's social objective requires primary devotion to medical care of the highest quality in order to bring to bear on the problems of illness the most advanced scientific facilities and services. It must also provide a place where physicians and health workers can be trained to the highest level possible. Moreover, the hospital must engage in multifaceted research to illuminate the innumerable unsolved problems of disease and health.

All these things Montefiore Hospital does and does well. No amount of concern with compassion in medicine — no amount of involvement with new methods of organizing and delivering medical care — no concern with broader opportunities to serve the community — can compensate for a deficit in the quality of patient care, of teaching, or of research.

## HOME CARE

After the Second World War, Montefiore Hospital was still devoted primarily to the care of the chronically ill. Its patients with heart disease, cancer, tuberculosis, and neurological disorders had very long hospitalizations, the average length of stay being about 200 days. At the same time, the waiting list of prospective patients lengthened. Not uncommonly, individuals were forced to wait six months before being admitted. This situation of people in need being denied admission while patients who had received whatever definitive care could be provided and continued to occupy beds, harassed the conscience of the professional and administrative staff. Dr. E. M. Bluestone, the distinguished Director of Montefiore Hospital, encouraged by some of the thoughts of the Chief of Medicine, Dr. Louis Leiter, decided that care in the home might solve some of the problems surrounding this dilemma. In 1947, with grants from the New York City Cancer Society and subsequently from other sources, notably the Commonwealth Fund, modern-day home care was initiated. The plan was that patients who still needed doctors' and nurses' care but who no longer needed the specialized facilities of the hospital would be returned to the home and cared for there. Not only would this benefit the patients but it would also make our beds more readily available for those who desperately needed the hospital's facilities.

The mechanical process, as well as philosophical content of the Montefiore Home Care Program, can best be understood by following a typical patient:

John J., in his fifties, had been having abdominal discomfort for some time. He had lost some weight and had blood in his stool. His physician sent him to Montefiore Hospital where he had a complete examination. X-ray examination revealed that he had a narrowing of the bowel which probably represented cancer. At operation, a cancer was found but it had already spread so far that ultimate cure was not possible. Therefore a procedure was done which would prevent him from having a bowel obstruction in the future. Here was a patient who was sick and would remain so as long as he lived. This might be three months, six months, or two years. During all this time he would require the care of a doctor and nurse and the support of social services and other personnel and facilities so that his life might be extended and made as comfortable and dignified as possible. Before home care, the hospital might have kept this patient for a very long period of time, for John J. was unable to use the out-patient department and was at that time considered too sick to be cared for at home. It is this enormous gap between the patient's ability to use ambulatory services and his need for in-patient services that home care fills with an appropriate and suitable mode of care.

Home care was founded on the cardinal principle that return to the home must be in the patient's best interest. To make certain of this two evaluations were undertaken: a medical one to determine whether the patient's medical needs were such that they could be adequately dealt with by the physicians, the nurses, and the others in the home; and of equal or even greater importance was the social evaluation of the patient by a skilled social worker. The patient's feelings about his illness and the effect of his illness on his relationship with other members of the family were studied. In turn the family situation was reviewed to see whether it had the will and capacity to care for the patient if he were to return home.

I was fortunate enough to direct the Montefiore Home Care Program at its inception and was both the physician and administrator during its early years. At that time I presumed that the medical evaluation was the critical one. I quickly learned that this was not the case. Experience clearly proved that the study of the patient's social situation was crucial and it was here that I, personally, had a learning experience which had not been made available to me in my previous medical school or hospital training. The contrast between caring for a patient in a hospital bed where he is cut off from all his usual familial and social relationships and caring for this patient within his home in his natural environment is extraordinarily striking.

Often the return of a sick person to the home represents a heavy obligation for the family. The fact that a husband and wife have lived together for 25 years and seemed to manage quite well does not necessarily mean that there are strong bonds between them. In some instances, the first flush of love has long since worn off and a new set of forces such as inertia, the pressures of social conformity, and the needs of children have kept these people together more as boarders sharing the same physical facilities than as people tightly tied to one another emotionally. We learned that unless there were reasonable and mutually shared feelings of respect and affection and love, return of the patient to the home would not be in his best interests or even, for that matter, the family.

In addition to the doctor and social worker, the third key member of the team was the public health nurse. She had long been working in the home and had great experience in dealing with families and patients under the special circumstances which the home provided. The Visiting Nurse Service of New York enthusiastically welcomed the opportunity to work with a doctor and a social worker in an organized fashion. In every instance, the visiting nurse was asked to evaluate the family even though initially we did not see any particular need for nursing care.

Other personnel were provided if need was present. There were physical, occupational, and recreation therapists to serve the rehabilitation needs of the patient. Appliances and equipment were also made available for immediate use.

The Montefiore Home Care Program has been fully described in a large number of publications from our own institution and from the many places in the United States where such programs have been developed in the last fifteen years.[1-6] There is no question that for the suitable patient home care is an ideal device. It allows the patient to be taken from the atmosphere of the hospital with its routines and inflexibilities. It returns him to his natural environment as soon as possible. For appropriate patients, the warmth, the flexibility, the therapeutic value of the home, is sufficient reason for a hospital to have an organized home care program.

Home care has many other important virtues. It is much less expensive than hospital care. Today, home care costs the hospital between seven and eight dollars a day. In-patient hospital costs in major New York hospitals are more than $50 for each patient-day.

In addition, it spares the precious hospital bed for use by those who need it most. Finally, it provides an unexcelled opportunity for the young physician in training and persons from other health professions to learn about patients and disease in the most appropriate and illuminating circumstances, within the home and within the bosom of the family.

## THE MONTEFIORE MEDICAL GROUP

Once the hospital's eyes were turned out into the home and the community we became aware of other problems of medical care to which the hospital's resources could properly be applied. Chronic diseases have replaced acute illnesses as a major cause of death and disability. Many of these illnesses have an insidious onset where the severity of illness is not forecast by the presenting symptoms. All too often these symptoms may be so innocent as to be readily overlooked and only become insistent when the disease is well advanced. Since, with almost all serious chronic disease the only chance to cure or arrest the illness is by early diagnosis and treatment, it is apparent that nothing must obstruct the patient's easy access to high-quality medical care.

The community must, in fact, organize and finance its medical care in such a way that it will encourage the patient to go to his doctor as early as possible and in turn allow the physician to use freely the laboratory and x-ray services he needs for early and accurate diagnosis. The removal of financial barriers is particularly important in view of the fact that since World War II medical care prices have been the fastest rising item in the consumers' price index.[7] Tragically, serious chronic disease can make paupers of many families.

Another major factor which demands a change in medical care organization is the development of specialization. Medicine has been making extraordinary advances and this has inevitably led to the growth of specialization because no one physician can master all the medical knowledge now available. Even within the specialties themselves it is becoming an ever-increasing chore for the specialist to keep abreast of all that is going on in his particular field. Specialization is here to stay; there will be more of it. And this is good, because it is a direct reflection of our increasing knowledge, understanding, and capabilities. However, the patient still remains physiologically, biologically, and psychologically a whole person and some means must be found so that all this fruitful specialization can be coordinated and integrated in a manner that does not fragment and depersonalize the patient's care. It was all of these considerations that led Montefiore Hospital in the late 1940's into an association with the Health Insurance Plan of Greater New York.

Briefly, this was a prepaid, group practice, medical care program providing comprehensive service directed toward prevention as well as treatment of disease. The plan was that there would be groups of physicians working in centers throughout the City of New York who would provide to the subscribers a whole range of diagnostic and therapeutic services in home, hospital, and office on a prepaid rather than a fee-for-service basis. Montefiore Hospital, as it surveyed its resources which were now focused on the inpatient and more recently on the patient in his home, saw that these same resources could be directed toward the general medical care of the community. In 1948 the hospital signed a contract with the Health Insurance Plan of Greater New York and the Montefiore Medical Group was formed. The hospital undertook to render this type of group practice as an integral part of its total responsibility to the community.

Today, in New York, the Health Insurance Plan has over 650,000 subscribers who are cared for by 31 groups of physicians. Montefiore is the only hospital in the city which is an integral part of this plan. The Montefiore group consists of 50 physicians who provide the total medical care for about 30,000 people in the geographical area in which the hospital is located. They are all employees of the hospital and one-third of them work full time on the project. The program was undertaken not only to render service to the people of the neighborhood but also to explore the use of one mechanism for meeting the changing medical care needs of the population. I stressed earlier the need for hospitals to develop and maintain the highest level of patient care services, teaching, and research. This would, indeed, be an ineffectual exercise if medical care cannot be organized, paid for, and delivered such that the skills we teach and the truths we uncover can be made available to the people that we serve. Montefiore has had fifteen years of experience with prepaid group practice in association with the Health Insurance Plan of Greater New York. In our view, this is an ideal way to meet the medical care needs of the community.[8,9,10]

Prepaid group practice enables the physician to practice the kind of medicine which he has been taught in our medical schools and teaching hospitals. In addition, it can provide for the doctor's professional satisfaction and growth. By working intimately with other physicians his level of competence is maintained. There is no single more important device for maintaining the quality of care than having a doctor share his care of the patient with other physicians whom he respects and whose respect he requires.

Not to be minimized when discussing prepaid group practice is the salutary effect of such programs on hospital utilization. Since the hospital now represents the community's most expensive medical care resource, its use should be limited to a sharp and circumscribed objective and that is, definitive diagnosis and treatment. Studies have on the whole shown that when, as in the Health Insurance Plan, extensive ambulatory diagnostic and treatment services are provided in a group practice setting, the use of in-patient hospital facilities drops. A survey done a few years ago indicates that HIP patients have 20 per cent less hospitalization than a comparable group in the general population.[11] Most of those concerned with skyrocketing hospital costs are searching within the hospital's operations for means of controlling these costs. It is my own view that while this approach is appropriate and will produce certain economies and efficiencies, the major determining factor in over-all hospital cost relates to how and when the hospital is used. It is the doctor's method of practice, his capacity to meet the patient's needs on an ambulatory basis, the manner in which he is paid, the kinds of medical and hospital insurance carried, and other such considerations which exert a major effect on hospital use. It is, therefore, the organization, delivery, and payment for medical care that presents us with the greatest opportunity to control hospital costs on a community-wide basis. The per diem rate will continue to rise inexorably in the foreseeable future at almost 10 per cent a year. Only by providing comprehensive, ambulatory, diagnostic, and treatment services and restricting the use of the hospital for "hospital sick" patients can we make progress in our attempts to control the total medical care bill of the hospital. Since most hospitalization is initiated by the doctor, study and research in all aspects of medical care are a timely and appropriate hospital responsibility.

## FAMILY HEALTH MAINTENANCE
## DEMONSTRATION

In 1949 the Montefiore Hospital undertook, in collaboration with the College of Physicians and Surgeons and the Community Service Society of New York, a sociomedical research and demonstration project entitled "A Family Health Maintenance Demonstration." The impetus for this project came from the Community Service Society, one of America's oldest and most distinguished family agencies. This group was painfully aware of the relative ineffectiveness of social work and other services when applied to families which had begun to disintegrate because of overwhelming internal and external pressures. It was obvious that at the existing level of social and psychiatric casework palliation was often the best that could be accomplished. Important persons in the Community Service Society and in the Milbank Foundation, which was very prominent in the society, were turning their thoughts toward the possibility of developing more constructive and imaginative social welfare services. Montefiore Hospital was then chosen to be the setting for an exciting demonstration project.

The program was begun in 1950. Briefly, it set out to determine whether the health of a group of average families could be favorably influenced over a significant period of time if the physician, public health nurse, and social worker were to apply their skills and knowledge in an organized way to these families. The services of these professionals would be rendered in an integrated fashion with the commanding emphasis on education and prevention rather than treatment. Since the Montefiore had an existing medical group with 4,000 families who were receiving comprehensive preventive and therapeutic care as well as a home care program that had already demonstrated the effectiveness of the health team of physician, nurse, and social worker, it seemed appropriate that this particular hospital collaborate in this unique experiment. The project was financed by the Community Service Society and the Milbank

Foundation and Columbia's College of Physicians and Surgeons provided specialized professional and technical advice.

The program was carried on for five years and much has been written about it.[12,13] Most recently a book entitled "Family Medical Care," written by Dr. George Silver, Montefiore's Chief of the Division of Social Medicine, summarized this very intricate and complicated experiment.[14] Among the specific objectives, we sought to determine how best the family can be motivated to make it seek health, to discover the range and kinds of services which are necessary in the encouragement and maintenance of health, and to determine objectively the difference in health of those families receiving care from the health team as compared to a control group of families.

The findings demonstrated that there is no clear formula which would show us how to achieve in any substantial way the broad goals of family health which we seek. We did, however, learn a good deal about the use of a team of physician, nurse, and social worker in the prevention of illness, and we developed some new and interesting thoughts about the role of social work in such a setting.

Of crucial importance to the developing program at Montefiore Hospital, however, was that the hospital became involved in a sociomedical program which had its accent on health and not on disease. We accepted a concept of health as being not merely an absence of disease but a state of mental, physical, emotional, and social well-being which enables the individual within his family to live a full and fruitful life within society. Montefiore Hospital, through this demonstration, continued its interest in the total needs of the patient and his family, and in fact at the present time is moving forward to new and more sophisticated research in this challenging area.

## THE COMMUNITY CENTER

One of the interesting by-products of the Family Health Maintenance Demonstration was the hospital's sharper recognition of the effect of planned leisure time on family health and well-being. It was, therefore, quite natural for Montefiore to give a portion of its property to the Associated Y's of Greater New York on which a neighborhood community center could be built. The center has been in operation for two years and there are several programs that have been developed jointly by the hospital and the center.

For example, a psychiatric group worker is employed jointly by the hospital's psychiatric division and the center. He works half time at the "Y" and half time at the hospital. The goal of psychiatric care is to enable the patient to return as soon as possible to the community. The group worker supervises a program designed to bridge the gap between hospital and community for the psychiatric patient. The patient, when ready, has recreation activity at the community center so that he is enabled to have an early living experience with his neighbors and his friends. This program has already achieved favorable results.

The center has been useful to the hospital in a very practical way. Montefiore, like many other institutions, is short of nurses and technicians. The center has created a Day Center for the children of our employees. Many of them who ordinarily would have to be at home caring for their children are now able to work at the hospital and be assured that their children are having a full day of supervised and worthwhile activity at the Community Center.

The hospital and the center are now about to initiate a joint project working with the Jewish Family Service to create a co-ordinated program of service and activity for the aged in the community. The hospital will provide the medical screening while the Jewish Family Service provides casework services and the Community Center supplies the recreation and leisure time activities. Many new joint programs will inevitably flow from the collaboration of the "Y" with a hospital which has broadened its horizon to include health as well as disease.

## THE LOEB CENTER

In the middle 1950's the directors of a convalescent home in the northern suburbs of New York began to question the social usefulness of their undertaking. They were seeking patients where once they had long waiting lists. They were suffering the fate of many such institutions removed from the urban mainstream of medical care. After a survey and negotiations, the directors of the institution agreed to recreate their facility as part of the Montefiore Hospital and to change their goals of treatment so that they could join with the hospital to introduce new concepts and set higher standards in the field of nursing home care.

As the hospital becomes more complex and costly and an aging population suffers more chronic illness, the nursing home becomes even more necessary as a resource for posthospital patients. Here the oldest, and most enfeebled, the most helpless, and the most impoverished segment of our society find themselves. It is in the nursing home that the community's effective concern for those who cannot help themselves should be demonstrated. In point of fact, however, nursing home care represents a most scandalous and heartrending crisis in our country's medical care. It has been estimated that we have a shortage of over 260,000 such nursing home beds and out of 307,000 existing beds 134,000 were found to be unacceptable.[15] The vast majority of nursing homes are under proprietary auspices and in my view such control represents a slender and faulty reed upon which to rest so heavy and critical a burden.

The nursing home is often without those very critical medical care skills and resources which the voluntary general hospital has in such abundance. Is it not proper and timely for the voluntary hospital to become more aware of its social responsibility and do something about the quality of care in these homes? A hospital can do as much for the community by helping to elevate the level of nursing home care as it can do by treating patients in its own facilities.

In mid-January 1963, the first patient was admitted to the Loeb Center for Nursing and Rehabilitation. This 80-bed unit is designed not as permanent placement for the long-term patient but as a halfway house where intensive nursing care will follow the definitive period of hospital care with the goal of returning the patient to the community within a period of days or weeks. Moreover, in the Loeb Center we are experimenting with a unique kind of nursing care which hopefully will enable patients to return to their homes sooner than heretofore. The Loeb Center is physically attached to the hospital. This permits the hospital to provide the medical and

ancillary services which in isolated nursing homes are either unavailable or must be created at great expense. We hope in this joint
venture to learn something about the role the general hospital can
play in nursing home care and also in turn to study the effect of
the nursing home on hospital operations and length of patient stay.
Blue Cross, which generally does not pay for nursing home care,
has tentatively consented to pay for thirty days of care in the Loeb
Home at a rate not to exceed 50 per cent of the hospital rate. They
have further agreed that the use of this nursing home benefit would
not in any way deprive the patient of the other in-hospital benefits
to which he is entitled. Needless to say, if it can be shown that this
program can significantly decrease the patient's hospital stay it will
have important and far-reaching economic consequences for the
community at large.

It has become clear that chronic disease, as it is characterized
not only by its long duration but by an acute, active, even emergency phase at one end and obdurate, slow moving, more or less
stable disease and disability at the other, requires a variety of medical care resources to meet patient needs at these various stages of
illness. It is our belief that the hospital as the hub of modern-day
medical care has a responsibility for the continuum of care the
patient requires. With the recent addition of the Loeb Nursing
Center and with the responsibility we have for the medical program of the Beth Abraham Home (a 500-bed custodial institution
ten minutes from Montefiore by car), we have developed or are
participating in the several resources and facilities needed to meet
the patient's changing medical care needs, which are: the general
hospital ambulatory services of the out-patient department and the
Montefiore Hospital Medical Group; the Home Care Program,
Loeb Nursing Center; and the Beth Abraham custodial institution.
It should be reiterated that under the hospital's medical care program the supporting resources make it possible for the patient to be
cared for in the facility or by the program suited to his needs. In
turn, these programs enable us to use the costly, complex, general
hospital in an appropriate manner.

## THE TEAMSTERS

Another program has been undertaken recently by Montefiore Hospital in collaboration with Columbia University and the Teamsters' Union. The Teamsters' Union has approximately 160,000 members in New York City. Several years ago, their Labor-Management Hospitalization Trust Fund, consisting of representatives of labor and management, evinced great concern over the continuous rise in the cost of Blue Cross Insurance. They went to Dr. Ray Trussell, Dean of the School of Public Health and Administrative Medicine at Columbia University (now on leave as Commissioner of Hospitals, New York City), and asked him to help them establish a group of hospitals in New York City which they were certain could be operated much more economically than the existing hospitals in the city. Dr. Trussell suggested that before undertaking so complex a project it would be prudent to learn more about hospitals. They did not care for this advice and left, only to return some months later to ask Dr. Trussell to develop an educational program for them. This was done. The course of study consisted of 16 half-day sessions over a 32-week period. Included in the curriculum were lectures, seminars, and field work at Montefiore Hospital.[16]

As these labor and management representatives developed increased knowledge of the hospital's activities and operations, they soon recognized that the medical care problems of the Teamsters who with their families numbered 500,000 persons, could not be isolated from those of the community as a whole. If they were to receive high-quality and more economical medical care, it was up to them to help achieve these goals for all of New York.

At the same time that this educational program was undertaken, a research group at Columbia University were engaged in a retrospective medical audit designed to evaluate the quality of care for some 400 hospitalized Teamsters. The results of this study were very disturbing not only to the Teamsters but to organized medicine and to hospitals; particularly the proprietary hospitals. There was evidence of serious errors of omission and commission in medical service with such significant frequency that all concerned felt that something had to be done.[17]

The management and labor leadership, as a consequence of their educational experience and the medical audit, abandoned the idea of new independent hospitals which New York City did not need and decided to give their support to any program which would make hospital and medical care as economical as possible and would give assurance of higher quality care. The immediate result was a tripartite contract between the Columbia School of Public Health and Administrative Medicine, Montefiore Hospital, and a segment of the Teamsters representing about 120,000 persons and their families.

The program consists of five parts, all fully financed by the Teamsters: (1) Columbia will continue to expand the medical audit and will attempt to develop new techniques to evaluate the quality of medical care. (2) A medical advice center was created where members of the union and their families could turn. It is our belief that if as a first step the Teamsters were directed to accredited hospitals and board-certified doctors, a significant improvement in the quality of their care would result. (3) Montefiore Hospital undertook, through a specially created Unit, to provide the Teamsters and their families with certain complex specialized diagnostic and treatment procedures such as neurosurgery and cardiac surgery. All these activities are housed in the Teamsters' Center at Montefiore and have been in operation since August 1962. (4) A long-range provision of the contract stipulates that the Teamsters will build at Montefiore Hospital a research hospital floor as well as a floor to house the present activities of the center. An additional floor will be built to provide space for a hospital and medical care research team. This group will use both the hospital research floor for pilot and experimental programs and the entire Montefiore Hospital as a field laboratory for research into every phase of hospital operations. (5) The Teamsters have also committed an additional sum of $200,000 a year for five years to initiate the research program. This will be a joint Columbia-Montefiore undertaking. It is planned to bring together a research team consisting of economists, engineers, social scientists, architects, and operations research experts. The task of this research unit will be to lay open all phases of hospital care and operation and to develop new programs for rendering high quality, economical hospital service.

The program is now underway, and it represents an enormous

challenge in many directions. The Teamsters as a whole spend more than $20,000,000 a year on medical care in New York City. The quality of the care which their members are receiving varies considerably. Their insurance coverage is often inadequate. It remains to be seen just what a coordinated effort by labor, hospital, and university can do to improve the situation.

There are, moreover, important long-range goals in working with this organized group of consumers. As they become knowledgeable and sophisticated they will become a potent force in bringing about the changes in medical practice that are vitally needed. It is of crucial importance that such potential fiscal and political power be guided by professional experts who understand medical care.

### THE MORRISANIA CITY HOSPITAL

Finally, some mention should be made of a new program of vital interest to the people of New York. Since the war the deterioration of those municipal hospitals in the city which had no medical school affiliation seriously affected the quality of care given the tens of thousands of patients who used these institutions. We at Montefiore had ample, high-quality, full-time, attending and house staff. Just fifteen minutes from us a once great hospital of about 400 beds, the Morrisania City Hospital, was deteriorating from the lack of such skilled people. The result, after years of effort, is a $3,000,000 a year contract between Montefiore Hospital and the City of New York for which we undertake to provide medical care at the Morrisania Hospital using full-time, part-time, and volunteer physicians. By July 1964 all intern and residency programs at the Municipal Hospital will be integrated into the Montefiore program. Within a few years we look forward to implementation of the city's commitment to rebuild the Morrisania Hospital at Montefiore, on land given by our hospital for this purpose. This will result in the full integration of the two institutions.

### SUMMARY

Montefiore Hospital has concluded that it must be prepared to consider carefully any undertaking that seems to have the potential for improving the health and welfare of the people of our community in which its resources, skill, and capacities might play a significant role. It is inevitable that the hospital will become the center of medical care activity within the community.

We have assumed that how doctors and hospitals are used, how medical care will be organized and financed, and how it will be brought to the people who require it are clearly within our framework of interest and concern. The hospital is a public and social instrument. I can visualize only disaster and disorder if these admittedly difficult problems are not dealt with by those institutions and those people who know most about such things and have such great stakes in appropriate solutions. One of Montefiore's interests in joining with the Teamsters was that we desired an opportunity to work with a consumer group which had an awareness and concern with the issues in medical care. Dr. Trussell was able to turn this interest and energy into productive and creative communal channels. It is our feeling that the decisions in medical care will be made by the organized consumer and not by the professional. Consequently, we professionals must make ourselves available to such interested and powerful consumer groups to advise and guide them to solutions which are appropriate to the needs of the people we serve and to the doctors and hospitals which provide the service. About a year and a half ago in Detroit in a paper delivered before the American Public Health Association,[18] I made this very statement, that the organized consumer would prevail. This aroused considerable reaction among various groups within the medical community. I was interested and not surprised when subsequently I read the following from a chapter written by Dr. Edward D. Churchill in 1949,[19] "It is important that as much as possible be learned about the hospital because the future of this institution will be determined by society, not by the medical profession."

The Montefiore Hospital program has imposed an extraordinary burden upon the hospital, its board, its staff, and its administration. Despite our weariness, the joy and satisfaction which come to an institution in successfully undertaking these community programs are fully equal to the feelings which the investigator experiences who successfully completes an experiment in his laboratory. Both are of equal importance to the community.

# THE PROBLEMS OF MAINTAINING
# QUALITY IN HOSPITALS

Ray E. Trussell, M.D.

No topic is more timely or more sensitive in the health services field than how to provide modern medical care to the public. Perhaps it is well to start with a common area of agreement on the part of all concerned, namely, that there are more and more advances in medical knowledge which, when made available, either prevent disease, shorten illness, or save life. The widespread public expectation of the best in medicine derives in large part from excellent science reporting through the press, radio, and television. Such science reporting is supplemented by enthusiastic publications from medical, hospital, and pharmaceutical organizations and, whether for public relations, fund raising, or enhancing sales the common theme is "have faith, all is well and getting better everyday." And, indeed, if people are asked in household interview surveys what they think of the care they have received, almost invariably they answer that their care was the "best" or "reasonably good." A very small per cent of the respondents say their care was "not good."

In the face of this harmonious situation, why then a Lowell Lecture? Why talk about quality if patients, doctors, and hospitals are happy? The answer to this question is manyfold but I would put two reasons at the top of the list: increasing costs and increasing research. In the past few years the apprehension over increasing hospital costs on the part of management and labor trustees as well as other consumers has generated confusion and criticism in several states, followed by demands for action on the part of hospitals and government, and finally, by studies usually made by a university group under official auspices and intended to bring fresh information and clarification to the public. In New York this process has just been completed and the results are not very reassuring. However, the studies have stimulated action, some constructive, some obstructive, and this will be discussed later.

Added to these "demand" type studies is a parallel and rapidly developing body of knowledge resulting from research sponsored by universities, foundations, government at all levels, and management and labor. While techniques in the field of medical care research do not have the precision of those in some of the biological and physical fields, they are being refined and extended. Many disciplines must be brought together to study medical and hospital care. A research team in this field may represent eleven or even more scientific and professional backgrounds. Further, in order to obtain answers, it usually is necessary to collect and analyze large volumes of data or to set up organizational attempts to do things better with concurrent evaluation, and either approach is expensive. Yet in relation to the billions spent annually on medical and hospital care in this nation, the amount of money allocated to research on the problems of providing such care is a drop in the bucket. We need more trained personnel, more resources with which to work, and many more research centers. Nevertheless, what is already known is not being faced up to adequately.

The discussion which follows is largely derived from an intensive personal experience during the past thirteen years — both in rural and urban settings. While it may be deliberately provincial, there is no question that the kinds of problems to be discussed exist everywhere. They differ in various locations only in a quantitative sense. Since in New York City rather sweeping moves are afoot, talking from a live, on-going experience is sometimes more rewarding than a theoretical exposition. The scope of the discussion is such that one can do little more than touch the high points.

At this point I come to the topic assigned: "The Problems of Maintaining Quality in Hospitals," in this case, urban hospitals. It is an unpleasant topic because there really should not be any major problems. In covering the assignment I will draw largely on our research experience at Columbia University and my current experience as Commissioner of Hospitals of New York City. At the moment (1963) I am in charge of 22 municipal hospitals, I license 37 proprietary hospitals, and authorize payment for care of the indigent or medically indigent in 82 voluntary hospitals.

## TYPES OF HOSPITALS

There are three types of hospitals at the service of the public:

First, voluntary nonprofit hospitals which range from a Massachusetts General Hospital or a Columbia-Presbyterian Medical Center, providing a broad range of constantly improving services to all segments of the community, with interlocking research and training, to tiny facilities with no training, no research, no accreditation, no professional strength, and no reason to exist any longer in urban areas where the trend is unmistakably toward fewer but larger and better hospitals. In between the very large and the very small is a large number of community hospitals, some of which are excellent, some of which have much room for improvement.

Second, proprietary hospitals built and operated for profit and which, in New York at least, are owned by physicians. These facilities provide care only to private and semiprivate patients and in New York City make up 25 per cent of the beds available to such patients. Training, research, ward care, home care, and clinics are not characteristic of such hospitals and if emergency services are provided they are usually minimal. In size the current building trend is toward the 200- to 300-bed group but there are many proprietary hospitals which are quite small.

Third, governmental hospitals, usually county or municipal, for those among the general public who must use tax-supported facilities for general care. Within this group there are wide ranges in size, distribution, and professional standing, depending on whether or not they are affiliated with a medical school or a strong voluntary teaching hospital and how realistically they are financed.

For the sake of completeness it may be useful to summarize one scheme for classifying hospitals in terms of their professional stature. The "unaccredited" hospital is a facility with 25 beds or more which does not meet the minimal standards of the Joint Commission on Accreditation of Hospitals. In the New York area, at least, the unaccredited hospitals are concentrated in the smaller size proprietary group although this picture is changing rapidly.

The "accredited" hospital is one which has been surveyed by the Joint Commission and has met its minimum requirements but has no other form of professional recognition. Some of these hospitals are well staffed medically; others have been demonstrated to be very weak in this regard.

In our research jargon the "approved" hospital is an accredited facility which is approved by the Council on Medical Education and Hospitals of the American Medical Association for the training of interns and/or residents, our future physicians. It is generally stated that the teaching hospital maintains a climate in which excellence of patient care can flourish because well recognized physicians are there teaching young doctors in a program approved by an outside agency. This "fish bowl" life, where everyone is constantly scrutinizing the work of others, may be confusing to the patient but it does help to maintain high standards of care. Every physician receives his training in such an environment. It is a sad commentary on how well or how poorly we are organized to provide health services in this country that once a physician is licensed and goes into practice he is free to do what he will to his patients unless he is a member of a hospital organized in such a way that privileges are related to qualifications and every physician's work is an open book. Unfortunately such a situation is not universal and where economic interests supersede ethical precepts the public interest is at stake and public action is required. Such action must be based, of course, on objective data. I will return to some examples of both public problems and public action soon.

Finally, the "affiliated" hospital is described as one manned by, or having very strong relationships with, a medical school. The Massachusetts General Hospital is a classic example. These hospitals by and large are not only great centers of education and research, but they are also the last court of appeal for life for the critically ill, the complex problem and the undiagnosed. The world and the medical professions owe such institutions a great debt and a free hand to grow and grow.

## THE COST OF MEDICAL CARE

This brings me to a practical consideration, namely, the cost of good hospital and medical care. No study in recent years concerned with the impact of hospital costs on Blue Cross premiums has failed to predict a continuing and in fact accelerated increase in costs per unit of service. There are three simple reasons: inflation, medical advances, and personnel wages and salaries. With 70 per cent of a hospital's budget attributable to personnel and with unionization extending to more and more hospitals, personnel costs are going up and rightly so. It is a ridiculous situation when in a wealthy society, hospital employees can hold full-time hospital jobs, yet be simultaneously on public welfare, a state of affairs which actually existed in a strike in New York City within recent years. America can do without this kind of philanthropy. Good hospitals are complex, constantly changing, improving, building, rebuilding, and expanding education and research, all for the good of the patient and at great expense. The deficits so accrued can no longer be carried adequately by endowment income and philanthropic giving. Such assets should be used to further the preparation of our future physicians, to experiment with better ways of providing care, to provide fiscal flexibility in an otherwise inflexible situation, and for a number of other worthwhile purposes rather than for the relief of the taxpayers' responsibilities as defined by their elected representatives.

There is a growing realization that good medical care in a good hospital costs money and that all people are entitled to modern medical care regardless of any other consideration. Hence, it is important that voluntary health insurance pay hospitals realistically and that government do likewise. In the New York area, for example, Blue Cross (the largest such plan in the world) now pays hospitals on the basis of audited costs and in relation to what they do for the community. The city administration has just announced a new scheme of payments oriented basically toward the same concept. Currently the city is paying voluntary hospitals in the fiscal year 1962–1963 about $55,000,000. In the next fiscal year (1964) a sliding scale from $30 to $36 per day of general care is to be introduced which will recognize in a substantial way the better institutions. The total cost is expected to be about $66,000,000.

By no stretch of the imagination have all local governmental agencies and administrations taken a realistic view of the cost of good care. Some pay full cost, some far less. However, there is no such thing as free care. The only questions are, how will care be paid for and at what level of excellence? If there is inadequate financing, only the patients suffer. It is of course quite clear now that without substantial governmental subsidy, voluntary health insurance could not survive, a view recently re-emphasized by the president of the largest Blue Shield Plan in the nation. It is equally certain that without the billions spent on voluntary health insurance the problems faced by individual families and in turn by government would be severe. Whether voluntary insurance and government can coexist peacefully remains to be seen. There is much to be said for such coexistence and the final choice will be made by the public with the quality of care issue being a major consideration along with the availability of care. Certainly, the mere possession of health insurance is no guarantee of good care in an adequate hospital. The trustees of health insurance plans can constructively influence the quality of care by administrative policies which reward better service and which do not encourage the development of more substandard service. Blue Cross is actively pursuing such a policy in New York. One could only wish that Blue Shield and other medical care plans would do likewise.

The subject of costs is not as simple as some would make it out to be. The intangibles in deciding what 24-hour stand-by services shall be available, at what level of excellence, and for whom, all affect cost. Unnecessary hospital use creates unnecessary cost, which is a drain on the voluntary health insurance subscribers' premium pool and on the taxpayer.

Another severe threat to the financing of good care is the impact of unnecessary construction. Every 100 beds built and standing empty drain off several hundred thousand dollars a year. Furthermore, if they are filled to 80 per cent occupancy, the added cost is well over a million dollars. Empty beds are an invitation to administrators and physicians to fill them in order to increase income. Recently a new hospital opened and the owners were so anxious to build a census of paying patients that they instituted an "emergency" admission policy whereby physicians not yet on the staff could admit and take care of patients and the "screening" of credentials came later. A more open invitation to poor care could hardly be conceived.

The basic authority for the control of unnecessary building rests with government but should be exercised in relation to sound community planning. There has been much activity in this area.

In New York, for example, a State Hospital Review and Planning Council was established by law, and regional councils were encouraged by executive action so that every part of the state is now covered. Yet these regional councils have no authority over construction and manifest little concern with the quality of care. Even proposed legislation which would subject questionable projects to a public hearing died in our state legislature this year, a failure for which a prominent labor leader has just taken our governor to task. As a trustee of a pension and welfare fund he had learned from our various studies and from Blue Cross that operating costs resulting from new hospital construction in the New York area will be increased by about $80,000,000, and that Blue Cross carried by his union members will pay much of the new burden. He also learned that too many beds invite more care, often of poor quality and patently unnecessary.

In an effort to deal with part of this problem I have, as Commissioner, referred all requests for proprietary hospital expansion within New York City to the local regional council. Taking their recommendations into account, several hospitals have been denied expansion under the licensing powers residing in the city charter. However, there is no such control on voluntary hospitals in New York City and on all types of hospitals outside of the city, all of which are under state control. When the next inevitable Blue Cross rate increase comes up for a public hearing some embarrassing questions are going to be asked as to why so many unnecessary hospital beds were permitted. While the anger will be generated by increased and unnecessary costs, the issue of good care is implicit throughout because some of the facilities being built are of the type which characteristically have weak medical staffs with little if any limitation of privileges.

## STANDARD SETTING

Many forces are at work, upgrading care in hospitals, among them medical advances, better trained personnel, and standard-setting agencies. Best known in the hospital world as a standard-setting agency is the Joint Commission on Accreditation of Hospitals. This voluntary organization sponsored by four important professional groups has stimulated large numbers of hospitals to self-improvement and has had a most significant impact throughout the nation. Yet the Joint Commission's standards are minimal in the final analysis and must be set at a level which can be achieved anywhere in the country. Recently I refused to relicense a hospital that had long-standing violations, mostly relating to fire and operating room hazards. Yet this hospital which is now closed had a full, 3-year accreditation. There also is a great need for the Joint Commission to pay more attention to the quality of medical care. To do so will require more staff, in part with different backgrounds. Certainly in urban areas, rich in resources, there is no excuse for an unaccredited hospital. Yet in 1960 in New York City alone, only 15 of the 40 proprietary hospitals were accredited and 70 per cent of Blue Cross payments to unaccredited facilities were to the proprietary group. Blue Cross is now bringing strong pressures to bear on this problem. Within the past two years also the Board of Hospitals of New York City adopted a regulation that licensure of proprietary hospitals after January 1, 1965, would be contingent on accreditation. Since then at least 13 more proprietary hospitals have secured accreditation. Further, a policy was adopted that the city would not pay for care of indigent or medically indigent patients in unaccredited voluntary institutions beginning January 1st of this year. Actually, this created no problems but the basic principle is sound and is being expanded in ways which I will describe later.

Before I go on, it should be stated clearly that there are in this country large numbers of excellent hospitals and there will be more. A truly good hospital cannot be contained in its professional growth and is a thrilling place in which to work. However, one of the problems facing the public as well as government is how to identify such hospitals. In some ways it is easier for government officials because we turn to panels of recognized experts to establish criteria by which we can designate approved centers or services in which we are willing to pay for the care of patients with certain kinds of complicated diseases. After our Interdepartmental Health Council adopts such criteria, the same nongovernmental experts inspect those hospitals which wish to be approved and those which qualify are so designated. There are professional and administrative obstacles to the full use of these approved facilities. Patients who would benefit by care in such hospitals are frequently subjected to surgery elsewhere to "enrich" the training of a resident, or for lack of referral by the private physician, or because of administrative failure to identify and arrange for transfer of the patient. Currently, a research group is studying our patients in both municipal and voluntary hospitals to provide a knowledgeable basis for administrative action to reduce these problems. Already, on the basis of advance information, one small voluntary hospital with an unapproved intern training program has been taken off the list of hospitals approved for city-pay patients. This promptly resulted in political pressure to rescind the order but the Mayor when informed of the issue supported my decision. Defenseless sick people should not be the victims of political friendliness and no public official with whom I have worked understands this more clearly than Mayor Wagner of New York City.

The most recently published list of approved services in New York City was for amputees, many of whom require an array of services not available in most hospitals. This month criteria for approval of neurosurgical centers or services were adopted and all hospitals are just now receiving these with an application form. After several months of inspections, the approved centers and services will be publicized. The Commissioners who constitute the Inter-Departmental Health Council will make maximum use of these facilities for patients for whom government has any direct responsibility: the municipal hospital patients, welfare patients, patients paid for by the city in voluntary hospitals, and patients picked up by the ambulances operated or paid for by the city. Such a program is intended to bring the best professional resources of the city together with patients who need them badly. The program will stimulate some hospitals to do better but it will also arouse professional resistance in others which do not qualify because any re-direction of patient flow, particularly of those patients involved in accidents, will affect the economics of certain segments of medical practice.

For the individual in the community securing his care through private physicians, the kind of hospital he enters is frequently based on where his physician has admitting privileges unless he is referred to another physician. As an example, in the New York area our data indicate that patients who seek care from certified specialists are much more likely to be hospitalized in the better hospitals. On the contrary, using surgery paid for through health insurance as an example, we recently demonstrated that one-half of the appendectomies and tonsillectomies in children under 12 done by physicians with no evidence of advanced training were in unaccredited proprietary hospitals. In the same study, it was shown that in large teaching hospitals all procedures paid for were performed by physicians with recorded evidence of training in surgery, whereas this did not pertain in small voluntary and proprietary hospitals, whether accredited or not. One, in fact, had a record of only five per cent of all surgery done by "qualified" surgeons.

These data were applicable to 1958. Recently, my staff took the ten proprietary hospitals with the poorest score in 1958 and repeated the study for 1962. It is interesting to know that the hospital with the five per cent score has now a 16 per cent record of surgery being performed by qualified surgeons. This represents a phenomenal improvement of more than two hundred per cent in five years leaving a mere 84 per cent of surgery performed by surgeons with no recorded evidence of surgical training on what some of my medical society critics refer to as "just plain folks." Eighty-four per cent is an incredible figure too. In the same study, the qualifications of the physicians who performed fifty per cent of the major surgery in the ten hospitals were also examined. There were only forty physicians and of these, fourteen had had advanced training.

Such data and other reports regularly available as a result of our own inspections and those of the Health Department have brought us to an on-going revision of the city code under which proprietary hospitals are licensed. This is being done with the assistance of an advisory committee of outstanding people including representatives from the local medical societies, the State Medical Society, and the New York Academy of Medicine. The greatest challenge as far as I am concerned is how to assure the patient entering a hospital which I license that the care he receives is from physicians qualified to handle his problem. Such a consideration cuts across areas such as professional pride, physicians' income, return on investment, physician-patient relationships, occupancy rates, the responsibility of government, the willingness of organized medicine to stand up for standards locally, and a host of other issues. I am sorry that the section of the code dealing with medical staff appointments and privileges has not been worked through yet because my presentation here would undoubtedly be more informative. The usual round of editorials and resolutions has already started, however, the first shot having been fired by the Bronx County Chapter of the Academy of General Practice.

Regardless of localized editorial criticism the fact is that we have in New York City a wonderful group of physicians, hospital administrators, and trustees who are trying to help resolve some of the problems I have touched on so far. Beyond these great resources there are two others: the free and knowledgeable press and the now organized interest of management and labor in avoiding poor care or unnecessary care and in controlling costs through limiting unnecessary construction. The recently created Labor-Management Council of Health and Welfare Plans comprises management, labor, and professional representation, and it grew out of the concern of the AFL-CIO labor union about the cost of care for more than three million people. (See Mr. Pollack's "Voice of the Consumer," p. 167.) We at Columbia also, in partnership with Montefiore Hospital, work closely with the trustees of the Teamsters' Joint Council 16 and Management Hospitalization Trust Fund. (See Dr. Cherkasky's "The Hospital as a Social Instrument," p. 93.) These trustees are concerned about a half million people and are not only trying to provide better services but also are financing medical audits and research in hospital operations.

## PROVIDING QUALITY

And this brings me to my final subject of this session — the problems of providing quality care in municipal hospitals. For the past 26 months I have been involved in a massive and exciting reorganization of our municipal system with the very strong support, both moral and financial, from our Mayor and his cabinet officials. We have a very large organization. Our annual budget is over $200,000,000 and our city hospitals admit 270,000 patients a year, deliver 36,000 babies, provide 2.7 million clinic visits, and 1 million emergency visits. Our ambulances make 435,000 trips, we have 2,100 people on home care, and two of our six psychiatric services have more admissions than 27 state mental hospitals.

The municipal hospitals vary in size from 200 to 2,800 beds and have had a multitude of problems which were perhaps highlighted most dramatically by house staff recruitment problems.

In 1959 the Mayor was convinced by some knowledgeable people that the city's health services might be deteriorating. Therefore, he appointed a Commission on Health Services, of which I was the part-time Executive Director. The commission produced a succinct report drawing attention particularly to the deteriorating, unaffiliated city hospitals, the shortages of house staff, the loss of interest, as well as members of attending staff, and a whole host of other problems. The Mayor assigned the report to one of his administrative staff groups and a few months later created a small group of citizens and public officials called the Mayor's Task Force on Reorganization of Medical Services to work with the problem. Subsequently I became Commissioner of Hospitals on leave from Columbia University. At the outset there were four general hospitals well staffed by medical schools and eleven unaffiliated general hospitals. One was so completely deteriorated that it had lost accreditation and every other form of approval. The plant was obsolete. The interns and residents had all failed the examination given by the Educational Council for Foreign Medical Graduates. An expert committee advised me that the place should be closed because of the poor standards of care. Yet, the proposed closing was fought by community leaders, one newspaper, and the medical board. However, after 17 days and with the encouragement of committees from labor and management and the Hospital Council the Mayor authorized my closing the facility, an action for which he received strong editorial support.

Next, an emergency appropriation was made to pay physicians to work on the wards of hospitals with inadequate house staffs. As a minimum requirement, these physicians must have completed an approved residency. One hospital immediately took on 68 community physicians. Others varied in their requirements. Money was secured to staff better our emergency rooms some of which were staffed by unlicensed physicians trained in other countries many years ago. More than 100 board-eligible or board-certified specialists have been recruited to date. We have also made direct appointments. These are noncompetitive appointments which have to be approved by the deans of the six local medical schools, so that I am spared any pressures for mediocre or political appointments.

Largely, however, we have approached the problem of upgrading our weaker city hospitals through the mechanism of extending affiliations with the full cost to be borne by the city. The Gouverneur Hospital Clinic and Emergency Service on the lower East Side is run by the Beth Israel Hospital. We have Chiefs of Service now in five of the major departments at Harlem Hospital and four of these five departments are under Columbia University contract with the city, with more pending. The Lincoln Hospital will by the end of the year be 80 per cent under the Albert Einstein Medical College. Morrisania Hospital is staffed completely by Montefiore Hospital. Greenpoint Hospital is staffed totally by the Mt. Sinai Hospital and still other affiliations are pending. These contracts are for total medical services on the wards, the clinics, the emergency room, the home care service, and the house staff. In dollar requirements for example there is a contract pending for affiliating an inadequate hospital of 440 beds with an excellent voluntary hospital which will be given $3,000,000 a year to staff that hospital, making appointments subject to the approval of one of our six medical school faculties. This is a professional merger only. The hospital continues as a municipal facility. There is no threat to the civil service tenure of the employees. However, we secure by this contract mechanism the prestige and excellence of medical schools or strong teaching hospitals whose professional strength is such that they can reach out and help us if the city pays full cost and makes it administratively palatable. The lump sum budget to be spent according to prevailing university practices is the best device yet invented to give maximum flexibility. There is a 2-way flow in this professional merger; we get better medical care for our patients and the university or teaching hospital has enlarged clinical, training and research opportunities with no added expense and no need to raise more capital funds. One possible obstacle was securing enough money, but the Mayor and the Board of Estimate have been very good about giving it to us so far.

It is also important to keep in mind the social significance of strengthening our best voluntary institutions. In New York we have enough hospital beds; we need replacement for some of our beds but we do not need more beds. Yet the professional programs in our good teaching hospitals continue to grow and grow. Capital funds are a real problem and when the city makes it possible for a good institution to help a city hospital they also make it possible for that institution not to have to raise capital funds to build unnecessary beds. Automatically through affiliation there is an immediate lateral extension into existing facilities. They immediately enrich their training program for the residents and interns because many hospitals do not have ambulance services whereas all municipal hospitals do. This whole concept is in keeping with long-range policies enunciated by the Hospital Council.

Providing quality medical care through this type of reorganization is a very exciting and rewarding job. It meets obstacles such as I mentioned, some by inference, some very obvious. Yet if there is understanding, support, and courage, much can be done. No one can afford to be against quality medical care when confronted with the issue.[1]

# GOVERNMENT AND HOSPITALS

## Jack Masur, M.D.

TWENTY years after these Lowell Lectures were opened to the public, the great English philosopher and economist, John Stuart Mill, wrote in 1859:

"Some whenever they see any good to be done, or evil to be remedied, would willingly instigate the government to undertake the business; while others prefer to bear almost any amount of social evil rather than add one to the . . . human interests amenable to government control.

"The interference of government . . . is with about equal frequency, improperly invoked and improperly condemned." [1]

In a similar vein, Abraham Lincoln wrote several years later:

The legitimate object of government is to do for a community of people whatever they need to have done but cannot do at all or cannot do as well for themselves in their separate and individual capacities. In all that the people can do as well for themselves, the government ought not to interfere.

When we speak of "government" we include the federal government, 50 States, 3,000 counties, 16,000 municipalities, and 17,000 townships. Thus, in the arcane complexities of health care, we have an indeterminate number of possible interactions with the 7,000 hospitals in this country — with nonprofit voluntary hospitals, tax-supported hospitals, and proprietary hospitals.

Much of what we say here will be concerned, first, with the citizen who serves as trustee or administrator or physician in the voluntary hospital and, second, with the government official engaged in the administration of a health-related program. Let us then generalize about these types:

## THE VOLUNTARY MAN

The typical voluntary hospital man tends to equate voluntarism with freedom of action, political immunity, local initiative, free enterprise — all amounting to noninterference by government in the fulfillment of the hospital's primary mission of caring for the sick. He is apt to look upon the government bureaucrat as an unpopular, unsentimental, unemotional, and unspectacular advocate of social experiments. The voluntary man has been brought up to be especially wary when the employees of the taxing machine set forth on a do-good campaign — "the insidious encroachment by men of zeal, well-meaning but without understanding."

The more conservative voluntary elements are convinced that planned social change by government results in clotting of local initiative and a bloated overhead in the cost of rendering services. And many of our colleagues are not about to rearrange their prejudices. They are convinced that the authority of bureaucracy is a corruption to be avoided like hospital infections.

## THE GOVERNMENT BUREAUCRAT

The average government bureaucrat strives to administer the law and to watch over the tax dollars according to the expressed intent of the elected representatives of the people. Like any administrator, he knows that the sure formula for failure is to try to please everybody. Nevertheless, sometimes when he is convinced that a health or welfare program is a sincere effort to express the social conscience of everybody he is dismayed by the resentment of some judges of public policy who do not feel themselves a part of our democracy. Too often the government official is confronted with the image of the citizen who shakes his left fist at the old devil government while holding out his right hand for larger grants-in-aid to implement a worthy program of social action. It would seem that many consider taking money from the government as a sinful dalliance, but a few practice abstinence.

In the course of time, some brooding bureaucrats begin to doubt whether righteousness will ever prevail unless it is assisted more vigorously by government.

## HOSPITAL CARE IN A GROWING NATION

Hospitals have an important role in building America's health and thus increasing the strength, productivity, and progress of our nation. We like to think these days that all members of our society are equal in a truly democratic sense and that we all share an entitlement to medical care of certified quality, available at the right time and place in the proper amount. How do we stimulate the growth of our gross national health product so that we shall have more and better medical care for each person of every age, race, color, and creed?

The dilemma is to find ways and means of achieving a more satisfactory balance between the quantity and quality of medical care, within the resources of personnel, facilities, and money we can afford in our national economy for the improvement of health. A major part of the quandary in our society is the quest for an increasingly effective collaboration between voluntary organizations and big government, without compounding the hazards of what some critics choose to call a perilous partnership.

During the past dozen years we have had a parade of national commissions, advisory committees, task forces, and work parties to study and to recommend answers to the health needs of the nation. There is abundant documentation of the demographic, social, economic, scientific, and political changes which make health care a major public issue today.

In the 1930's our population increased by 9 million; during the 1940's we grew by 20 million; in the 1950's we added 30 million more; in this decade we shall increase by 33 million, so that by 1970 the population of the United States is expected to reach 214 million. As people tend to concentrate in cities and suburbs, more than two-thirds of our population will reside in metropolitan areas. With higher standards of living, better education, and a greater voice in the organization of health affairs, more people will look to hospitals to facilitate the provision of a wider range of services for the young, the middle-aged, and the old.

The rapid growth of a population eager to use more health services compounds the frustrations of existing shortages of physicians, dentists, nurses, dietitians, social workers, and other health personnel. Our capacity to recruit and train the necessary professional and technical man power is urgently in need of expansion and greater support — the disparity between supply and demand for high-level skills has already distorted many professional, administrative, and economic problems in health care.

The phenomenal growth of hospital prepayment and insurance plans which now provide financial protection to two-thirds of our people has made hospital care more readily available. Last year we admitted 25½ million patients to hospitals. In fact, the total days in hospitals per capita has increased by 50 per cent in the last three decades. During the same period, however, average costs have gone up from 9 dollars a day to 36 dollars a day in voluntary general hospitals. Although the American people want the best that modern medicine can provide, many of them do not accept the fact that higher quality of hospital care justifies today's higher costs.

These are but some of the issues which have been dealt with in the large stack of reports by presidential commissions, surgeon general's committees, and congressional surveys.[2-9] These issues relate to the national interest; they are issues of public and personal concern; they will receive more and more scrutiny by both political parties. Under these circumstances, there will be many who will "see good to be done" and "evil to be remedied"; they will, therefore, "instigate the government to undertake the business."

## GOVERNMENT HOSPITALS

There are about 1,670,000 hospital beds in this country, comprising a multibillion dollar personal service industry. Some of the facilities are operated by government; some of them are operated for government; all of them are operated within a system profoundly affected by government support and regulation.

The hospital beds operated by government make up two-thirds of all hospital beds in the United States. City and county governments provide about 200,000 beds for the sick poor. State governments furnish about 700,000 beds for long-term mental illness and tuberculosis. The acceptance of responsibility by the states for the mentally ill dates back to the beginning of our country and continues as a recognition of the lack of capacity by philanthropy to cope with a problem of this magnitude. The federal government administers an aggregation of about 180,000 beds in Army, Navy, Air Force, Public Health Service, and Veterans Administration hospitals (of which about 120,000 beds are in the Veterans Administration for the use of veterans with service-connected and non-service-connected illnesses — particularly mental illness and tuber-culosis).

These hospitals, owned and operated by different levels of government, range in quality from poor to excellent. Many of them at the local and state levels suffer from skimpy budgets, intrusive politicians, the dead hand of bureaucracy, and isolation from progressive professional attention. They are rarely supported with reasonable finances — the appropriations are frequently controlled by non-health-oriented officials who often seem to have the mentality of Mr. Scrooge, knowing the price of everything and the value of nothing. There are two outstanding examples of tax-supported excellence on a large scale in medical care: the medical centers of state universities and the postwar programs of the Veterans Administration hospitals. Most of these state and federal hospitals have well-designed facilities and very competent professional, administrative, and technical staffs. They provide high-quality medical care for a large group of government beneficiaries and engage in first class teaching and medical research. The experiences of the state-financed university hospitals and the Veterans Administration medical care system reaffirm the conviction that it is extremely difficult to sustain high-quality patient care in a tax-supported hospital without the benefits of an active affiliation with a medical school — an arrangement which is mutually advantageous in patient care, in research, and in medical education.

## GOVERNMENT DOLLARS AND REGULATION

There are about 450,000 beds in voluntary, nonprofit hospitals; they took care of most of the 25½ million patients admitted to hospitals last year. Throughout the operations of voluntary hospitals in the treatment of patients, in educational programs, and in research programs, there are interwoven a great many relationships with all levels of government. In general, there are three areas of involvement:[10] financial assistance, purchase of care for specified beneficiaries, and regulatory requirements.

The greatest government dollar impact on voluntary hospitals has come from the two billion dollars paid by the federal government to subsidize the construction of hospitals in the Hill-Burton program, and the several billions of federal tax dollars provided to the medical schools and teaching hospitals for biomedical research.

The exemption from taxation of nonprofit institutions and the tax allowances for charitable donations represent significant, indirect forms of support which have an important bearing on the responsibilities of voluntary hospitals in matters of public policy.

Many of the beds maintained by voluntary hospitals are operated *for* government in the sense that local, state, and federal governments buy hospital services for certain people unable to pay and for groups of patients with special entitlement.

The federal government pays voluntary hospitals directly for hospital treatment of dependents of the uniformed services, veterans eligible for the "hometown program," and federal employees injured in line of duty. It also shares with state and local government in the cost of care of public assistance recipients, and the welfare categories of dependent children, blind, and totally and permanently disabled persons. Similarly, the state agencies utilize federal grants-in-aid in buying services from voluntary hospitals for the diagnosis and treatment of special groups such as crippled children and handicapped persons in vocational rehabilitation. The Social Security Administration estimated that, in 1961, 56 million people, comprising almost a third of our population, were eligible for some medical or hospital care at government expense, regardless of ability to pay. The largest group included 44 million wage earners entitled to health care benefits under workmen's compensation programs. Other major groups included about 5 million employees of the federal government and their dependents; 3½ million military dependents ("Medicare" program); 2½ million military personnel; and smaller numbers of Indians, merchant seamen, state employees, and so on.

## REIMBURSABLE COST

A major cause of disquiet in the relationships of government and voluntary hospitals has been the way in which tax dollars are spent in procuring hospital care for the indigent sick. Many city, county, and state government officials have been reluctant to pay full costs of hospital services for which they contract. They offer a hatful of excuses, but the real reason is usually the lack of sufficient appropriated funds to discharge their official obligation of providing medical care for the sick who are unable to provide it for themselves. The hard-pressed county commissioner or state legislator yearns for the old bountiful days when the voluntary hospitals with endowments could afford to mix sweet charity with poor cost accounting and accept discount payments from welfare boards. I have heard local and state government authorities argue loud and long that they would be derelict in their sworn duty if they spent the taxpayers' money in payment of full costs for the hospital care of beneficiaries of their programs. They were positive that the teaching hospital admitted some patients unnecessarily, kept many patients in the hospital too long, and did a lot of extra laboratory tests solely for the instruction of student nurses, medical students, interns and residents — and perhaps even for clinical research. The most prevalent rationalization for failure to pay full cost to all voluntary hospitals is that the best free enterprise device to hold down the per diem expenses of patient care is to fix the income at as low a level as possible — which is reminiscent of the old story of the farmer who tried to hold down expenses by feeding his mules more and more sawdust every day; he saved money, but the mules got skinny and eventually died. The daily operation of every voluntary hospital is almost entirely dependent on income from the care of in-patients and out-patients. When a government agency pays a hospital less than the real cost of care for a beneficiary, it transfers the burden to other patients. This is a sorry device to redistribute wealth at the local level. It is certainly not a sound mechanism to cope with the troublesome problem of rising hospital costs. Underpayment to voluntary hospitals by government has a deleterious effect on the quantity and quality of care of all patients in all hospitals.

There is a consensus that, whenever feasible, it is preferable for local, state, and federal governments to purchase care for their beneficiaries in nongovernmental hospitals, rather than to establish and operate more government institutions. Thus, government officials must have a realistic understanding of the economic facts of life which confront voluntary hospital authorities who must meet the payroll. The contractual arrangements must be fair. Government agencies have a public obligation to pay voluntary hospitals full costs for the care of approved beneficiaries; the basis of reimbursement must be the real cost, audited regularly, based on accurate analyses, uniform accounting, and sound statistical records.

There is, of course, a reciprocal relationship in the methods of payment by government and by other third party payors for service. A reimbursable cost formula mutually agreeable to government, prepayment and insurance plans, and hospitals, and subject to regular review, is a consummation many of us are devoutly wishing for.

In order to achieve this objective, it is imperative that all hospitals move forward even more rapidly in the utilization of uniform accounting and statistical reporting systems which have been developed and advocated by the national and state hospital associations. There has been gratifying progress in several states where certified uniform cost reports are being utilized by all government agencies, but we have a long road to travel throughout most of the country.

## COST, QUALITY, AND EFFICIENCY

In the expenditure of hundreds of millions of dollars of tax funds for the direct procurement of care for beneficiaries in voluntary hospitals, government at every level has a stake in satisfying itself as to quality and efficiency, as well as cost.

There is, moreover, growing evidence of more active involvement of government in the relationships of voluntary hospitals and third party prepayment plan and insurance company payors. Some of the State Commissioners of Insurance are on the march with orders for broad studies of hospital practices, and intimations of more standard setting by government agencies. Similarly, federal officials have had to learn more about the business relations of hospitals and prepayment and insurance. Three years ago the Government of the United States assumed the combined role of contributor and negotiator for the world's largest employer-sponsored health insurance program, which supplies voluntary coverage for 2½ million federal workers and 2½ million members of their families. There is also a good deal of legislative interest now in the utilization of Blue Cross, Blue Shield, other nonprofit prepayment agencies, and commercial insurance as the "chosen instrument" in administering the financing of government-supported health care of the aged and other potential beneficiaries, particularly in the underprivileged groups, such as low income wage earners and the temporarily unemployed. All of this reflects the prevailing attitude of some government officials that the people need to have these things done but cannot do as well for themselves in their separate and individual capacities.

## REGULATION

The third area of involvement between hospitals and all levels of government is in regulatory requirements. These run the gamut of licensure, fire safety, water supply and sewage disposal (including radioactive wastes), newborn nurseries, drug control, labor relations, and broad aspects of hospital organization and services.

One of my colleagues, a hospital superintendent in New York City, has counted up the number of licenses, permits, certificates, reports, and inspections which are required by public regulation from the voluntary institution over which he presides. He complained that the total submitted to various government bureaus was 105: 65 city, 29 state, and 11 Federal. I am constrained to remind him that with respect to the federal government, at least, he is a little better off than the salmon swimming up the Columbia River to spawn, which passes under the jurisdiction of 12 federal agencies.

## VOLUNTARISM AND HOSPITALS

Most of our interest here is in the principles underlying the relationships of government and voluntary hospitals. As part of the perspective, I quote sections of a statement approved by the Board of Trustees of the American Hospital Association in 1961:[11]

The hospital system in the United States has a long precedent of creativity through voluntary action. Its distinguishing feature is its dependence in large part upon the voluntary principle — that principle which emphasizes the individual rather than the crowd; that stresses freedom of choice rather than compulsion; flexibility rather than rigidity; quality rather than quantity; that provides a place for charity as well as duty; that is in essence freedom and, in sum, the aggregate of free choices made by individuals through all other means than increasing the powers of government, which involves the use of involuntary taxing and police powers.

. . . . . . . . . . . . . . . . . . . . . . . . .

We believe that the hospital system in the United States is a system in which the voluntary principle is the primary influence and is held by the majority to be the principle which assures the highest quality of result to the largest number of people, now and for the future.

. . . . . . . . . . . . . . . . . . . . . . . . .

The voluntary principle is most manifest and society is best served when the following criteria are most fully met:

1. The individual hospital has autonomy and local nongovernmental control.
2. The hospital is responsible for its own financing and receives its support from those who use it and from those who donate funds or services for its continuation and improvement.
3. The hospital is not operated primarily for profit.

. . . . . . . . . . . . . . . . . . . . . . . . .

In our opinion, the voluntary principle reaches its maximum development in the private nonprofit hospital and these hospitals should remain the predominant influence in the hospital system in the United States.

In order for the voluntary principle and the voluntary nonprofit hospital to survive as the predominant influence in the hospital services in the United States, the following conditions must be met:

. . . . . . . . . . . . . . . . . . . . . . . . .

Demonstration of the ability of the hospital system to deal adequately with the coordination and availability of services to all segments of the community in addition to maintaining and improving quality of care.


## TWO CASE HISTORIES

John Stuart Mill's classic paper on Liberty estimated that the interference by government was improperly invoked and improperly condemned with about equal frequency. In thinking about some examples to illustrate various facets of "too much government" or "not enough government," I too have had some trouble in rearranging my own prejudices. I have chosen two case histories to present and will leave to your judgment the assay of propriety in terms of the public interest.

## Government versus the Profession

Last year we witnessed the sad Saskatchewan episode[12] which epitomizes the conflict between a government determined to carry out what it considered the mandate of the people and an organized profession equally determined to protect what it considered its freedom to practice as it wished. The hospitals were caught in the middle, with some incidental anxiety about the ultimate impact the example of the doctors' collective action may ultimately have on the no-strike position of workers' unions in hospitals.

Since July 1958, all of Canada has had a national hospital care insurance program which pays most of the patient's hospital charges, a share of his drug bill, but no doctor's fees. In the province of Saskatchewan, however, the government-supported hospital insurance system dates back to 1947. Early in 1962, Saskatchewan enacted a Medical Care Insurance Act which represented North America's first plan for universal, compulsory, tax-supported, comprehensive medical service insurance under government auspices. As the time for implementation approached, relationships between organized medicine and the government authorities in the Western province deteriorated rapidly. The Canadian Medical Association declared that the type of plan passed by the legislature in Saskatchewan was neither necessary nor desirable in Canada; the association expressed its support of the decision of the Saskatchewan doctors to strike. In July 1962, the 925,000 citizens in that province were confronted with the alarming fact that their 750 practicing physicians had walked out on the new medical care program of the government. About a third of the physicians volunteered to staff emergency stations part time at 34 hospitals; most private offices were shut down with signs stating that the doctor could not and would not practice under the government plan; 113 hospitals were unable to accept patients. Accusations flew back and forth in newspapers, magazines, radio, and television. Some physicians moved away from Saskatchewan; a few physicians were threatened with reprisals by families of sick patients. The medical profession denounced the government for arbitrarily imposing a scheme of state medicine; they vehemently asserted that they were fighting for minority rights in a democracy where the tyranny of the majority had, by popular vote, imposed involuntary servitude on the minority. The government spokesmen countered with the charge that the real reason for the rebellion was the doctors' fear of loss of income. The president of the provincial medical society retorted that the socialist government bore the complete responsibility for introducing a plan which drove a free profession to the stand it had taken:

. . . On the one side we have those who believe in control by the state and on the other side we have those who believe that the state should not interfere when the individual is adequately looking after the problem. To many doctors and patients the basic issue is freedom . . .

The Premier called the revolt further evidence of a calloused disregard for the welfare of the people:

What is at issue is whether a special power bloc can use its monopoly of skills to frustrate the will of the people expressed through legislative action. The doctors who have been boycotting the plan have challenged the right of government to legislate.

In the midst of the controversy Canadian newspaper editors sadly observed that both the government and the doctors were failing the people they were dedicated to serve.

After 23 days of rancor the controversy was finally settled with some outside help in negotiating concessions on both sides.

In discussing this hazardous aspect of government control of personal and professional matters, in the light of the Saskatchewan impasse, a historian friend drew an analogy with the Whisky Insurrection of 1794 in Western Pennsylvania. During attempts to enforce the new excise law on domestic spirits, several federal revenue officers were tarred and feathered. Following the arrival of a force of federal militia, the rebellious Pennsylvanians submitted without bloodshed. My scholarly associate informed me that one of Alexander Hamilton's letters suggests that his object in proposing this excise law was to provoke just such local resistance as would enable the central government to demonstrate its strength. My lesson in comparative history of North America was concluded on the note that politically this show of force in the Whisky Insurrection proved to be a mistake, because so many people were aghast at the ruthless power the Federalists in charge of government chose to wield.

Whatever conclusions may be arrived at concerning the doctors' strike in Canada last year, the fact remains that the physicians chose not to obey the law of the land and by concerted action abandoned their patients. It was a contest in which there was much at stake: the results were that the government lost, the physicians lost, the hospitals lost, and the public lost.

## Hill-Burton: Government-Voluntary Collaboration

The second case history is a happy example of fruitful collaboration of federal government, state government, local government, and voluntary hospital agencies. The popular Hill-Burton program for the construction of hospitals and health facilities has operated in this country for 15 years and we have much to learn from an objective appraisal of its long-term achievements and shortcomings. Even more significant may be the lessons to be gained eventually in a critique of its impact on our thinking about the obligatory symbiosis of government and hospitals.

During the prosperity of the 1920's, we gave little attention to the development of hospitals in many parts of the country. At the end of the decade, there were 1200 counties, comprising a population of 15 million people, with no hospital facilities. During the depressed 1930's, we made do with what we had, and there was no hospital construction. In the war years, we built a small number of simple hospital structures to deal with the emergency requirements of communities crowded with workers in shipyards, airplane factories, and industrial war plants.

In 1942, the American Hospital Association and the U.S. Public Health Service joined forces to establish the Commission on Hospital Care, with financial support from several foundations, to study this crucial public problem and to make recommendations for national action. In the summer of 1946, congress enacted the Hospital Survey and Construction Act which incorporated the major recommendations of the Commission on Hospital Care: to provide for orderly planning of a system of hospital services by the states; to furnish government financial subsidy through the states for planning and for the construction of needed public and voluntary hospitals and public health centers.

The Hill-Burton program was structured as an idealized federal-state relationship, including the use of national and state advisory councils with consumer and professional representation. Moreover, the provision for implementation (Hospital Survey and Construction Act, passed August 6, 1946) sought the ideal goals of the following: comprehensive approach to relieve the shortage and maldistribution of facilities through coordination by regional planning and integration of special services (mental, tuberculosis, chronic disease) for in-patients and out-patients in the community general hospital; formulation of standards of need for acceptable facilities through the mechanism of surveys and the use of bed ratios as criteria; promulgation of standards for quality of construction; compliance with state minimum standards for licensure, operation, and maintenance of hospitals; provision of administrative hearings and appeal to the courts for contesting decisions; establishment of flexible and equitable allocation of federal funds through a formula to favor the poorer states; choice of variable matching formulas for projects in the states; and, last, what was considered the all important, prohibition of governmental interference in the operation of hospitals, stating "Except as otherwise specifically provided, nothing in this Title shall be construed as conferring on any Federal officer or employee the right to exercise any supervision or control over the administration, personnel, maintenance, or operation of any hospital, diagnostic or treatment center, rehabilitation facility, or nursing home, with respect to which any funds have been or may be expanded under this Title." [13]

The 1954 amendments provided categorical support for constructing nursing homes, diagnostic and treatment centers, chronic disease hospitals, and rehabilitation facilities. They also made grants available for research and demonstrations relating to the effective utilization of hospitals.

The nation has been well served by the Hill-Burton program in many ways. The federal government has furnished almost 2 billion dollars to match about 4 billion dollars of sponsors' funds in order to build more than 6,700 projects involving 285,000 hospital beds and 1,880 health units of various types. In accordance with one of its major objectives, this grants-in-aid device has satisfied the demand for hospital beds in many rural areas. More than half of the hospitals constructed with Hill-Burton support have been in areas that had no hospitals. About one-fourth of the Hill-Burton projects have been in areas that previously had only unacceptable hospital beds. There has been an improved distribution of doctors and nurses. Through its technical services activities, the Hill-Burton administration has greatly improved the average level of architectural and engineering design of hospitals throughout the country.

In four-fifths of the states, the health departments have been given responsibility and financial support for systematic survey and inventory of hospitals and for licensure, with at least some minimum standards of operation and maintenance. Of considerable importance in terms of public administration is the fact that enabling legislation at both federal and state levels has brought representatives of consumer and community interests as well as nongovernmental hospital officials into the policy-making structure of state health departments.

These have been gratifying achievements. There have been some failings, some deficiencies. In a program of this size and complexity, some of the wide variations in performance by state governments in a federal-state program have slowed progress: there have been insufficient staffing of some state Hill-Burton agencies, *pro forma* inventories, and occasional rigidity in administration of the program. The stress on rural needs in the genesis of the legislation led to the building of many small hospitals — three out of five new general hospitals constructed with Hill-Burton subsidy have less than fifty beds. Many small communities have insisted that a hospital, however small, was a necessity, like a school or a fire department, if the town was to continue to exist as a viable economic entity. Very small hospitals may be convenient, but often they are not competent to provide modern medical care.

We have learned too that the fixed bed population ratios are not adequate for interpreting the multifaceted needs of hospital and health care. More sophisticated guidelines must be developed to take into account the dynamics of population growth and movement, local economy, the utilization of existing facilities and services, and changes in professional practices. Under stimulation of Hill-Burton research grants, the growing capacity of some of the universities to engage in research in the administration of health and medical care activities will improve our rate of progress in establishing better data for planning and management.

We know, too, that we have arrived at the time when we ought to shift the emphasis in construction from rural to metropolitan

areas. The great teaching hospitals, especially the university medical centers, are urgently in need of more financial support from
government. They have fared well in grants for clinical investigation and for laboratory construction — without too many cries of
anguish about government interference with the freedom of research — but we are long overdue in modernizing the patient care
and supporting service facilities of these centers of leadership.

We still have large unmet needs in the number of acceptable
long-term care institutions, community mental health facilities, rehabilitation centers, and medical group practice facilities for ambulatory care.


## REGIONALIZATION

As we ponder those things we have left undone which we ought
to have done in the Hill-Burton program, the most notable deficiency is in area-wide planning. The concept of regionalization was
first applied to public health activities in this country about forty
years ago. It was devised as a process for the organization and coordination of health services in a well-defined area in order to improve their quality, efficiency, and availability.

The first significant application of this idea to hospital services
in the United States was the regional pilot program of New England, begun in 1931 by the Bingham Associates Fund. It was intended to ameliorate "the plight of the rural physician . . . cut off
from the stimulating and developing contacts which his urban
brothers enjoyed in . . . progressive medical societies, hospitals,
clinics, and medical school teaching."

Following the recommendations of the Commission on Hospital Care, the plan for a coordinated hospital system through regionalization was written into the Hospital Survey and Construction Act of 1946. The assumptions were that most patients could
receive care in a hospital with certain basic services, a small proportion of patients would require more complex professional services, and a smaller percentage would need the most comprehensive
care of a great teaching center. Thus, in the best of all hospital
worlds, patients would be distributed among affiliated community,
regional, and base hospitals in order to furnish the types of care

needed by sick people, without duplication of facilities and services. But the trouble with regional planning, even in its simplest
form, as described in the Hill-Burton scheme, was that it was too
logical. Regionalization has been balked by factors of self-interest,
medical economics, professional chauvinism, civic pride, and institutional autonomy. Until such time as we can attain real area-wide
integration of hospitals and their services, we shall continue to
struggle with difficulties in striving for a more efficient over-all
utilization of beds, improvement in the quality of care in small
hospitals, and much-needed programs for the continuation of education of practicing physicians. There is, moreover, a growing conviction that the promotion of interchange of services among hospitals will do much to bring the benefits of our vast medical research programs earlier to patients in all hospitals.

The President's Commission on Health Needs of the Nation in
1952 described a much wider range of goals for regional systems
of health services. These objectives would entail a heavy commitment of the medical schools, university hospitals, and schools of
public health in extension services, postgraduate education for all
levels of health personnel, appraisal studies, and sharing of medical,
technical, and administrative resources. The current stresses in the
adjustment of universities to their burgeoning research programs,
the shortage of teachers, and the traditional reluctance of many
faculties (even in state medical schools supported entirely by tax
funds) to project their services beyond the campus, all lend little
encouragement to hopes for a realization of this grand strategy.

We all say that we are in favor of regional planning, whatever
that means. But thus far the record shows minimal results by both
voluntary and governmental agencies. If a coordinated system of
health services is indeed the best way to provide the greatest good
for the greatest number for the longest time, we shall have to find
some way of adding more authority and much more money to the
devices we have been experimenting with.

One of the cynics among the philosophers defined "experience"
as: "the wisdom that enables us to recognize as an old acquaintance
the folly we have already embraced."

This is a little bitter for my taste, but it is worth remembering
as we ruminate on some of our difficulties. It may be disconcerting
for many to speculate on whether we can actually achieve united

voluntary action on certain long-standing challenges which have now become public issues. Is it likely, for example, that we shall be able to control regional planning through collective self-discipline of nonprofit agencies? I have heard it said that men of small vision hold on to what they think they have and take small measures which can only end in the assumption of more authority by government. One old timer suggests that imposing sanctions in a matter such as area-wide planning is an onerous task which many folks will finally relegate to officials of government with a sort of none-too-reluctant acquiescence. The history of regionalization efforts will provide a fascinating chapter in the Lowell Lecture of 1975 on the subject of government and hospitals.

## PUBLIC UTILITY — NEW GOVERNMENT AGENCY

Hospitals represent a "public utility" as some people think of the role of hospitals in providing services to the community. But, technically, as Harrison[14] points out, the term describes a profit-making business in which service and profits are controlled by the government as a condition of the right to operate in a certain area as a monopoly. None of this fits in with our cherished concept of a nonprofit, voluntary hospital. But more importantly, Willcox[15] stresses that the designation of hospitals as public utilities with a rate-setting mechanism established in the state government could effectively reduce our best hospitals to a level of mediocrity.

Harrison has proposed the establishment of a new type of public agency at the level of state government which would bring together many statutory objectives: encouragement of planning and utilization of hospitals on a community or regional basis, elimination of substandard or unnecessary hospitals, stimulation of higher standards of care, development of practices to limit costs without impairment of quality, approval of health prepayment plans, and promotion of public understanding of hospital problems. The creation of this type of state governmental unit dealing with so many ramifications of hospital administration, prepayment, medical care, and the health professions is an interesting possibility. Certainly it would require clear legislative authority, high-quality administration, adequate budget, and the sustained support of good citizens dedicated to the improvement of the health of every community.

## GOVERNMENT AND BUSINESS

We in the health field are not alone in the confusing debate over the proper role of government in support of the public interest. Our total economy becomes increasingly dependent on business with the government and for the government. Twenty years of hot war and cold war, the expenditure of 12 billion dollars of tax funds this year (and 15 billion dollars next year) in research and development for promotion of the nation's economic growth, the rising competition for world markets — all are factors in the United States that force the blending of our public and private economy. Raskin[16] and other economists have stressed that the need for new instruments of cooperation between government, industry, and labor is evident in the lobbying struggles over atomic energy power plants and space communications and in the rash of strikes afflicting the airlines, railroads, newspapers, and missile plants. Just as there are some of us who believe that government has a greater role to serve in health, so are there many who look to government to assume a more active part in fostering maximum employment, production, and purchasing power.

## BEWARE OF THE GOVERNMENT

There are those who believe that the voluntary system can only avoid the compulsion of government by staying one jump ahead. Throughout the literature of hospital administration and medical economics we find examples of the "beware of the jabberwock" school. The most popular choice of exhortation is to urge the immediate organization and expansion of voluntary controls in cooperation with trustees and medical staffs to forestall the imposition of further government regulation of the hospital. This type of *caveat* suggests a portion from a less well known work of the author of "Through the Looking Glass":[17]

He thought he saw a banker's clerk
Descending from the bus.
He looked again and found it was
A hippopotamus.
"If this should stay to dine," he said,
"There won't be much for us!"

I commend to you for careful reading the Lowell Lectures of 1948, a published series of eight remarkably good dissertations by members of the staff of Massachusetts General Hospital and the faculty of Harvard Medical School.[18] In an excellent essay on "The Development of the Hospital," Dr. Edward D. Churchill points out that those responsible for our social institutions are continuously searching for a course of action that will safeguard those things that are essential and yet be sufficiently elastic to accommodate the changing needs and moods of society. He predicts the increasing participation of government in the managerial and financial affairs of hospitals, on the principle that the more useful and vital a service becomes in the social order, the more certain it is to become identified with the functions of government.[19]

## GOVERNMENT AND RESEARCH

In our consideration of that aspect of voluntarism which connotes freedom from constraint by government, let us look at one other analogy. At the time the Lowell Lectures of 1948 were presented, the federal government was subsidizing biomedical research in the universities with grants amounting to several million dollars a year. At the present time, the federal government supports biomedical research in the universities with well over a thousand million dollars each year devoted to research projects, research training, and research facilities. My colleague at the National Institutes of Health, Dr. Charles V. Kidd, devoted a year of study at Harvard, under a Rockefeller Public Service Award, to the effects of federal financing of all types of research (biomedical engineering, social sciences, and the physical sciences — including chemistry, physics, mathematics, and others) upon the operations of universities and upon the relationships between government and universities.[20] In his examination of the consequences of government support through billions of federal dollars, on the kind and quality of research done, the freedom of scientists, the quality of teaching, the administrative structure, and other elements of university function, Dr. Kidd emphasizes that the single most important factor in maintaining the independence of the universities is the effectiveness with which they negotiate for suitable terms and conditions in carrying out what needs to be done for the good of society with government support. This incisive review of a massive government subsidy program which has become a permanent part of university life offers encouragement that we can avoid the undesirable aspects of government control with "the development of a sound set of guiding principles with extensive help from nongovernmental advisory groups, a pragmatic administrative approach, maintenance of diverse sources of support, and powerful sources of independent responsible criticism." The voluntary hospitals too can accept much-needed support from government without losing their independence and initiative by negotiating terms and conditions in carrying out their missions of caring for the sick, training health personnel, and conducting research.

## CONCLUSION

In much of the contemporary writing on medical care there is a recurrent note that we are not yet providing to enough of our people what they deserve in health services. The best planned, best operated system of hospital care for this country will not be accomplished by government alone or voluntary enterprise alone, but by joint effort with mutual respect and mutual confidence. Large grants from the federal government are indispensable if we are to marshal the resources necessary to carry out what needs to be done in the urgent future. The real challenge is to the disciplined organization of the voluntary institutions rather than to the logistics of the bureaucrats of local, state, and federal government. Each generation is given its own chance to develop a constructive collaboration with government. In these troubled days when our nation is in a position of world leadership, we have a special obligation to channel the power and resources of our government in vigorous, effective support of the affairs of business, educational institutions, hospitals, and other social agencies vital to our society.

Last year an editorial in a Washington newspaper, a city in which editors and readers worry about the way government fits into our lives, observed:

> Every well regulated democratic society is an on-going compromise of conflicting interests reconciled to each other in a nicely balanced equilibrium arrived at by a long process of trial and error, maintained only by continuous thought and attention and restored only with difficulty when it is once disturbed.
>
> The point of balance is not fixed by considerations of pure logic or absolute morality but is determined more by experimental pragmatism — by finding the point at which conflicts can be reconciled and put to temporary rest; by the exercise of art as much as by the application of science.[21]

# MEDICAL CARE RESEARCH:

## COUNTERBALANCE TO OPINION AND HABIT

Osler L. Peterson, M.D.

It will perhaps be useful to begin by making a distinction between medical science and medical care to explain today's subject. The biochemist who studies an enzyme, the clinician who tries a new drug, and the surgeon who works out a new technique are all concerned with medical science. Medical care, as an academic subject, is concerned with the problems of organization, functions, and economics that are involved in the application of medical science to a patient.

Why should one study medical care? Although I propose to cite a number of examples of studies in this field that have contributed important knowledge, it is best to start with a general justification. First, medical care is important and expensive. This country spends nearly $30 billion every year on doctors, hospitals, medicines, and health services. In 1960–1961, this amount constituted 5.7 per cent of the nation's Gross National Product, or about $1.00 of every $18.00 produced.[1] Of this $30 billion, almost one-quarter is spent by governments in providing and purchasing medical care and health services. It is good common sense to spend a small fraction of this amount to find out how and how well these monies are spent. The United States spends more of its Gross National Product on health than do many other countries. England and Wales spend about 4.5 per cent and Sweden 3.5 per cent.

Economics and health have always been closely connected. A high standard of living has been accompanied by low death rates. The United States undoubtedly has one of the highest, if not the highest standard of living in the world. But, there are a number of countries that have a lower infant mortality rate than the United States. Among them are England and Wales, Holland, Iceland, and the Scandinavian countries. Our death rates are low, but the lower death rates of other countries raise the question of whether our monies can be spent more effectively.

Just as research in the medical sciences is related to scientific knowledge and to clinical practice, so medical care research is relevant to such questions as hospital organization and financing, the number of doctors needed, the distribution of doctors, and other issues that impinge strongly on public policy and are often controversial. Questions of public interest will be mentioned today because medical care research may produce information that is important to their resolution.

While research and study can provide information, they cannot solve medical care problems because these are problems which involve social issues. Information may narrow the argument, but decisions on social questions are part of the political process. The current debate as to whether Social Security should be used to pay the hospital bills of retired persons is a case in point (see Dr. Schottland's lecture on "The Social Security System and Medical Care," p. 201). Information dealing with this question is voluminous, but obviously it is interpreted quite differently by different people.

In discussing medical care today, three of its aspects will be considered. The first deals with the economics of medical care; the second is concerned with how medical care is delivered, that is, with its organization and functions; the last deals with its result. The result consists of two parts — the first, which is how much medical care is given, is relatively unimportant, and the second is how good this medical care is.

## ECONOMIC STUDIES

The United States is one of the few, if not the only, well-developed nations that does not have a large measure of government support of health insurance. Practically all European governments subsidize health insurance. Virtually all hospital care in Canada is now tax-supported. With the organization of a new congress (1964), there will apparently be further debate in this country on the question of provision of medical care for the aged through Social Security. Because the economic aspects of medical care have long been under intensive investigation, we have more information about medical care in the United States than in any other country — possibly with England excepted.

A few figures will illustrate the type of information available. Figure 1, taken from Dr. Odin Anderson's studies, shows an im-

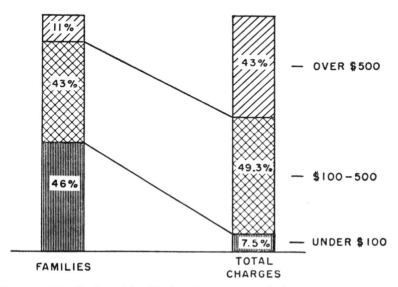

*Figure 1. Distribution of families by charges for medical care, 1953.*

portant and basic fact which tells us why paying for medical care is a problem.[2] The left-hand column shows percentage of families and the right-hand column illustrates the breakdown of their medical bills. Nearly half of all families have small bills, less than $100 a year. Forty-three per cent of the families have a small to moderate sized bill, here defined as $100 to $500. The most important fact illustrated is that 11 per cent of the families had an annual bill in 1953 of over $500 and incurred 43 per cent of all the charges for medical care incurred by all families. In other words, the medical bill is very irregularly distributed. This result is apparently constant. The Committee on the Costs of Medical Care found in 1930 that 10 per cent of the families incurred 40 per cent of all charges.[3] The small group of people for whom illness is likely to be a problem is probably a group which changes from year to year. The fact that for some people the bill is high and cannot be anticipated is the reason why any sensible person wants health insurance.

Figure 2 was also prepared by Dr. Anderson, and shows the average size of a medical bill incurred by persons according to their family income. The sample is further broken down into those with and those without insurance. It is clear that the bills of persons with insurance are generally higher than those of persons without

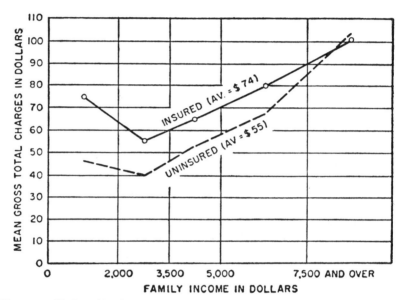

Figure 2. Nationwide charges for personal health services.

insurance. Presumably people who prepay their medical care through insurance are prone to use more medical care. There is another income-related effect. Members of families with incomes below $2000 per year incur higher bills than members of families in the next income group of $2000 to $3500 per year. It is possible that people with very low incomes have more sickness because they are poor, or are poor because they have more sickness. For the remainder, as family income rises, people incur greater charges. However, in 1952 when income rose above $7500, the charges incurred were no longer influenced by having or not having insurance. People in this range perhaps had sufficiently high incomes so that medical care was obtained whether or not insurance was available to pay the bill.

Figure 3 shows the percentage of people discharged from hospitals who had part of their bill paid by insurance. There is a dip in proportion insured when children reach 18 and coverage as a dependent is lost. As young people enter employment, coverage increases and remains high until the middle years. The probability of having one's hospital bills paid by insurance diminishes sharply

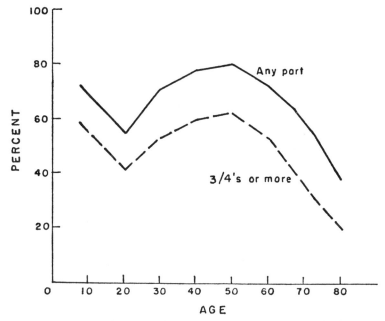

Figure 3. *Hospital discharges with some insurance payment of the hospital bill, United States, July 1958 to June 1960 (in per cent).*

and steadily as middle age is passed. There is ample information available on the frequency of doctor visits among retired persons as well as the whole population. The size of their medical, hospital, and drug bills is known. The incomes and assets of the aged have also been well described. In the present debate on the administration's proposed medical care program, investigators have left us with no dearth of information. To some people this information obviously connotes an acute and demanding problem for which the solution is prepayment into the Social Security fund during working years to assure payment of hospital bills upon retirement in old age. To others an expanded relief program is needed. The facts about income, health, and use of doctors and hospitals are not disputed. These are available as a result of research, but there is no consensus about their meaning.

## ORGANIZATION STUDIES

The organization of medical care is being recognized increasingly as a fruitful subject for study. Within this large industry, hospitals are popular subjects because they are complex, interesting, and costly. About one-third of each medical care dollar is spent on hospitals, a proportion that is increasing rapidly and steadily.

Group practice is another attractive institution for study, particularly when group practice is combined with health insurance. There are many strategic reasons for examining this American invention. In the past three decades the proportion of general practitioners has declined from 90 per cent of all physicians to less than 50 per cent. Groups, which provide a sensible alternative to family doctors, have increased to the point where they include about 15 per cent of all private physicians.

Like the hospitals, the group practice is an inviting research target. One of the first groups to include prepayment for doctor bills was the Health Insurance Plan of Greater New York (Table 1) hereafter referred to as HIP. Provision of physicians' care, com-

TABLE 1. HOSPITAL ADMISSION RATES PER 1000 ENROLLERS IN HIP AND OTHER POPULATIONS IN NEW YORK CITY

| Insurance plan | Rate |
| --- | --- |
| HIP — Blue Cross, 1955[a] | 81.1 |
| N.Y.C. Blue Shield — Blue Cross, 1955 | 93.9 |
| HIP — Blue Cross, 1959 | 63.0 |
| GHI — Blue Cross, 1959 | 110.0 |
| HIP — Blue Cross, 1958[a] | 64.3 |
| Clerks' Union, 1958 | 63.9 |

[a] Adjusted for Age and Sex.

bined with Blue Cross hospital coverage, makes very comprehensive insurance. HIP enrollees obtain care through group practices from whose members they select a personal physician. The groups are paid a capitation fee for each enrollee and this income is shared on any plan that the group may devise. Patients are not charged for individual services. Several years ago, Dr. Paul Densen, Director of Research at HIP, and his colleagues began to publish a series of studies illustrating some aspects of HIP's performance. Table 1, taken from one of his studies, shows the hospital admission rates of HIP enrollees and other defined populations. For the first comparison he selected people in New York City who had the same Blue Cross hospital insurance as HIP enrollees plus a Blue Shield contract to pay physicians' and surgeons' charges.[4] It can be seen that the hospitalization rate among the HIP subscribers was lower, that is, 81 as contrasted with 94/1000 annually among persons with Blue Cross-Blue Shield policies. The HIP population and New Yorkers holding Blue Cross-Blue Shield insurance differ in many ways, so this is not an ideal comparison. However, Densen and his colleagues were able to identify the diseases — respiratory infections such as colds, influenza, and pneumonia — which accounted for the greatest difference in hospitalization rates between the two groups. These are diseases in which there is often an option between home and hospital treatment, an option that can be exercised without danger to the patient.

The second two lines of Table 1 represent a second study done by Dr. Odin Anderson of the Health Information Foundation by a different technique.[5] Members of three New York City unions have a choice as to whether they will insure themselves in HIP or in Group Health Insurance (GHI). GHI also provides comprehensive care, but provides its doctor care by paying fees to any New York physician selected by the patient. In performing this study Dr. Anderson found union members with each type of insurance who could be matched by age, sex, and family size to assure comparability before examining their hospital use. This rather elaborate study revealed a sharp difference in the frequency of hospitalization, that is, 63 HIP against 110 GHI enrollees per 1000 insured. These two studies taken together were widely interpreted as evidence that group practice strongly influences hospitalization rates. The problem is obviously more complex than this, since there are also differences in the methods of practice and in payment of doctors. The HIP physicians are a selected group and hence possibly quite different than the doctors in New York whom the GHI patient employed. The many administrative services in HIP probably have a tendency to encourage judicious use of hospitals. Specialist use is also encouraged in HIP and a readily available specialist may effectively substitute for hospitalization.

The last comparison in Table 1 shows the 1958 hospitalization experience of the clerks' union.[6] This union is a relatively small, somewhat paternalistic organization that provides its members with an option between receiving medical care through HIP or through its own self-insured fee-for-service care. Extensive programs of worker education are undertaken to encourage "necessary but conservative use of the health benefits available." Equally important perhaps is the fact that this union also tries to educate doctors to use its insurance carefully. Since the experience of this union with its own fee-for-service insurance is no different than the experience of HIP, it appears that administrative action can control hospital use.

Another study of the steel workers union has added similar evidence.[7] This union is a large one and includes men who mine, smelt, or fashion steel and other metals in all parts of the country. Its health insurance is purchased from many different Blue Cross, commercial, and other insurers. Table 2 shows the vastly different

TABLE 2. STEELWORKERS' HOSPITAL EXPERIENCE UNDER
SEVERAL INSURANCE ARRANGEMENTS (1957–1958)

| Utilization | KFHP | Blue Cross plans | Six commercial contracts |
|---|---|---|---|
| Admissions per 1000 insured | 115 (90) | 135 | 150 |
| Range | — | 110 to 181 | 124 to 182 |

experiences of the locals in relation to the insurance carrier. In the right-hand column is shown the experience of six large steel unions whose health insurance was provided by commercial insurance companies. These companies provided comprehensive health insurance that was similar or identical to Blue Cross.

Hospital admission rates under commercial contracts were high. The lowest rate in any area, 124/1000 population, is equal to the average for the United States in the year under study. The hospitalization rate of workers insured under the Blue Cross-Blue

Shield plans was also above the United States average. The left-hand column entitled KFHP (Kaiser Foundation Health Plan) represents the experience of steelworkers who received their medical care from an organization very much like HIP. This care is given through group practices staffed by salaried specialists. The higher rate, 115 admissions, is for workers in the Kaiser Steel plants. The lower rate of 90 admissions/1000 population is for steelworkers in other plants who receive their care through the Kaiser Foundation. The Kaiser employees have a generous insurance plan which includes care for dependents both young and old. These age groups are hospitalized more than the rest of the population so that this provision presumably explains the higher rate of Kaiser employees.

It is difficult to conjure up a logical explanation why hospitalization should differ under similar commercial or Blue Cross policies or why variation within each type of insurance is so large from area to area. Certain of these areas have high hospitalization rates year in and year out, whereas others usually have lower rates. The low rate, associated with coverage by the Kaiser plan is presumably related to the control of admissions which specialists in group practice can exercise when out-patient care is a logical and feasible alternative to hospitalization. *It is very doubtful whether there are differences in illness that can account for this varied experience.*

A series of studies in England has further confounded the question of numbers of hospitalizations. In that country there is a waiting list for elective surgery. Under the stimulus of the Nuffield Foundation several different groups have tried to determine the numbers of additional beds required to clear this waiting list. When this number is calculated, it is always found that the additional number needed is a very small fraction of the existing number. More important than the determination of this critical number is the appreciation of variation in hospital use. In the Oxford area, for example, there are 4.8 surgical beds per 10,000 population, whereas the Newcastle area has 7 beds. Though one region has nearly 50 per cent more beds than the other, their waiting lists are about the same. R. F. L. Logan, who performed these studies, concluded tersely "the number of beds is the number available." [8]

If one region within England can make do with two-thirds as many beds as another, it would seem wise to look closely at the hospital for an explanation. Professor McKeown did this several years ago when he examined the patients in a chronic disease hospital in Birmingham.[9] On the basis of their medical and nursing requirements he concluded that one-fifth of the patients needed general hospital care. Another fifth, he felt, should have been in psychiatric institutions or in other places where they could receive the supervision required by their abnormal mental states. Three-fifths of the patients could have been cared for in their own homes by general practitioners and visiting nurses, or in institutions other than hospitals where these frail people could have help with domestic services.

This led to further studies of the "unnecessary hospital admissions" in England. During one investigation of the critical bed number, Dr. Logan of the University of Manchester found that there were substantial numbers of patients in hospitals who did not require hospital facilities for their care.[10] His estimate varied from a low of 9 per cent on surgical services to a high of 40 per cent among women admitted to medical services. As a result of another study, Crombie and Cross of Birmingham reached the conclusion that about 25 per cent of patients had no diagnostic or treatment need requiring hospitalization, or needed only out-patient laboratory studies.[11] Professor McKeown seemed to find these conclusions a bit strong.[12] He reviewed the records studies by Crombie and concluded that the unnecessary admissions were lower than Crombie had estimated. However, McKeown did state that some 13 per cent of patients had their discharge delayed, meaning that he found this proportion of patients hospitalized who no longer needed to be so. It is clear from all three studies that many patients who do not need hospital care are there because there is no one to care for them at home or for other social reasons. This type of admission should not be criticized unduly, but it does suggest that there are better alternatives than the expensive hospital bed.

Lest this may lead to the conclusion that the several British studies merely reflect the errors of socialized medicine, I should like to point out several things:

First, the hospitalization rate in the United States is nearly 50 per cent higher than in England and Wales. Since death rates at almost any age are lower in England than in the United States, one cannot impute any serious consequences to less frequent hospitalization. Furthermore, if one examines hospitalization in the two countries more closely, one finds that patients with head injuries or appendicitis, conditions that are always treated in the hospital, are admitted at about the same rate in both countries. In other diseases such as hemorrhoids or respiratory infections, in which there is a choice between home and hospital care, the admission rates in the United States are higher. Proportionately more patients with cancer are hospitalized in England and a greater proportion of all patients die in hospitals. Hospitals are being used very differently in the two countries. The reason for England's low hospitalization rate is its salaried full-time specialist staff. An independent specialist staff can readily control the number of admissions. Since these specialists have been chosen on the basis of their good judgment, their selection of patients for hospitalization should reflect this good judgment.

Lastly, mention should be made of a study conducted by Dr. Harry Becker for the Michigan Medical Society and the Michigan Blue Cross.[13] Becker and his coworkers concluded that 36 per cent of Blue Cross admissions and 28 per cent of all patient admissions in Michigan contained some element of "misuse" or "faulty use," that is, the admission was unnecessary or the stay was prolonged. He stated that one in eight Blue Cross admissions was for laboratory or x-ray studies that could as well have been done in the out-patient department.

The role of custom in influencing hospital admissions is illustrated by Logan's previously cited studies.[14] He observed that patients with certain diseases would be hospitalized routinely in one region of England whereas in another the same condition would be regarded as suitable for home care. Hospital administrators in this country are also aware of the fact that local custom may govern the decision as to home or hospital care for patients with certain diseases. Another example is supplied by the practices respecting delivery. In America, hospital deliveries have become virtually universal. But in Holland, two-thirds of babies are born at home. Home confinement has no apparent detrimental effect since Holland's infant mortality is the lowest in the world.

We thus find from medical care studies that hospital needs are rather indefinite characteristics related to the number of beds available, local customs, and to the organization of medical services.

In the earlier part of the century an interesting surgeon, E. A. Codman of the Massachusetts General Hospital, was obsessed, or as he described himself, "riddin . . . by the end result hobby." [15] Codman felt that a hospital should account for services rendered annually as it did for monies spent. How many nurses and physicians were trained? How many appendixes were removed when a renal stone was causing the difficulty? Somewhat quaintly he inquired how many patients had a good excuse for dying. Codman unfortunately did not develop these interesting ideas. He did stimulate Dr. George Grey Ward of the Woman's Hospital in New York to prepare graphs to illustrate the performance of surgeons by showing which of them had high postoperative infection rates and which of them had high care fatality rates. The graphs of these very final end results must have been striking and painful exhibits.[16]

The outcome of surgery in terms of its success as measured by death or survival, cure or failure to cure, is an ideal measure of quality. A few examples of its recent application indicate that it may occasionally be a discriminating tool to use, even though death rates are low and death from surgery rare. A few years ago Shapiro, Wiener, and Densen employed perinatal mortality to study medical care given by HIP physicians in New York.[17] Perinatal mortality is a measure of infant deaths between the 20th week of pregnancy and the first 7 days of life. It is well recognized that miscarriages, still-births, and death of the very young infant can be influenced by the skill of the obstetrician and pediatrician. In this study, Shapiro *et al.*, compared the perinatal mortality among HIP patients with that of other New Yorkers. Table 3 shows the results of this

TABLE 3. PERINATAL MORTALITY RATES PER 1000 LIVE BIRTHS
PLUS FETAL DEATHS, BY ETHNIC GROUP (1955)

| Ethnic group | New York City | | |
| | Total | Private physicians | HIP |
|---|---|---|---|
| White | 32.4 | 29.3 | 20.5 |
| Nonwhite | 64.3 | 51.2 | 35.8 |
| Puerto Rican | 49.9 | 31.7 | qns. |
| Total | 40.3 | 30.0 | 22.7 |

study. Since it is known that this mortality rate is very much influenced by race and social factors, it was necessary to separate the population into the white, nonwhite, and the Puerto Rican, and private and charity patients. It can be seen from this table that the white infant mortality is better than the Puerto Rican's which is in turn better than the Negro's. In the New York City sample, the group who used private physicians had lower mortality rates than the total group. Pregnant women who received care through HIP, whether Negro or white, delivered infants who had a lower perinatal mortality than infants delivered by private doctors. These figures are undoubtedly an end result, but an end result caused by a complex of factors of which HIP's group organization may be most important. Of the HIP women, virtually all received their care from specialist obstetricians. The proportion of New York City women who received care from specialists is not known, but it is almost certainly less. Another factor that may play some part in these different rates is the educational effort made by HIP to acquaint mothers with the need for early and frequent prenatal care and with the advisability of having the infant supervised by a pediatrician from birth. Thus the better record of HIP probably represents a sum of results that can be attributed to patient education, an organized medical care program in which special medical skills are made freely available, and lastly, the special medical skills themselves. It is a virtue of HIP that it does assure these advantages to its patients.

A second type of end result study has come from England. Dr. John Lee has investigated the case fatality rates of surgery in various types of hospitals.[18,19] For this purpose Dr. Lee selected certain types of serious diseases in which the probability of death was high by modern standards. Table 4 shows his comparisons. A ruptured

TABLE 4. CASE FATALITY RATES (PER CENT) IN TEACHING AND NONTEACHING HOSPITALS, ENGLAND AND WALES (MALES)

| Disease | Teaching hospitals | Nonteaching hospitals |
|---|---|---|
| Appendicitis with peritonitis (1951–1953) | 3.3 | 6.6 |
| Perforated peptic ulcer (1951–1953) | 7.2 | 9.7 |
| Hyperplasia, prostate (1953–1954) | 4.1 | 7.6 |

appendix is far less lethal today than it was in the 1930's, but it is still dangerous. As can be seen, the case fatality rate in nonteaching hospitals in England was twice as high as in the teaching hospitals. The perforate peptic ulcer is another grave disease. In this disease the different case fatality rates in the teaching and nonteaching hospitals are neither large nor significant. The third disease, hyperplasia of the prostate, again showed a definite difference between the teaching and nonteaching hospitals. One may easily conclude that the teaching hospital results stem from superior medical staffing. Dr. Lee, however, pointed out that the teaching hospitals had more staff surgeons, more house officers, and more nurses than the nonteaching hospital. It is possible that the better results of surgery in teaching hospitals may be related to a complex of factors, rather than to any unexplained general factor under the broad heading of goodness.

## QUALITY OF STUDIES

Studies of the quality of medical care *per se* have become a field of research only recently. This is a type of study which has received the greatest attention in the United States. In most of the economically developed countries with which the United States can be compared, the medical profession is divided into two parts — a well-trained, selected medical elite which controls admissions and care in hospitals, and the others who care for patients outside of the hospital. The European argument for this organization rests on the assumption that seriously ill patients should be in the hospital, attended by a competent specialist. Under this organization, the general practitioner has only to recognize that a patient is sick and send him to a hospital. In the United States through custom the hospital doors have been kept open to all types of doctors. It is common for a man of very little training and a man of superb training to be caring for patients of the same type in adjoining beds. Under these circumstances it is important that there be a way of measuring doctors' skills in the patients' interest. Our practice is justified on the basis of the good that it does for the medical profession. It is generally agreed that doctors will be better doctors for having rubbed shoulders with colleagues, for having attended the conferences and meetings that have become such a universal feature of hospital life, and lastly for having some attention directed to their weaknesses and shortcomings.

We went to some pains to point out in the previous section that the end result, which is in one sense a measurement of quality, is not a direct and sole consequence of the quality of medical care given. The favorable perinatal mortality rate of HIP patients may be a consequence of the organization giving medical care, administrative action, patient education, or lastly, the goodness of the obstetrical or pediatric care itself. In discussing studies of quality of medical care hereafter, the focus will be on direct measures of the skills which doctors apply to the resolution of a patient's problem and disease.

Preoccupation with the excellence of medical performance is becoming a commonplace. Medical schools undergo periodic scrutiny in order to maintain their accredited status. The same is true of hospitals and of nursing schools. Approved internship and residency programs for surgeons, obstetricians, psychiatrists, or internists must meet standards. If hospitals are to maintain an open door to all kinds of doctors whatever their qualifications, this process will have to be extended to an examination of the individual physician's performance to ascertain that the patient is cared for by the right doctor. Some hospitals now employ an audit to monitor the doctor's work. The audit is still at an early stage and rests upon a few easily obtained observations such as: does the patient with heart disease have an EKG done or does the patient with pneumonia receive a chest x-ray?

The history of serious attempts to measure the quality or skills of doctors is relatively short. A decade ago my colleagues, Dr. Andrews, Dr. Spain, and Dr. Greenberg and I undertook to study the performance of general practitioners in North Carolina.[20] From preliminary studies we knew that these North Carolina physicians see a great variety of illness. The general practitioner of course has a great responsibility in determining which patients are seriously ill and which are not. In other words, his first responsibility is to make a diagnosis. The time-honored process of reaching a diagnosis consists of a systematic history of the patient's illness, a thorough physical examination, and lastly, the laboratory. If these are applied systematically, a doctor will in most instances arrive at his goal. The family doctor must daily discriminate between serious and trivial illness. The general practitioner who is confronted by a bouncy adolescent who states he fell in a poison ivy patch does not need to apply the systematic method to reach a diagnosis. There are many patients who have complaints which suggest the need for careful study such as the patient who has lost weight, or suffers unusual fatigue, or who has pain, or is bleeding, or who discovers a lump, or who has had unusually persistent headaches. My colleagues and I spent a year watching 88 doctors, each for about one week. We found that with sufficiently prolonged observations we could give a highly reproducible description of many details of the doctors' diagnostic process. For example, patients who have high blood pressure, pregnant women, and patients with headaches should have the retinas of their eyes examined with an ophthalmoscope. About one-third of doctors used this instrument when it was indicated. The patient who complains of chest pain when he exercises should have a careful study of his heart. About one-fifth of patients had a fully satisfactory examination. From many items we could build up a composite picture of how well each doctor performed. At the very best they were doing work that would have been quite acceptable in university hospitals — where we think we do quite well. At the other end of the scale, the care given patients was quite poor.

Since we completed that study in 1954 there have been two further applications of the technique which we developed. Dr. Kenneth Clute has recently completed a study of general practice in Canada for the College of General Practitioners.[21] Since his results are almost identical with ours and are far more recent, I prefer to read a few of his conclusions. "The quality of practice observed by us varied from excellent to extremely poor. Both in Ontario and Nova Scotia some of the practices that we visited were considered definitely satisfactory and some so unsatisfactory as likely to expose the patients to serious risk. The differences that we observed in the practices did not relate to recent discoveries or rare diseases, but to the fundamentals of clinical medicine." Since the problems of psychiatric illness will be discussed later (see Dr. Lindemann's "Health Needs of Communities," p. 271), his opinion about their treatment by Canadian general practitioners is worth quoting. "After observing the handling of many patients, we were left with the impression that the general practitioners in dealing with the patient's emotional problems were basing their practice on their personal experience rather than on any professional preparation that they had had for such practice . . . it appeared that apart from advice about physical matters, a clergyman or a lawyer, if he had been as well disposed as the doctor, if he had had as many years' experience as had the doctor, would have been able to counsel as effectively as most practitioners; and some psychiatric social workers are probably a good deal more effective in this."

The third study using this technique was done in Australia under the auspices of the Australian College of General Practitioners by Dr. Clifford Jungfer, a distinguished physician.[22] (One might parenthetically remark that these general practitioner organizations require considerable courage to expose themselves to this type of scrutiny.) Jungfer, like Clute and ourselves, found that the skills that doctors brought to their patients were variable. Of the poorest, Dr. Jungfer says, "Grade I practitioners were quite unsuitable for general practice." In both the North Carolina and Canadian studies the amount of internship and residency training obtained by the doctor correlated with his skills; that is, the more of such training, the better the doctor. In Canada training obtained in a teaching hospital had a significantly greater effect than that of a nonteaching hospital.

Although the burgeoning middle class of the United States seeks "specialist care" with the same avidity as purchase of a second car, there is no real evidence that patients are able to judge the skills of their doctors. Dr. Clute found that the very good and the very poor doctors in Canada were equally busy. The same observation in North Carolina forced us to the conclusion that the patient is a very poor judge of his doctor's skills. The fact that the patient cannot make this judgment places a responsibility upon medical educators and the profession to ascertain that all doctors are as skilled as education and training can make them.

Dr. Fremont J. Lyden. formerly a member of Harvard's Department of Preventive Medicine, undertook to find out why some doctors prepared themselves well for practice whereas others were satisfied with the barest minimum of preparation. Table 5 is taken from Dr. Lyden's study of nearly 2000 recent graduates of 12 medical schools in the United States. Shown here is the type of

TABLE 5. FIELD OF PRACTICE BY CLASS RANK
(distribution for each third of class, 1950 and 1954 combined, in per cent)

| Field of practice | Five public schools[a] | | | Six private schools | | |
|---|---|---|---|---|---|---|
| | Lower third | Middle third | Upper third | Lower third | Middle third | Upper third |
| GP | 43.5 | 38.2 | 17.9 | 16.9 | 11.1 | 4.6 |
| Medicine[b] | 7.1 | 11.8 | 25.8 | 15.6 | 15.9 | 25.3 |
| Surgery | 15.9 | 10.5 | 14.3 | 25.2 | 24.2 | 19.8 |
| Teaching/Research | 4.6 | 6.3 | 10.7 | 8.6 | 15.3 | 21.9 |
| Psychiatry | 8.4 | 5.5 | 7.1 | 10.6 | 6.1 | 5.2 |
| Pediatrics | 4.2 | 7.6 | 4.0 | 6.0 | 10.5 | 7.7 |
| OB-GYN | 6.3 | 5.9 | 5.2 | 6.6 | 5.1 | 4.6 |
| EENT | 5.4 | 5.5 | 4.8 | 2.7 | 2.5 | 3.1 |
| Other | 4.2 | 8.4 | 9.5 | 7.0 | 6.4 | 6.5 |
| Not in practice | 0.4 | 0.4 | 0.8 | 0.7 | 2.9 | 1.2 |
| Total | 100.0 | 100.0 | 100.0 | 100.0 | 100.0 | 100.0 |
| Number of respondents | 239 | 238 | 252 | 301 | 314 | 324 |

[a] One school is eliminated from these tabulations because rank distribution not given by thirds.
[b] Includes Dermatology and Neurology.

practice selected by doctors who graduated with different academic records. Also, in both the public and the private medical schools the men who went into general practice came much more often from the bottom third of the class than the top third. Most of the men who went into general practice normally prepared themselves with only a rotating internship, usually in a nonteaching hospital. This is in marked contrast to the men who went into specialty practice, who on average obtained three years of further training after internship. This then is a situation in which the medical students with the poorest records are selected for the internships which have the weakest educational programs. These internships are likely to be dead-end jobs that lead directly to practice. The more able students train in teaching hospitals where the educational resources are far more extensive and the training programs longer. This selection gives the teaching hospitals very bright young men to run their services. The fact that the least able are quickly shunted into general practice following a poor internship will assure the continued existence of the poor practices which Clute described so frankly.

Many phases of routine administration in hospitals such as the Massachusetts General are being turned over to computers. It is very probable that they will shortly be applied to monitoring the patients' temperature, blood pressure, and in making other routine observations. There are already quite a few hospitals that audit and continuously scrutinize the work of their physicians. It is easy to speculate on the contribution that the data-handling capacity of computers may make to this self-examination. Instead of reminding the doctor that he forgot to have white blood cell counts on two patients last month, as the present audit does, a future audit might note the presence of certain symptoms, physical abnormalities, and laboratory results, and then suggest, "You had better get a chest x-ray, Doctor; this might by Kartagener's Syndrome!"

The possible role of the computer is highly speculative and may seem to combine elements of both science fiction and Alice in Wonderland. Modern data processing does nevertheless provide us with great opportunities for handling very complex questions and large amounts of data. If we seriously address ourselves to questions of continuously scrutinizing work being done in hospitals, there is no doubt that the computer will make it possible to do jobs which at the present time are too complex and too cumbersome to be worthwhile.

## CONCLUSION

I would like to summarize briefly the points that have been covered today and from these draw a few general conclusions.

In the first section, which dealt with economics, a few examples of the information available about the economics of medical care were shown. It was pointed out that this is a field in which there is much information available. As the debate on hospital insurance for the aged through Social Security is resumed in congress, as one presumes it will be, the decision will be difficult to make not because of any deficiency in information, but because the issue touches upon public policy and raises questions which sharply divide men.

In the second section, in which group practices and hospitals were discussed, an attempt was made to illustrate the contributions of medical care research to an understanding of institutions and their functioning. Examples were given showing how organization and administration affect the outcome of medical care and hospital use. The argument dealt at some length with the frequency of hospitalization to show that hospital need was an indefinite quality that is subject to many influences in addition to the patient's illness.

An attempt has also been made to show that when the Blue Cross director periodically appears before the insurance commissioner and requests a rate increase, he should not be the target for criticism. If there is serious concern about the increased cost of health and hospital insurance, attention should not be directed to the man who gets the bill, but to the hospital organization and staff that determine the way our hospitals are used. Hospitalization can be restricted, but such restriction will involve changes in our philosophy and practice, rather than blaming Blue Cross.

Last to be presented was some evidence of the quality of medical care in America. In this we have tried to be good doctors and we have tried to diagnose the cause of unsatisfactory practice. Although the medical schools are always very concerned about the quality of their instruction, they suffer from a peculiar educational myopia at one point because they are not concerned about whether certain graduates are ready or unready to enter practice. Russell Nelson has proposed that all internship and residency training should be under university supervision.[23] (See Dr. Nelson's "The Hospital and the Continuing Education of the Physician," p. 237.) I would like to add to Dr. Nelson's suggestion. Several years ago a statement by the Association of American Medical Colleges recognized the fact that graduation from medical school does not prepare a man for practice. The graduate's theoretical background is an adequate basis for the internship and residency training which does get him ready for practice. The time has come for medical schools to ascertain that each of their graduates receives enough of the right kind of hospital experience so that each one will be a competent doctor when he finally takes full responsibility for his patients.

It is to be hoped that these many examples of medical care research will have demonstrated that systematic study and investigation can produce good and worthwhile information, and that we should spend some small fraction of the millions that are poured into medical care on study of the industry and in measuring its results.

# THE VOICE OF THE CONSUMER:
## COST, QUALITY, AND ORGANIZATION
## OF MEDICAL SERVICES

Jerome Pollack

THE voice of the consumer is heard increasingly in the affairs of medicine. His presence is felt questioning, criticizing, arguing, judging, and acting in a field to which consumers were previously inattentive and in which their competence was often challenged. Medicine had long been attuned to its transactions with the patient and accustomed to his voice. Now, however, care is purchased increasingly by a consumer who is not sick, but well; not dependent, but resourceful. The new payments come usually from companies and unions that are establishing a new economic relationship with medicine. They bring not only new funds but a new influence. They contemplate health care from a perspective beyond the immediate pressures that concern the patient. They consider the cost of care and the methods of financing, the adequacy of man power, the quality of practice and its organization, as well as other matters of medical policy. The new consumer already pays for most private hospital services and will probably play an expanding part in the economy of most medical care. The new financing has helped sustain the largest increase in expenditures for health care in the nation's history. Though voluntary and evolutionary, it is profoundly restructuring the economics of medicine. And, although the new consumer has thus far accepted much of what he has found, he is beginning to exercise independent judgment. His could be the decisive influence in medical policy.

## CONSUMPTION OF MEDICAL CARE

In theory, the consumer might be expected to have his way. The classical economists placed the consumer at the center of the economy. Adam Smith declared, "Consumption is the sole end and purpose of all production." The interest of the producer, he said, "ought to be attended to, only so far as it may be necessary for promoting that of the consumer." [1] This maxim he regarded as "so perfectly self-evident, that it would be absurd to attempt to prove it."

The supremacy of the consumer, however, was short-lived, for in the very next sentence Adam Smith hastened to observe that: "the interest of the consumer is almost constantly sacrificed to that of the producer." Production, and not consumption, is considered "as the ultimate end and object of all industry and commerce."

The relationship between consumer and producer remains ambiguous and the search for the articulation of these two essential elements of the economy continues. In few endeavors are consumers and purveyors placed in more exacting circumstances than in acquiring and providing medical care. Yet in few activities do they seem less equipped to find the answers.

Few civilizations have entrusted the distribution of medical services entirely to the workings of the market. Medical transactions have been characteristically modified. In the ancient world, the healing arts were often practiced outside of a market system. As medicine turned from its roots in magic and faith to naturalistic and surgical methods, it became more expensive and corresponding changes came about in the mode of payment.[2] Medical fees, unlike those for other services, were graduated according to social status and ability to pay, an ancient practice that undoubtedly preceded its mention in the diorite entablatures of Hammurabi nearly two thousand years B.C.[3] Even graduated fees remained beyond the means of many until religious precept insisted that no one was to be deprived of care through inability to pay. To achieve this, care was provided to many as beneficiaries rather than as consumers.

Today the medical arts are again involved in a great advance that history may find to be as sweeping as the turn from magic to science. Again changes in the financing and organization of medical care are occurring. A new urgency has descended on the social adaptations of medical care. The further the capacity of the economy advances, the greater is its obligation to promote human welfare. The further medical care advances, the less can society countenance its unavailability to people who may need it. Consumers are insisting on greater assurances than ever of access to contemporary care.

As primary consumer the patient has most at stake. His needs again appear so perfectly self-evident that it would seem absurd to attempt to prove them. He needs an adequate supply of well trained and well motivated physicians and technicians practicing in well-equipped and logically ordered facilities, keeping abreast of their field and attuned to the total technology. He needs a means of distributing the cost of such a medical system that can support it without inhibiting access to care.

As an individual, however, the patient is unable to act effectively on any of these requirements. Vital as they are to him, he does not pursue them actively nor does he comprehend them competently. The planning of medical care is not his role in society.

The patient's knowledge of medical care is inescapably limited. He does not know what the physician is inquiring, looking, and probing for and he lacks criteria to judge the appropriateness of the therapy or its cost.

Plato spoke of the empirical physician who, on encountering "the gentleman physician talking to his gentleman patient . . . beginning at the beginning of the disease and discoursing about the whole nature of the body . . . would burst into a hearty laugh — he would say, 'Foolish fellow, you are not healing the sick man, you are educating him; and he does not want to be made a doctor, but to get well.' " [4]

Nor have we since made doctors of patients. In spite of vast advances in education and an avid popular interest in health, today's patient may be even less able to judge health care than yesteryear's. Medical knowledge is outrunning popular understanding and the physician has neither the time nor the opportunity to close the gap.

Life is pursued with a strange mixture of reason and unreason. Great contrasts exist of unprecedented enlightenment and unprecedented quackery.[5] The finest of clinical care coexists with the worst of self-medication. Many millions resort to self-prescribed analgesics, tonics, vitamins, cough and cold medicines, laxatives, digestion aids, skin compounds, sleeping and reducing pills, and other proprietary medicines for conditions requiring medical attention.

The boundaries of care are ill-defined. The patient often does not know whether or when to approach the doctor and whom to approach. In this medical maze the average person is not only poorly informed; he often is wrong.

Patients increasingly come to the doctor self diagnosed. One recent survey reported a 45 per cent increase over ten years in the number of patients who advance their own diagnoses and an even greater increase — 89 per cent — in those who demand specific drugs and therapies.[6] Although the patient's interest and participation need to be enlisted, most physicians believe that to carry this initiative to the point of diagnosis and therapy is, on the whole, undesirable. The patient wants quick and sure relief and is as susceptible to strong therapy as his ancestors were to the therapeutic excesses of their time. He may ask for injections, antibiotics, steroids, and other treatments held to be strong and effective. He judges adversely doctors who withhold them. He may request unwarranted hospitalization rather than treatment at home. When he backs up such demands with economic pressures on the doctors, his influence is not invariably salutary. He may even withdraw his patronage from the physician who resists his demands.

The patient's perspective is understandably personal and not concerned with policy. Most frequently he criticizes doctors for not showing enough interest, for not listening to his troubles, or for making him wait too long in the reception room.[7] He does not consider that his is one of nearly a billion visits a year to physicians whose shortage is now becoming increasingly apparent.

Once in the waiting, examining, treatment, or operating room, the patient is limited by what he finds there. It is then far too late and far beyond his capacities to correct deficiencies in the number of doctors, dentists, nurses, and other personnel or to do anything about the methods of practice and organization of care. He might refuse to pay if the physician does not do well by him but this would probably put him in wrong with the law. For a serious lapse of care, he might sue for malpractice, but this requires evidence that the patient does not easily acquire and at best may bring indemnification rather than correction.

No amount of health education will produce a patient able to deal effectively with medical policy. The important and effective expressions of consumer interest have come when the individual began to purchase care as a prospective patient and together with others entered into a continuous and collective relationship with medicine.

## THE FINANCING OF MEDICAL CARE

Efforts in America to share the cost of care and arrange for its availability can be traced back for over a century.[8,9] Some of these efforts attained a comprehensiveness as yet generally unmatched. But until very recently such ventures did not flourish in American soil.

Trade union membership, one of the major vehicles for the eventual spread of health benefits, remained small and unstable until the mid-1930's. Employers provided care for the occupationally disabled and occasionally for other employees, but usually in such industries as mining, lumbering, and railroading, where the employees were isolated and care might not have been otherwise available. Industry generally did not welcome a liability to provide such benefits. The medical profession, after an initial period of interest, then neutrality, resisted both public and private health insurance.

As late as 1940, fewer than one in ten Americans had any hospitalization insurance and fewer than four in a hundred had any surgical or medical protection. Hopes for health insurance gravitated toward legislation. A *Fortune* survey revealed that almost three-fourths of the people believed that the federal government should collect enough taxes to provide medical care for all who need it.[10]

Not until disaster struck was large-scale action taken to provide for the social financing of health care. Until the mid-1930's, personal financing was buttressed only by philanthropy, a graduated fee system which had never been adequate to provide care for the underprivileged, and a commitment to provide charitable care under a poor relief system that was collapsing.

The depression of the 1930's lashed the unprotected financing of health care with a fury that storms reserve for the unprepared.

Faced with economic disaster, the hospitals took the initiative in establishing prepayment plans to restore occupancy. For a few additional years medical societies opposed such "social experiments," even in voluntary form. Sooner or later, the House of Delegates of the American Medical Association warned, insurance would spread to medical care and result in an "inevitable deterioration in the quality of service." [11]

It soon became apparent, however, that if voluntary action did not come, a governmental program would be enacted. Medical societies entered prepayment hoping to avert legislation. Insurance companies, likewise fearing governmental action, entered health insurance with considerable misgivings over the insurability of health care.

The medical economy more than recovered. Voluntary health insurance grew to governmental proportions in the number of people it covered. From near bankruptcy at $2 billion, private expenditures for health services regained the $3 billion level and rose eightfold to nearly $24 billion this year. Sustained by the new financing, the volume, standards, and costs of care all soared.

The unprecedented increase in expenditures occurred without a shift from private to public financing. The bulk of health care remained in the private sector of the economy which accounts for about three-fourths of all expenditures. Since 1949–1950, expenditures in the private sector increased from 3.4 to 4.1 per cent of the gross national product while public expenditures remained at 1.3 per cent and, as a proportion, had decreased in the interim. [12]

Although public financing was averted, social financing was not. The voluntary system grew mainly because of the assumption of responsibility for the financing of care by the organized consumer, chiefly by labor and management. Of the 136.5 million people having hospitalization insurance at the end of 1961, 106 million — 41 million employees and 65 million dependents — were covered by arrangements arising out of employment. [13] Of the nearly $5.7 billion paid in benefits for hospital and physician services that year, $4.5 billion came from employee benefit plans. [14]

These contributions above all sustained the voluntary system. Indeed where the employee relationship is breached or doesn't exist, there is a precipitous fall-off both in the volume and the quality of protection. There is, in fact, little to the voluntary system apart from the funds it expends on behalf of management and labor. If these purchasers are showing an increased interest and initiative in health care, the reason should not be obscure.

The allocation of wages for health care which supported the spectacular growth of voluntary health insurance came about because of a remarkable confluence of favorable circumstances. Labor had succeeded in organizing basic industries and had attained stability and strength. It had achieved wage levels that made a turn to other benefits feasible. It was able to pursue the necessary negotiations and litigation to establish by law an employer responsibility to bargain over health benefits. Direct wages were for a time unobtainable but health benefits were permitted. The postwar economy was revealing unanticipated strength. There was a desire for labor peace and industrial stability. Health insurance was needed and in one form or another could not be put off much longer. By regarding the contributions as an allocation of wages rather than quarreling over the respective rights and responsibilities of labor and management, the acceptance of a commitment to contribute was greatly facilitated. Employers who might otherwise have long disputed a liability to contribute for off-the-job illness or toward care for dependents began to contribute very materially for health insurance. Thus on a largely unanticipated scale, labor and management first initiated and then enlarged their contributions toward health care.

In the process, contractual commitments were developed to provide health benefits as a matter of right that resemble in form and content the statutory requirements of social insurance. They made it possible to accomplish privately what elsewhere had required government.

But the metamorphosis from a lesser evil to an adequate system of financing health care has only begun. If the horizontal growth of prepayment has been unexpectedly rapid, its vertical dimensions remain shallow. Health insurance has only entered the second quartile of consumer expenditures for care. In all, between one-third and two-fifths of expenditures regarded as insurable are covered.[15] That much more needs to be insured is evident.

Once the economic crisis passed, however, hospitals have shown conspicuously less disposition to continue pioneering. Many of their prepayment plans appear to be concerned mainly with preserving a degree of peace and quiet that the rising cost of hospital care is not likely to grant them. Once the threat of national health insurance abated, many physicians relaxed what earlier had been a reserved support of their prepayment plans. The tempo of development has slowed down with the course only partly run.

The initiative has been assumed by the former have-nots of the voluntary system: by producers whose services are only little or not insured who also want to bolster the financing of their work, such as internists, general practitioners, dentists, optometrists, and pharmacists; by insurance companies who originally followed but now lead in senior partnership; and by consumers who increasingly find that their needs and interests are not yet adequately and equitably served.

## WEAKNESS IN THE FINANCING OF CARE

The consumer was initiated and educated in prepayment by the purveyor. He came to the purveyor's household as a foster child. The purveyor had created one of the principal instruments of consumption and if the consumer had been more sophisticated he might have questioned the medical interference in lay affairs. But he didn't. He observed the rules of the household and was indoctrinated in his manners at the purveyor's table. It was repeatedly stressed that there must be a complete separation between payment and practice. This was one of the covenants insisted on vigorously by the physicians. Only later was he to learn for himself that such a separation was literally impossible. For payment does influence practice: whether certain services are performed, where they are performed, when they are performed, by whom they are performed and, to an extent, how they are performed. Through these insurogenic influences laymen, expert and otherwise, some with less at stake than the consumer, are practicing medicine almost as predictably as if they admitted the patients or performed the surgery themselves. Ignoring these influences does not eliminate them. The consumer increasingly finds it necessary to recognize them and employ them constructively.

The consumer's political tendencies were feared as a force once committed to governmental insurance, and there was concern over his economic aims, that he might support competing medical and hospital plans. He was largely read out of influence in policy-making and given only token representation on the governing councils of prepayment.

The consumer in fact proved less rebellious than had been feared. He went along with most of the rules and even the preferences of the purveyors. But his independent judgment became necessary.

Benefits had been hastily designed and uncritically accepted when any protection was preferable to nothing. Hospitalization came first largely because hospitals acted first. By a logic that was not too carefully scrutinized, hospitalization was considered not only worthiest of insurance, as the site of the most important and expensive care, but also as a way to police other benefits and make them more insurable. As a result, needless resort to hospitalization is stimulated as patients seek to acquire and physicians to provide benefits not otherwise available. A maldistribution of insurance over the spectrum of care is distorting medical practice.

Surgery was overemphasized not because it is necessarily more insurance-worthy but because it is more easily verified. As a result, caring for an in-grown toenail is a commonly insured procedure while cancer and heart disease are often ignored until the patient needs to be hospitalized. Other specialties and segments of health care are largely underinsured. Consumers see the underdevelopment and frequent omission of diagnostic services and often wonder whether, if these had been covered first, the impact on practice would not have been better.

The functions of health insurance are undergoing a necessary reappraisal. Expenditures for health care cannot be taken solely as losses to be replaced by insurance: once such benefits are used to pay for most hospital care they must be regarded as a major instrument not only of loss replacement but of financing care. The consumer wants to use his benefits as an aid to health and not merely as an economic resource in illness. He wants and will probably win the prepayment of preventive services.

The prevalent indemnity form of benefits for medical care is grossly defective, reflecting a lack of medical commitment to prepayment. Without assurance of what physicians will charge, insurers protect themselves by setting limits to their payments. This leaves the insured to pay a remainder that has no predetermined ceiling and exposes him to a burden that could have been borne by insurance. The ambiguity of allowances toward fees traditionally set according to ability to pay and the susceptibility of such transactions to abuse are producing poor value for consumers and undermining their confidence in the conduct and integrity of health insurance.

The consumer is not trying to drive a hard bargain. He agrees that physicians should be well paid in accordance with their responsibilities and that hospitals should be fully reimbursed for their costs. But he is faced with subscription rates for hospitalization and some other benefits that have gone into a steep and relentless ascent, for which he holds prepayment plans partly responsible. Consumers believe that prepayment is reducing or removing incentives to contain costs and they fear the collaboration of purveyors and their plans in imposing cost on the public. Labor and management do not feel that prepayment plans have given them sufficient assurance that unwarranted elements of cost are being scrupulously resisted.

The justification presented in support of increased cost in many instances is defective. Fearing a hostile public and mistrusting the adjudicative procedure of regulatory agencies, the plans request more than they expect to receive, and thus introduce spurious factors into their presentations.

The consumer perceives a lack of vigor and motivation on the part of prepayment plans to bargain with hospitals on behalf of purchasers; he sees signs of indulgence of medical societies over excessive fees; he sees hospital accounting that is far from adequate to sustain proper charges or reimbursable cost formulas; he sees evidence of faulty utilization of hospitals and ominous increases in the utilization of some physicians' services; he sees lack of balance in the composition of the governing boards of prepayment plans; he sees the inadequacy of direct controls and the temptation to resort to controls at the expense of the patient. In all, these lead to a growing belief widely held by the principal payers of health care that costs are insufficiently in hand.

The financial commitment on which the voluntary system so largely depends rests on less stable foundations than are generally perceived. Contributions have been set by pattern rather than policy. Few purchasers have committed themselves to pay for benefits irrespective of cost. Variations in the level of contributions and of benefits exceed almost any rational standard. Some employers pay all, others part, and some still pay nothing. Some pay for a given level of benefits; others a fixed monetary amount. There are no agreed-upon standards either for benefits or for contributions. In the less affluent industries, employers contribute less and their employees receive less. There is reason for uncertainty over the consequences of a continuation of the steep and sustained rise of cost on such an uncertain structure.

Health insurance is contributing toward higher cost and more intensive patterns of practice. Its impact is suffused throughout the medical economy and not called off for persons who have little aid from an employer or none at all, for those who have less efficient or less economical protection, or who may be totally uninsured. So far, the have-nots have tried to run in an unequal race, but those who are falling behind are beginning to question whether they can stay in such contests without some compensation of their handicaps.

Prepayment plans had earlier attempted to provide uniform benefits at uniform cost to all in their communities. Under unrelenting competition the ability of the voluntary system to share the cost is being undermined at the very time when it needs strengthening.

America is again facing the future with a mode of financing care that at best is in a precarious equilibrium with the present, but is as ill-prepared for what lies ahead as it was in the 1930's. The voluntary system faces serious crises over the justification of cost, the distribution of cost, and in deciding the respective roles of public and private financing. If the drop of one-third in consumer expenditures produced one kind of crisis, the subsequent eightfold increase is generating an even more severe crisis. We simply are less attuned to recognizing the crises of affluence and we have not yet learned how to anticipate what certainly lies ahead.

## THE ORGANIZED CONSUMER AND THE
## QUALITY OF CARE

The patient's interest in the quality of care is universally conceded. Indeed, it is often argued that the quality of care is best protected when he is able to bring his person and his fees to physicians of his choice. Such arguments would make the individual consumer final arbiter over the quality of care.

But what is conceded the individual is denied the organized consumer. The third party is regarded as a threat to quality. Most health insurance plans have gone to great lengths to assure the separation of payment and practice. For a time purchasers generally went along with this philosophy and few even attempted to observe the quality of care rendered.

Evidence that the quality of care purchased might occasionally be wanting intruded itself in instances brought forward by the beneficiaries. These involved not subtleties of medical judgment but simply poor, negligent, and at times inexcusable practice.

The course of events is well illustrated by the United Mineworkers Welfare and Retirement Program. The fund started out with free choice of physician and a reliance on existing safeguards of quality. After encountering many instances of grossly inadequate care and insufficient corrective action by medical societies and hospital staffs, where practicable, the fund began to require consultation with an appropriate specialist before hospital admission. It ruled that, if feasible, major surgery be performed by "broadly competent and responsible surgeons according to criteria established by the American Board of Surgery or the American College of Surgeons." [16] It refused to pay individual physicians for services of inferior quality as judged by qualified consultants.

More recently, a labor-management welfare fund in New York arranged through Columbia University for a medical audit of hospital records to ascertain the quality of care received by its beneficiaries. The results, published together with other indexes of quality, have brought into sharpest focus the association between prepayment and quality.[17] Evidence was found of fair and poor care and some held to be unnecessary. The widely publicized results have made consumers aware that medical care can be assayed.

They have led to a program of continuing appraisal not only by the welfare fund itself but by the state health department under legislation just passed.

One of the chronic arguments against attempting to enforce standards of quality is the difficulty in measuring or determining it. However, once formal accreditation of hospitals was established, a minimum standard for hospital care had been set. A study of hospital prepayment by Columbia University commissioned by the New York State Health and Insurance Departments recommended payment only to accredited hospitals: this recommendation is now in process of adoption.[18] As other measures are developed and standards are set their application to prepayment can be expected.

As yet, most purchasers are not consciously committed to the pursuit of quality, but it is inherent in their purchase. Consumers want good care; that is partly why they are purchasing protection.

They cannot themselves initiate standards of care, but they can encourage their development and application once available. They can employ professionals who know quality and who can measure it. The organized consumers will insist increasingly on quality controls, with which they are familiar in industry, and they will exercise a fiduciary responsibility, to which they are accustomed in finance, with the funds entrusted for the purchase of health care. They will try to influence the professions and hospitals and prepayment plans to institute quality controls. More studies, investigations, audits, and other measures can be anticipated. Rather than causing a deterioration of quality, the third party is coming forward in support of higher standards.

## JOINT OPPORTUNITY

The consumer is conceded a legitimate concern with questions of cost, but when he moves on to consider quality of care and when he presumes to judge how care should be organized, his authority is likely to be challenged. Lay interference is resisted by medicine. A vivid local example goes back to the 1870's when President Eliot of Harvard tried to reform medical education and provoked a professor of surgery to denounce both the Harvard Corporation and lay interference in these terms:

Does Mr. Lowell know anything about medical education? Or the Rev. Dr. Putnam . . . Why, Mr. Crowninshield carries a horse chestnut in his pocket to keep off rheumatism! Is the new medical education to be best directed by a man who carries horse chestnuts in his pocket to cure rheumatism? [19]

When laymen less revered than the Harvard Corporation are involved, such as labor leaders, there is even greater acrimony and they may be accused of carrying something other than chestnuts in their pockets. Such conflicts evoke subterranean springs of resentment that the patient, whose limitations no one knows better than the physician, will eventually determine how medicine shall be practiced. If the patient is ill-informed, is his business agent or foreman any better equipped to set policy for physicians and hospitals? Medical education was eventually reformed by a layman and a foundation which supported a work so monumental that it was impossible to question whether Abraham Flexner knew anything about medical education. The reform of medical education has receded in time and Flexner's Bulletin Number 4 is regarded as a great classic.

The reorganization of medical practice is a current problem about which perspective has yet to be achieved. It is widely realized that changes are necessary, yet efforts to initiate substantial modifications in practice or payment have encountered bitter resistance. The old precepts of medical economics and organization were regarded as endowed with eternal verity. Alternative methods of organizing and paying for care were denounced as harmful and heretical. In a settled period, doctrinal clashes may be taken with good grace; in time of stress, heresy is taken seriously.

Just as the fears and prejudices of the public against dissection impeded the development of anatomy and pathology, as the fears of vaccination and, more recently, of fluoridation, have retarded public health, so, too, the fears of physicians of economic change have inhibited steps necessary in the financing and organization of health care — not only the fear of socialized medicine, but of closed panel plans, salaried practice, corporate practice and even the less ominous implications of third-party payment.

Bitter struggles to extirpate closed-panel plans form a dark and damaging chapter of recent medical history. This was a social phenomenon not unlike the breaking of machines by workingmen who had found themselves similarly threatened. Attempts to arrange and to pay for care other than through fee-for-service paid solo practice usually meant entering into serious conflict. Physicians risked their careers to participate: threats would often be enunciated and sometimes carried out. The counterpressures were often sufficiently strong to assure the failure of such ventures. Even now that the legitimacy of such efforts is generally acknowledged, they still are undertaken to a very large extent as an adversary proceeding. The warfare produced casualties on both sides. It placed organized medicine in a role of resisting important innovations. It brought into leadership the more combative and less reflective elements of the medical profession. Reciprocally, the closed panel plans were formed under conditions hardly conducive to success. They faced serious difficulties in recruiting both physicians and patients.

The adversary relationship has been harmful to organized medicine and it has done much to undermine public esteem for the physician. It greatly hampered the development of independent medical service plans. Its greatest casualty was to distort the whole concept of the changing organization of medical care, making it a matter of warfare and putting partisan connotations on features of medical practice and payment that need to be freely experimented with in a wide variety of ways.

Just as purveyors once intervened in consumer affairs to establish prepayment plans, so consumers have on occasion intervened to support and occasionally to establish group practice prepayment plans. If such arrangements had awaited medical society approval, we would not have valuable plans now conceded to be a valid part of the voluntary system. If hospitals had capitulated to campaigns to limit their practice many outstanding institutions would not exist today.

Consumers are by no means committed to the overthrow of existing plans and arrangements. By and large they respect the profession and have no desire to wage war against it. They will, however, support physicians who want to try new methods of practice and they will continue to establish some group practice plans themselves.

The American Medical Association's Commission on Medical Care Plans has made a valuable contribution in urging tolerance and objectivity and in conceding the right of independent plans to exist. Although lingering encounters over hospital privileges and some coercive practices are continuing, the right to attempt other methods of organization and payment is acknowledged. The rigidity that reigned till recently is now a rear-guard rather than a dominant position.

The overnight abolition of solo practice by consumer pressure is not imminent. Nor is fee-for-service payment in immediate peril. If anything, some of the independent plans need to revive their earlier aspirations. Inhibited by opposition and organizational obstacles they have tended to practice conventional medicine under a common roof and to forego a truly creative use of group practice.

In a more benign atmosphere, hospitals might venture more boldly into becoming the community health centers which they have so often aspired to be. Medical clinics might find ways of participating in prepayment, and medical societies could experiment with combining some capitation and fee-for-service payment, to offer truly comprehensive medical services. Many similar pragmatic steps can be taken.

If there is indeed a remission in the restrictiveness which previously inhibited experimentation, our country might be ready to make one of its greatest contributions to medical care the world over. Ours has not been a position of leadership in advancing methods of financing. In technological advance and in industrial organization, however, we stand unrivaled. The government health programs of other nations, many of which were developed at an earlier stage of medical technology, tended generally to incorporate what they found in medical practice and are susceptible to the criticism that they may have frozen organizational patterns. One of the great advantages of a voluntary system of financing is the latitude it offers for wide experimentation in evolving new organizational patterns. Ours may be the best opportunity of evolving better relationships of personnel and institutions, of family physicians, specialists, and other personnel in the new medical technology.

A near-classical clash of Utopian and laissez-faire doctrines is now drawing to a close. Utopia literally means nowhere. Its advocates had advanced measures that would require nothing less than a complete reorganization and regeneration of physicians; while the laissez-faire camp fought any change. The Utopians have been bruised by the unreadiness of American society to adopt grand and sweeping schemes with universal application or to reorganize care radically. The laissez-faire advocates have been equally pained by the stubborn refusal of Americans to stay put. Once reformers act with realism while conservatives accept the inevitability of change the outlook for progress is very good.

## FINANCING CARE FOR THE AGED

We are now in the late stages of a bitter contest over how to provide health insurance for the aged. (See Dr. Somers' "Private Health Insurance," p. 187, and Dr. Schottland's "The Social Security System and Medical Care," p. 201.) The struggle has become so polarized that instead of the clarity that should exist, there is confusion, and only with difficulty can the real issues be extricated from the slogans and campaign speeches. Some assert that any governmental action would be irreversible, harmful, sinister, and unwise; others believe that resort to government is needed when private action is inadequate or unavailing. Some regard any governmental action as an inevitable prelude to its eventual expansion to cover all health care. Others claim that government can complement private effort without engulfing it. Some have concerned themselves with the convolutions of the conflict and see conspiracy where there may be merely controversy. And there are insistent pleadings that what is at stake is a bilateral struggle between good and evil, responsibility and neglect, or freedom and compulsion.

The underlying issue is more simple. It inheres most of all in the reliance of the voluntary system on contributions from employment that are not sufficiently available for the aged.

Labor tried to negotiate for health benefits for the aged and generally found it to be either unobtainable or unmanageable. Without an opportunity to accumulate reserves over the employees' whole careers, employers see an unwarranted burden in having to cover increasing numbers of aged and provide them with lifetime benefits of indeterminate and increasing cost. The advocates of additional legislation are not engaging in a tactical first move to overthrow the voluntary system. They are looking for a solution to a specific problem which existing sources of financing have failed to solve. In keeping with American customs they will accept an interplay between private and public financing as they have with unemployment, retirement, disability, and other benefits.

There is today an unacknowledged consensus that further public financing for the aged is needed. That consensus is bipartisan although there is disagreement on the manner, purpose, and agency to be employed. Just as the position of those who wanted a total governmental program for all has become untenable, those who want an entirely nongovernmental solution are equally untenably situated. The forces of compromise are at work. But in looking for a formula to break a political deadlock, a solution that could be unsatisfactory seems most likely to succeed.

In spite of all the debate, there is little clarification of the fundamental question: Are we in America merely in an earlier stage of the same course that led the major industrial countries to governmental financing of basic health care or are we on another course that will lead to a new kind of program? If we are on the usual path but merely late in schedule, it is largely a matter of time. We have generally copied such programs from abroad, often with amazing conventionality. Disability benefits were added to social security in 1956 after a fight resembling the current struggle over health insurance for the aged. When it was enacted, in spite of all delay and the possibility of doing something much better in an age of advanced medical care and rehabilitation, the law in all of its essentials could have been written by Chancellor Bismarck. If we continue to establish such programs in the manner that has characterized not only this but the whole succession of conflicts, we are bound to arrive repeatedly at a stereotyped solution.

René Dubos has commented with amused pathos at the wild west gun battles so popular in our folklore and so characteristic of medical policies. The hero blasts out the desperadoes who have descended on the frontier town. The story ends happily but in reality the fundamental problems are unsolved. The conditions that had opened the town to the desperadoes will soon allow others to come in. The hero, says Dr. Dubos, moves out of town without doing anything to solve this far more complex problem. In fact he has no weapon to deal with it and is not even aware of its existence.

The very succession of battles in medical social-politics, over voluntary and compulsory insurance, over disability benefits, over the cost of medical care, over the rights of closed panel plans to exist, over the corporate practice of medicine, and now over health insurance for the aged, called one of the deadliest challenges ever to face the profession, suggests that as with the wild west hero, the basic problems have been left unsolved and not even understood. There will be other battles. We can readily foresee a Forand Bill for the unemployed. And if we are unable to evolve a more rational way of settling these problems, we are likely to wind up with a patterned rather than a reasoned answer. The past suggests that such a course of events is most probable, but it is not predestined.

America could develop a unique program of care and financing based on its own needs, resources, and state of medical and social development. It could embrace an apparently American talent for ingenious combinations of public and private effort. This is what we should do. It holds forth the greatest promise but is not strongly advanced nor even aspired to by any major force in medical care today.

## THE FUTURE OF THE CONSUMERS
## AND PURVEYORS

What does the rising influence of the consumer signify and what does it portend? The consumer's relationship to medicine is now fundamentally and irreversibly altered. He pays for an increasing proportion of his care as a prospective patient. Even when the employer seemingly makes the payment, the employee has set aside a portion of his wages that he might otherwise have received in cash. He has placed these wage allocations and direct contributions for health care in trust with the employer, union, or welfare fund. As yet, that trust has rarely been fully realized or assumed. The consumer's education is still not completed. Medical care poses difficult and perplexing problems in a field that is not his own. A deep involvement is a time-consuming activity that taxes the talents and resources of even the largest corporations and their corresponding unions and is out of the reach of most companies and unions. Only the exceptional consumer is well informed in the ways of physicians, hospitals, and insurance carriers and only the rarest have gone beyond what exists to consider what should be. Even when the labor or management official acquires knowledge it is difficult for him to effect change. He may be tempted to conclude that he is not in the health or in the insurance business and fail to devote serious attention to what in many cases are still regarded as fringe benefits.

But there is a greater likelihood that the new consumer will play a larger role. He cannot withdraw from participation without replacing his present activities. In discharging the trust that has been assigned to him he will be drawn into responsibility for care on a large and continuing scale. He will purchase benefits more carefully. He will not limit his horizons to financing. He will look at the care that he purchases and the hospital and the physician will increasingly face a consumer who will deal with them in a state of parity. The consumer is approaching a position of greater effectiveness and influence in medical policy. He will probably change the balance of power. If policy continues to be set in conflict, more of the decisions are likely to fall to the consumer.

However, the consumer is but one of the components of society; the producers are another. Between them they are obligated to find a rational way of arranging for care. Some conflict is inevitable, inherent in the relationship, and will undoubtedly continue. But consumer and purveyor are not irrevocably opposed. Both can indeed benefit from a more advanced method of providing and financing care. The issues may have been made unnecessarily combative by a philosophy that too readily resorts to conflict, by a brand of economics that too uncritically extolls the commercial in the transactions of physicians and consumers, and by a lack of channels and agencies to plan, coordinate, and reconcile what could be cooperatively determined.

Labor and management are looking for less combative ways of settling their differences. Even nations of diametrically opposed views are looking for some accord and are installing a telephone line to be sure they talk before they fight; in medical care combat has often preceded conversation. The technology that has produced the multimegaton bomb is essentially the same as that which enables our scientists to study and manipulate the large molecules of life. The same imperatives that are now inspiring another look at war call for another way of approaching matters of medical policy.

# PRIVATE HEALTH INSURANCE:

## PROGRESS AND PROBLEMS

Herman M. Somers

How odd it now seems that only three decades ago private health insurance was highly controversial and attacked as a restraint on personal liberty and the unfettered practice of medicine. Its initial acceptance by the medical profession was a lesser evil compared to the threat of public health insurance, but the high status it has achieved since then is a product of spectacular success.

Health insurance grew more rapidly than even its most enthusiastic supporters expected. In 1948, it collected only $858 million, representing only 11 per cent of all private expenditures. By 1961, it was a $6.7 billion business which accounted for almost 32 per cent of all private medical care expenditures in the United States. Of the 1961 business, Blue Cross and Blue Shield accounted for 42 per cent; group insurance carriers, 36 per cent; individual insurance carriers, 15 per cent; and all others, 7 per cent.

Of course, all forms of expenditure for health services, private and public, were expanding with unprecedented speed during this period, but health insurance was growing fastest of all. At the end of 1961, about 73 per cent of the population held some kind of insurance. Management, labor, government, and the general public all appeared to agree that private health insurance is a necessary and desirable American institution which has made a significant contribution to the nation's medical care.

History, however, disconcertingly demonstrates that achievements have an uncomfortable way of bringing in their wake new problems, oftentimes more intractable than those which were solved. Paradoxically, the success of health insurance has brought forth the major difficulties which now challenge the industry. By helping make more people acquainted with the wonders and value of modern medicine, by opening wider the door of access to such care, and by making the public aware of what is potentially available through improved financial and organizational mechanisms, it has greatly increased public impatience with the remaining bars to protection for those who have none and to more adequate protection for the others. Health insurance has been a major contributor to the well-known "revolution of rising expectations," expectations which will have to be satisfied. The industry appears quite aware that to the extent it fails to satisfy these demands, other instrumentalities are likely to be propelled to fill the gap.

However, it should not be thought that the increasing demand for health services has been artificially stimulated or is unwarranted. It is, after all, a major function of health insurance to organize the financial means to enlarge access to medical care. Having just completed a world-wide tour to observe medical institutions in many nations, I can testify that burgeoning demand is a universal phenomenon whether health insurance does or does not exist. It is a product of rising educational levels, higher incomes, increasing industrialization and urbanization, greater life expectancy, and, above all, the scientific advance of medicine which has given it unprecedented preventive and curative powers of which the public is increasingly aware. Rising demand for medical care all over the world is not capricious, and it is unlikely to abate in the future.

Available data in this country make it clear, however, that in the necessity to increase its benefits and enrollment, health insurance faces extraordinary and mounting difficulties. Most of the scientific and technological factors which have contributed to forcing up premium levels at a rate of 7 to 10 per cent per annum, and to making costs a national issue, will continue to operate, probably at an accelerated pace. Even more predictably, changes in demographic and morbidity patterns will cause a greatly expanded, and more expensive, rate of utilization of medical goods and services, pressing against limited facilities. Those people without current insurance protection are exceptionally difficult to cover and are becoming more so. Let us look more specifically at some of these problems.

## DEMOGRAPHIC FACTORS AND
## HEALTH INSURANCE

The insistent demand that health insurance offer broader protection and provide for payment of a larger share of the medical bill faces some hard demographic facts. First is the rapid growth of population. Within this decade we will be adding some 35 million to our population; by 1970 we will have about 215 million persons. The pressure of this growth on existing medical institutions will be relentless and, since there is little likelihood that supply will keep up with demand, price inflation will be given considerable stimulus.

Within this enlarged population, important shifts will continue to take place. The big bulges will be seen at the top and the bottom of the age scale. The very young and very old require much greater than average amounts of medical services. Much justified attention has been centered on the increasing number of aged, but they represent only part of the difficulty.

As we preserve life at all ages, there is more illness and disability for the population as a whole. The near-conquest of bacterial disease has been accompanied by a vast increase in the demand for facilities and personnel for chronic and mental illness. The great progress in control of infant mortality, plus the recent explosion in the birthrate, results in an extraordinarily higher proportion of young children in the population. The combination of these factors places an increasing proportion of the population, already about one-third, the aged, young children, and those with some significant disability, in categories requiring relatively large amounts of medical care.

The figures also indicate that in this decade the number of persons in the generally dependent age groups, those under 20 years and the aged, will increase about twice as rapidly as the number in the productive age groups from 20 to 64 years old. They will represent half the population by 1970. It should be clear that such increase in proportion of dependents has serious significance, over and above implications for individual utilization rates, for future premium levels.

Many additional factors will also press in the direction of expanded rates of utilization, which will affect costs. For example, there is the steady increase in industrialization and urbanization. The city man uses more medical care than the rural; the industrial worker more than the farmer. The narrowing differential in life expectancy between whites and nonwhites indicates a vast market for medical services among Negroes whose needs were once relatively ignored. The increasing proportion of women in the population also presages increasing demand. Women use far more physician services than men.

The financial and organizational implications of this demographic change are almost as great as that of the scientific revolution. This has been indicated during the past two or three decades, when, for example, hospital admission rates were increasing three times as fast as the population. There is no sign of abatement of this trend and it could become more dramatic. In 1948, payments for physicians' services was almost 50 per cent greater than for hospital care. By 1961, they were almost identical, each consuming 27.6 per cent of the private medical care dollar.

I need hardly remind this audience that the remarkable progress in medical science, with its inevitable accretions of expensive equipment, more intricate diagnostic and therapeutic procedures, increased specialization in medical and paramedical personnel, all of which has made medical care infinitely more valuable and far more costly, is not subsiding. On the contrary, the men in our research laboratories throughout the country inform us that the pace is accelerating. They assert that we can confidently look forward to control of an increasing number of today's incurable diseases as scientists master the fine structure of cells with the aid of the electronic microscope, the mechanism of metabolic pathways governed by the enzyme, the factors which cause cells to multiply widely, and so on. These are most welcome humanitarian prospects, but they also augur enlarged financial problems.

Moreover, our population data and medical education figures make clear that a decrease in the ratio of practicing physicians to population during the next decade is now virtually inescapable.

These trends, and others which could readily be added, tell us that in the years immediately ahead private health insurance is going to have to run fast in order to stand still, let alone meet the challenge of enlarging the range and extent of its benefits. Although health insurance benefits (exclusive of administrative and overhead expense), as a proportion of the nation's private medical bills, moved from a mere 8 per cent in 1948 to 27 per cent in 1961, the rate of expansion had begun to decrease perceptibly by 1956. It is apparent that as the base figure gets larger, it becomes progressively more difficult to maintain the rate of increase.

What do people mean when they demand "comprehensive coverage" by health insurance? This is a widely used, but quite imprecise, term. It does not, of course, mean 100 per cent protection. It rather signifies an aim for quantitative adequacy, an over-all benefit-expenditure ratio that will reduce the average consumer's out-of-pocket expenses to more feasible proportions. This means that health insurance benefits, in conjunction with manageable out-of-pocket expenditures, should be adequate to promote individual health and family welfare. It involves two related steps: (1) extension of coverage to many of the components of care now generally omitted, such as drugs, dental care, and psychiatric care; in 1961, insurance met about 1.5 per cent of consumer expenditures for medical care other than hospital and physician services, but the feasibility of such extended protection has been amply demonstrated in many experiments during recent years. (2) A balanced increase in protection among the major components so that the result does not favor excessively one form of service over another and cause an "unmedical," as well as uneconomic bias in utilization as appears to have been the case in the past.

This is obviously a goal that can only be approached in easy stages, each related to other factors, such as availability of facilities and other supply and demand elements. In *Doctors, Patients and Health Insurance*,[1] Anne Somers and I explained why we believe that for the immediate future satisfactory progress demands a 10 per cent annual increase in the benefit-expenditure ratio, gradually moderated as the base figure gets larger. We believe this can be done despite the fact that the average rate of increase has been less than 5 per cent in recent years (but in 1961, the last year for which data are available, the increase exceeded 7 per cent). The ultimate goal, which appears both necessary and feasible, as we first asserted two years ago and has since been endorsed by other authorities, should be to reach a ratio of about two-thirds within fifteen years. This is a practical goal for private health insurance within its natural orbit of business, mainly the productive age categories of the population and their dependents.

The second urgent issue facing health insurance lies in the fact that almost 50 million people, about 26 per cent of the population, still have no health insurance protection of any kind. Employee status is the single most important determinant of health insurance coverage as most insurance in this country is obtained through group policies in employee-benefit plans. Thus the bulk of the un-enrolled tend to be among the unemployed, the disabled, the aged, and rural residents, characterized generally by lower than average income and education. The difficulty of selling insurance at a feasible price to most of these people is obvious.

It is easy to see only the growth of enrollment has tapered off. Nonetheless, if economic conditions remain favorable, private insurance may be able to give some measure of protection to perhaps 80 per cent of the population. Public expectation is likely to find a 20 per cent gap too large, especially if concentrated in groups whose need for protection is greatest and who are becoming increasingly articulate. Moreover, the "uncovered" are not a static group; for longer or shorter periods many more people move into and out of the zone of the unprotected, as employment fluctuates or as people move into advanced retirement ages. If a man has already had insurance and then is deprived of it, his resentment is understandably great.

In view of the modern significance of medical care, its costs, and our knowledge of what can be done with insurance, an adequate public policy goal requires health insurance protection for around 90 to 95 per cent of the people. The notion, once widely accepted, that a substantial portion of the population is not insurable does not stand up to close examination of experience, although some unconventional devices may have to be employed to complete the job.

There are perhaps 5 to 10 per cent of the civilian population which cannot be reached by any form of insurance. On the basis of present knowledge and experience it appears quite feasible to bring coverage to the remainder, although it is unlikely that private insurance can reach the 90 to 95 per cent goal unaided. Yet, unless the coverage is somehow achieved, private health insurance will bear the brunt of public discontent.

## THE PROBLEM OF THE AGED

The aged are far the largest and most definable group among the uncovered. The issue of the aged has received such wide attention that it does not require detailed exposition before this audience. In briefest summary, for insurance purposes the decisive fact regarding them is that they are no longer in the labor force. Less than one out of four persons, 65 years and over, receives any income from employment, including women who are not themselves employed but are married to earners, a high proportion of whom are in agricultural or casual jobs. This means that only a small fraction are in jobs that provide health insurance, the vehicle through which three-quarters of all Americans with protection are insured.

This means that, in the main, if the aged are to achieve insurance protection they must purchase it for themselves, under circumstances which have an ironic twist. Their medical needs and their utilization of health services are obviously far greater than the rest of the population. Despite their holding current assets which on average exceed those of younger families, their financial resources for meeting such needs are much smaller, and they have far less access to the financial advantages of group coverage. They are what the industry knows as "substandard risks" without the money to balance this handicap.

Considering that medical costs for the aged average around one-third of their incomes, it is hardly surprising that health insurance has thus far failed to make a major contribution toward meeting these costs. In response to various pressures, insurance companies have in recent years undertaken some vigorous measures to enlarge enrollment of the aged. Even such imaginative measures have, after some years, resulted in only half of the aged having any form of protection, and most of this is confined to relatively meager hospitalization and surgical expenses. This is no fault of the industry. It is ingenious enough to devise almost any kind of policy, at any level of benefits, that people are able and willing to buy. But adequate coverage for the aged cannot be offered at an actuarially sound price that most aged could afford to pay. Given the circumstances, what has been accomplished is a tribute to hard work and resourcefulness of the industry.

It is a fundamentally intractable situation for private insurance which will get even more difficult. The long-time trend of decline in labor force participation for older men is still continuing. Moreover, those reaching 65 years of age no longer represent a single category of aged. The problem is far more difficult for those in the more advanced years, say 75 and over, than among those 65 to 74 years old. Mercifully a far higher percentage of the latter category have insurance than the former. But the aged over 75 are increasing far more rapidly than the total aged. Life expectancy for the more advanced ages is increasing at a surprising rate. The average number of years spent in retirement is increasing much faster than the average number spent working. As Professor Joseph Spengler has pointed out, "Whereas in 1900 an American male did about fourteen years work for each year spent in retirement he may by the year 2000, if present life-expectancy and retirement trends continue, be doing only about five years of work for each he spends in retirement."

It is clear that reasonably adequate health insurance for the aged requires either a subsidy from the premiums paid by the rest of the community or payment of premiums in early years loaded to provide for coverage in later years. The experience of Blue Cross and of other experiments demonstrates these are impractical measures for voluntary and competitive insurance carriers.

That is why the proposal for providing basic protection to the aged through a governmental social insurance program has such practical appeal. Such a program represents neither a criticism of nor a threat to private insurance. The assumption of responsibility by government for this minority group of poor risks will greatly improve the industry's chances of successfully meeting the challenge of a more acceptable benefit standard in the vastly larger and more profitable market of the employed population and their dependents, and assure private health insurance of privacy in financing prepaid medical care.

The probability of such a development appears to be only a question of time. An increasing number of doctors are aware that they have been misled by allegations that social insurance somehow means greater intervention in medical practice by government than do means test programs, which the medical societies have been supporting. All experience indicates the reverse is more likely to be true. It is also more widely understood that social insurance is financially more conservative and controllable than noncontributory financing from general revenues. (See Dr. Schottland's "The Social Security System and Medical Care," p. 201.)

## RISING COSTS, CONSUMER QUESTIONS AND THE PROFESSION

A major obstacle complicating the challenge of enlarging the scope of benefits, as well as enrollment, is the relentless and dramatic upsurge of medical care prices. According to the Consumers Price Index, prices of medical care services have been increasing three times as rapidly as the general price index. It has been calculated that of the enormous increase in per capita expenditures for medical care since 1948, only about one-third reflects the increase in per capita volume of utilization of medical care, and about two-thirds can be attributed to the rise in prices. Without doubt, a portion of the price increase is caused by technological advance, involving fantastically expensive new equipment, but there remains a very substantial portion which can only be attributed to price inflation. In any case, the cost of health insurance has been rising fast and significantly, while objections have been mounting in volume.

Americans have demonstrated their willingness to pay more for better medical care. Private expenditures for medical care, which exceeded $21 billion in 1961, more than doubled over the previous decade, at the same time that government expenditure for medical care also increased about 100 per cent. On a per capita basis private expenditures went from $66 in 1952 to $117 in 1961, an increase of 77 per cent. Incomes were not going up nearly so fast. Private medical expenditures represented 4.2 per cent of all personal disposable income in 1952, but 5.8 per cent in 1961, a proportionate increase of 38 per cent in ten years.

Americans have also indicated that they regard insurance as the most effective method of financing such care. Each year a higher proportion of medical expenditures moves through these channels. Employers have indicated awareness of their stake in medical protection for workers and are paying a steadily increasing share of premiums. The growing resistance, and even resentment, to increased costs appears to be based on: the widespread feeling that most of the increased price represents inflated costs of the same product; frustration over the fact that this is a field with almost complete absence of cost control; and a growing concern with quality of care.

About 50 per cent of all health insurance premiums in the United States appear on management's books as a labor cost. As those who pay the premiums, the large organized buyers among unions and employers and associations of employers have developed increasing experience and sophistication in medical care financing, they have become sensitive to the vast differentials in the quality of medical care a given dollar may buy. They are also aware of the influence of quality upon cost, that poor quality also turns out to be more expensive, and that insurance itself may have an effect upon quality. They know also that results do not rest entirely in the lap of fate, and that there are methods for determining and controlling quality as well as costs.

A recent internal "white paper" prepared in one of the country's largest corporations pointed out that medical care benefits for employees was the only important area of substantial expenditure in which the company had nothing to say about specifications, productivity, and costs. The author, one of the top executives, argues that in the interests of productivity alone, not to mention other advantages, his company ought, in association with the union, to set forth on the path of developing group practice to provide comprehensive care as a condition of their prepayment program.

An executive of American Motors publicly expressed his concern for the quality and cost of his employees' health care program. He reported that a joint company and union study found that there appeared to be excessive use of hospital and surgical services in programs which required hospitalization for collection of benefits. At about the same time, a Ford executive reported his company's concern with employee dissatisfaction with quality and availability of service under present arrangements and with the need for more comprehensive care.

Two recent widely-publicized studies by Columbia University's School of Public Health and Administrative Medicine, independently commissioned by the New York State Insurance and Health

Commissioners, and by the Teamsters' Joint Council and Management Hospitalization Fund in New York, documented that considerable money was being spent in New York City on unnecessary or incompetent medical and hospital treatment. It was asserted that the medical profession is "doing little" about disciplining the quality of care. The study director, Dr. Ray E. Trussell, director of the school and New York City's Commissioner of Hospitals, urged, "The organized purchasers of medical and hospital care can be the strongest arm of the community in upgrading standards, and it is in the best interests of organized medicine and hospitals to work with them."

Dr. Trussell appears to exaggerate the powers of buyers and consumers in this field. Their concern is real and growing, but aside from commissioning reports and protesting volubly for action, they appear relatively powerless. The insurance industry, with its very large stakes in the results, is also in a relatively weak position on this score. Quality standards and controls are issues almost wholly in the hands of the medical profession.

Regulation of medical practice can be successfully performed only by doctors, even though the stimulus may well come from outside pressures. The task is difficult and doctors are notoriously reluctant to undertake programs for effective professional self-regulation. There are signs here and there of the profession succumbing to accumulating pressures.

Most recently, medical review committees, established under the leadership of hospitals and Blue Cross organizations, have demonstrated that they can be effective instruments for reducing improper and expensive hospital utilization. Doctors themselves have been articulate in castigating unnecessary use of hospitals, but have blamed it on patients. However, as Robert Sigmund, of the Western Pennsylvania Hospital Council, has trenchantly stated, "It is not entirely accurate to say that patients utilize beds. Physicians utilize beds; patients are in them." A patient cannot have the privilege of lying in a hospital bed unless ordered to by a physician. Patients can, of course, bring pressure on physicians to admit them, but the decision rests with the physician. Similarly with discharges, the physician makes the decision that determines the end of the bed utilization episode. Patients can bring pressure to delay discharge, but again the decision rests with the physician. And even patients' attitudes toward such matters are often conditioned by their physicians.

An area in which other community forces may be more influential is in the need for more regionalization of physical facilities, particularly support for effective hospital planning at metropolitan and regional levels, the avoidance of unnecessary or uneconomic structures, the elimination of duplication of costly equipment, and the minimizing of the extravagance of low occupancy rates.

More basic and significant than any particular measures is, however, the problem of the organization of medical services. Here the profession itself is sharply divided on issues which are fundamental to the future of costs and quality. Medicine has long ago passed out of the stage when there was organized resistance to new scientific findings. It has successfully absorbed the scientific revolution which involves realization that today's truth may be tomorrow's falsity. Men of medicine are aware that much, if not most, of what was taught in medical schools 25 years ago is irrelevant to their present practice and they are prepared for the possibility that today's teaching and knowledge may, in large degree, appear equally inconsequential 25 years hence.

But this acceptance in science has not yet transferred itself to the newer technological and organizational revolution which is transforming medical practice from a private relationship between two individuals into a medico-social institution, vastly and intricately interdependent, which makes it possible to provide better care to more people than ever before. This is the overriding development in medical care in all countries regardless of differing economic and political systems, just as it is in education, industry, and government. It is the dislocation accompanying this movement which is at the root of the present conflicts within the profession.

Much conflict is illustrated in the increasing number of medical service plans of the medical schools and the increase of ambulatory medical care by hospitals. As the schools employ more full-time faculty and attempt to develop economically viable clinical services for paying patients, utilizing the resources of their teaching hospitals, a conflict with the practicing profession frequently emerges. Rising costs of medical education, increased hospital deficits, especially in connection with OPD's, the astronomical costs of in-patient care, the resulting mounting pressure to keep patients out of the hospital and to provide more acceptable ambulatory services, growing articulate consumer concern for quality of care, and the need for new types of patients to provide a better balanced population for teaching purposes; all these developments are forcing hospitals, especially the better teaching institutions that have traditionally assumed the burden of unlimited indigent care, to think in terms of completely reorganizing their ambulatory services. Such reorganization can hardly fail to come into conflict with some of the current dominant patterns of medical care.

The controversies directly or indirectly involve questions of salary versus fee-for-service remuneration, full-time versus part-time educators, closed versus open hospitals, quality controls, attitudes toward research and education, and a host of related issues that go to the heart of the existing organization of medical care.

The controversies extend to such related issues as federal scholarships or "nonrefundable grants" to medical students and schools, in order to increase both the quantity and quality of medical students, which virtually all medical educators support and organized medicine opposes; the legislation in almost half the states which effectively prohibit the establishment of prepaid group medical plans; and the annual battle over the inadequate number of young doctors to fill 13,000 approved internships and additional thousands of residencies, which has thrown into question the traditional financial and professional relationship of the practicing physician to the hospital and to the apprentice doctor, as well as the educational value of internships in many hospitals, particularly the nonaffiliated.

It is not widely enough recognized that the outcome of the present controversies going on within the profession over the organization of medical services may in the long run be far more significant for the community's concern with quality and cost of medical care, and thus to the future of health insurance, than the more publicized battles over financing. Obsolete organizational structure in medicine which results in unnecessarily high costs as well as poorer quality is a drag and a challenge to both private and public instrumentalities. Adequate financing, which the American community is willing and able to furnish, cannot alone guarantee adequate access to the quality of care we now know how to provide. It is in this area that doctors hold the key to the future.

They would do well to consider the relevance to the organization of medicine of the recent castigation of American education by John Gardner, president of the Carnegie Corporation of New York. He declared it monumentally ineffective because it put a premium on stability at a time when the only security lay in mobility and innovation.


## SUMMARY

Private health insurance is clearly a vigorous, competitive, and healthy institution. But as it grows and matures its problems multiply and become more complex. Its present challenges lie in meeting the demands for more comprehensive benefits and enrollment which are basically related to quality standards and costs of medical services. The industry has demonstrated considerable resourcefulness, but answers to its present and impending problems lie in substantial measure in other hands. The future of private health insurance, as indeed the health of the nation, rests in large degree with the decisions of the medical profession.

# THE SOCIAL SECURITY SYSTEM

## AND MEDICAL CARE

### Charles I. Schottland

CONTRARY to opinions still held in some quarters, social security in the United States did not spring full-grown from the New Deal womb. Its present status is the result of a long historical development going back several hundred years; its future will be influenced by this past as conditions dictate changes and modifications.

The past twenty-five years have witnessed a fantastic growth in social security programs throughout the world. Practically every industrialized country protects its gainfully employed and their families from loss of income as a result of old age, unemployment, disability, and death of the wage earner through some type of social insurance or social assistance program. In the foreign programs, the medical care component looms large and in most countries, health insurance and medical care are an important part of the social security system. Fifty-eight countries provide benefits for permanent disability or invalidity through their social security programs; fifty-nine countries provide cash payments for temporary illness and maternity care or have some type of health and maternity insurance or related program; and many countries finance medical services through the social security agency.

The growth of social security in the United States during the past twenty-five years likewise has been phenomenal. In November 1962, over 24,969,000 persons received benefit payments from public social insurance and assistance programs at a cost of $2.69 billion or an annual rate of over 30 billion dollars.

Workmen's Compensation, the earliest of our social insurance programs, now provides medical care in addition to cash benefits, in every state. Four states provide cash benefits when the worker is unemployed because of sickness; our public assistance programs will spend several hundred million dollars for medical care through the five public assistance categories under the Social Security Act; tens of thousands of persons receiving disability insurance under Old-Age, Survivors and Disability Insurance will receive examinations by physicians and some will receive medical treatment and rehabilitation services through state vocational rehabilitation agencies.

This mere recital of some of the social security programs which touch medical care indicates the growing relationships between social security and health and medical care services.

Our task today is to survey the past and present program of social security, speculate as to its future, and explore the implications of the growth of social security to medical care services.

## HISTORY OF SOCIAL SECURITY

"Social security," as we shall use the term in this discussion, refers to a variety of social insurance and public assistance programs designed to maintain income when such income stops by reason of old age, disability, death, or absence of the wage earner. In this sense, social security is a significant factor in the economic security of the gainfully employed. Throughout history, man has been concerned with his economic security and has devised various measures to cope with this problem. The huge granary reserves built by Joseph in Egypt were an attempt to make life more secure by storing food during years of plenty and distributing it during years of food scarcity. The extended families in more primitive societies were also a method of "spreading the risk" in that a large number of persons would have collective responsibility for the well-being of all of its members. This responsibility was later assumed by the tribe or other social unit.

Organized methods of providing some measure of economic security took very simple forms in primitive societies. Food storage, following the seasons, and migration as practiced by nomadic peoples — these and other simple measures were society's answer to the problem of securing the basic necessities of life. Although these primitive methods were frequently ineffective, they did serve to alleviate some hardships in an agrarian and uncomplicated society.

Furthermore, the prevailing belief until the nineteenth century, which considered poverty to be the result of improvidence, vice, and laziness, worked against man's attempts to deal more realistically and effectively with the problem of economic insecurity.

The Industrial Revolution highlighted the problems associated with economic security. The change from a rural, agricultural, barter economy to an urban, industrial, money-wage economy resulted in dramatic and serious poverty when money wages stopped by reason of old age, unemployment, death, sickness, or other reasons beyond the control of the individual. The modern family in an urban setting tends to be a parent-child family, with less close ties than in a rural economy to grandparents and grandchildren, uncles, aunts, nieces, and even adult brothers and sisters. The large extended family has virtually disappeared. Economic insecurity, in the modern sense, was relatively unknown in primitive societies. However, as we conquered nature, developed industry, and an increasing proportion of our population became gainfully employed, the economic security of most persons and the necessities of life which could be purchased began to depend almost entirely upon the amount and steadiness of money income. Any interruption, stoppage, or reduction of income raises serious problems.

Such stoppage of income is a result mainly of five basic causes: old age, unemployment, industrial accident and disease, permanent disability and temporary illness, and death of the family wage earner. To maintain income when these risks occurred, a variety of programs were established by industrial nations long before social security was a commonplace word in our vocabulary. Prior to the beginnings of social insurance in 1880, three major efforts were instituted by the industrial nations to protect workers from destitution.[1] These methods included a variety of savings plans, employer's liability, and private insurance. However, they proved entirely inadequate to keep workers from destitution and as industry expanded and unemployment, old age, death, disability, and sickness continued to cause serious hardships among workers, a variety of plans involving "pooling the risk" emerged prior to the twentieth century. These early plans came to be called "social insurance."

The first comprehensive plan of social insurance began in Germany in 1883. The growth of industry was bringing wealth and power to the German nation; but at the same time the workers felt increasingly discontented with the recurring stoppage of income as a result primarily of unemployment, sickness, and old age. This discontent expressed itself in the rise of the Social Democrats and opposition to Bismarck. The "Iron Chancellor" saw in social insurance an opportunity to halt the rising tide of socialism by yielding to the workers' demands for income protection and, at the same time, to strengthen the central German government as opposed to the states and local governmental units. He proposed a national plan of workmen's accident insurance in 1881, and for the next seven or eight years, Bismarck's proposals covering other risks were vigorously debated in Germany and, indeed, throughout the world.

In 1883, Germany adopted a program of compulsory insurance against illness; accident insurance followed in 1884; and compulsory invalidity and old age insurance was begun in 1889.[2] These German programs laid the basis for the later developments in the United States and other countries.

Prior to 1930, the pressure to insure against the risks of unemployment, old age, and sickness was not so great in the United States as in European countries. The American frontier kept expanding during the entire one hundred years of the nineteenth century. Land was given to settlers by the government either free or for a very nominal charge. The frontier was opulent. Rich forests, minerals, and agricultural lands provided the American worker who left the industrial Eastern seaboard with his "social security" for over a century.

While the frontier provided great economic opportunities, the city worker began to feel the insecurities of unemployment, old age, and sickness. Mutual aid societies and fraternal orders sprang up, offering to their members funeral, sickness, and old age benefits. These efforts served a useful purpose but were ineffective in solving the problems presented in the rapidly industrializing and ever-expanding economy of the United States. As a result, many writers and students of the problem began to advocate more effective measures.

The lack of a comprehensive public program or plan to provide economic security was not a result of neglect or indifference. It reflected an important and affirmative American philosophy: a philosophy which placed on the individual the responsibility for his own welfare. A man was supposed to save for his old age and for unforeseen emergencies, and the expanding economy did make it possible for many persons to do so. Nevertheless, the facts of economic insecurity and the clear evidence of poverty and suffering were shattering the faith of many in the ability of persons to take care of themselves, and various social insurance and social assistance schemes began to appear in the early 1900's.

Social insurance programs received great impetus in the United States through the work of a physician. In 1912, Dr. I. M. Rubinow, a Doctor of Medicine and the chief statistician of an insurance company, was asked to give a course in "Social Insurance" at the New York School of Philanthropy. Although the subject of social insurance had been discussed in courses on labor problems, social reform, or other related courses, this was probably the first time in the United States that a course was devoted entirely to this subject. Following Doctor Rubinow's initial effort, several courses appeared under this title in American universities. The next year, Dr. Rubinow published the first comprehensive American study of social insurance. His interest in social insurance grew out of his work in the field of private insurance.[3] He became convinced that the principles of voluntary insurance had validity also in a public insurance program.

Following Dr. Rubinow's work, the movement for social insurance grew and today social insurance is a firmly established political and economic institution in the United States as it is in almost all industrialized countries. Under one piece of legislation, the Social Security Act, the United States has established programs of old-age, survivors, and disability insurance, unemployment insurance, federal grants to the states for public assistance programs to assist the needy aged, blind, dependent children, and disabled, and federal grants for child health and welfare services.

Although the European programs of social insurance preceded those of the United States, it is interesting that the term "social security" first appeared prominently in the United States Social Security Act.[4] Its use spread rapidly throughout the world and mention of social security in the Atlantic Charter of 1941 gave further impetus to its use.[5]

## THE SOCIAL SECURITY ACT OF 1935

The Social Security Act was born in controversy and this controversy has continued to the present time. When the bill was introduced in 1935, feeling about it ran high. Congressman Fuller of Arkansas hailed the bill as "the greatest humanitarian measure ever presented to an American Congress," [6] while Congressman James W. Wadsworth of New York saw in its provisions "the entrance into the political field of a power so vast, so powerful, as to threaten the integrity of our institutions and to pull the pillars of the temple down upon the heads of our descendants." [7] When Congressman Mitchell of Tennessee declared that the bill "meant a new outlook on life for the aged" which was clearly "a responsibility of government," [8] Congressman Reed of New York proclaimed that "it means absolute regimentation" and "was a program of Karl Marx from beginning to end." [9] While Senator Wagner of New York maintained that "the care of the old cannot be left indefinitely to the miserably weak pension laws which exist in only thirty-three states," [10] Senator Hastings of Delaware replied that "we do not have the right to force any such plan as that upon the states of this Union." Senator Harrison of Mississippi asserted with pride that "it is a pleasure for me to champion this bill," [11] but Congressman John Taber of New York proclaimed in alarm that "never in the history of the world has any measure been brought in here so insidiously designed to prevent business recovery, to enslave workers and to prevent any possibility of the employers providing work for the people." [12] Congressman Vinson of Kentucky hailed it as "pioneer legislation," while Charles Denby, Jr., of the American Bar Association warned that "sooner or later [it] will bring about the inevitable abandonment of private capitalism." [13] Congressman Higgins maintained that "unemployment insurance is a necessity in our modern industrial life," [14] but a former President of the American Bankers' Association characterized unemployment insurance as "merely an industrial dole." [15] Business leaders generally saw in old-age insurance the destruction of "individual initiative and thrift" while supporters of the program saw in it a new "happiness in old age for America's aged." Opponents of unemployment insurance feared that "no one would work" while proponents maintained that it would save American industry from collapse. The violence of the controversy highlighted the fact that the United States was embarking upon a new phase in its history.

Just consider the social, economic, political, and philosophical distance traveled between 1887 when President Cleveland vetoed a bill providing seeds for drought-stricken areas with the statement, "I can find no warrant for such an appropriation in the Constitution, and I do not believe that the power and duty of the General Government ought to be extended to the relief of individual suffering," [16] and the words of Justice Cardozo in declaring the Social Security Act constitutional.[17] Said Justice Cardozo: "Nor is the concept of the general welfare static. Needs that were narrow or parochial a century ago may be interwoven in our day with the well-being of the nation. What is critical or urgent changes with the times." Asserting that the problem of the aged is "plainly national in area and dimensions" and that the "laws of the separate states cannot deal with it effectively," the court contended that "Congress may spend money in and for the general welfare" and that "only a power that is national can serve the interests of all."

With this decision a new phase began in the history of the federal government's activities to relieve destitution and establish social welfare programs. It involved a major change in United States policy and a significant break with past restrictions and inhibitions.[18] It laid the ground work for the gradual development of the largest public welfare program of the western world.

## OLD-AGE, SURVIVORS, AND DISABILITY INSURANCE

The largest and most important of our social security programs is Old-Age, Survivors, and Disability Insurance. When the average person talks about his "social security" he usually means Old-Age, Survivors, and Disability Insurance, a program covering almost all of America's gainfully employed, making monthly payments to more than 18 million persons, and paying out in benefits over one and a quarter billion dollars monthly.

Although Workmen's Compensation and Unemployment Insurance are large and important programs, and the public assistances under the Social Security Act care for seven million persons, our discussion today will center around Old-Age, Survivors, and Disability Insurance, which has become the basic program of social security and income maintenance in our country. This was a conscious and deliberate policy of congress. Prior to 1950, congress faced the issue: Was the social insurance system to become the nation's basic income-maintenance program or was major reliance to be placed on a combination of other approaches such as a broad public pension program, public assistance, and private pensions? [19]

The report of the House Ways and Means Committee in 1950 re-established congressional policy. It stated:

... There are indications that if the insurance program is not strengthened and expanded, the old-age assistance program may develop into a very costly and ill-advised system of noncontributory pensions, payable not only to the needy but to all individuals at or above retirement age who are no longer employed. Moreover, there are increasing pressures for special pensions for particular groups and particular hazards. Without an adequate and universally applicable basic social insurance system, the demands for security by segments of the population threaten to result in unbalanced, overlapping, and competing programs. The financing of such plans may become chaotic, their economic effects dangerous. There is a pressing need to strengthen the basic system at once before it is undermined by these forces. Once the basic system is firmly established, any remaining special needs of particular groups can be assessed and met in an orderly fashion.

The time has come to reaffirm the basic principle that a contributory system of social insurance in which workers share directly in meeting the cost of the protection afforded is the most satisfactory way of preventing dependency. A contributory system, in which both contributions and benefits are directly related to the individual's own productive efforts, prevents insecurity while preserving self-reliance and initiative.

The 1950 amendments to the Social Security Act expanded and improved the social insurance system to the end that it would offer basic economic security to most of the nation's working people and their families when income stopped by reason of old age or death of the wage earner. These amendments and the accompanying reports of congressional committees established as national policy the Old-Age, Survivors, and Disability Insurance program as the basic system of social security.[20]

This huge program may best be described briefly by nine main characteristics.

## Coverage Is Almost Universal

A basic premise and goal of the Old-Age, Survivors, and Disability Insurance program is that all persons who work, regardless of income level, type of employment, citizenship, age, or other special characteristic, should be covered by the system. This goal of universal coverage is on the way to achievement. Nine-tenths of all gainfully employed persons are covered or could be covered by election. All self-employed persons are covered or could be covered by election. All self-employed professional groups are covered except doctors of medicine. Doctors, by their own insistence, do not have the protection for their children and other survivors, nor for themselves in old age or disability, afforded to lawyers, dentists, accountants, and others. Nor do they pay the taxes imposed on other gainfully employed Americans. This uncovered group remains "unfinished business" in achieving the goal of universal coverage.

## The Right to Benefits

Benefits are paid as a matter of "right." This is a fundamental element in the Old-Age, Survivors, and Disability Insurance program. Benefits do not depend upon the discretion of administrations or a determination of "means." The right to benefits is a statutory right which can be enforced by the courts.[21] Furthermore, it is a right which arises out of covered work and the payment of contributions out of the earnings from that work.

## Integrated Protection Is Provided Against
## Three Major Risks

Benefits under Old-Age, Survivors, and Disability Insurance provide protection against the risk of income loss resulting from old age, disability, and death. A person who has attained "insured" status may receive retirement benefits for himself and dependent's benefits for his spouse and children. Survivor benefits are paid, when the insured dies, to the surviving spouse, dependent parents, and children. A lump sum payment is payable upon the death of the insured worker to the surviving spouse if he or she lived in the same household; if there is no such spouse, it may go to pay for unpaid burial expenses, or to reimburse the person who paid the funeral expenses. For the insured person, disability benefits are available if the insured is too disabled to work; dependent's benefits are then available for his wife and children.

These three basic benefits, old-age or retirement benefits, survivors benefits, and disability benefits are administered as a single program. Old-age benefits are payable to persons who work in covered employment for the required period of time and who retire from gainful employment. The full benefits are payable at age 65 and reduced benefits at age 62.

Survivor benefits are payable to the widow and children of a deceased worker. Disability benefits are payable to persons seriously disabled and unable to engage in any gainful occupation. In November 1962, 730,000 persons received disability payments. This program, established in 1956, has significant implications for medical care. For the first time in the United States, practically every seriously disabled person will undergo a complete examination by a physician in order to qualify for disability payments. We now know more than we ever did about the characteristics of our most seriously disabled. The close tie of Old-Age, Survivors, and Disability Insurance program to the federal-state program of vocational rehabilitation makes possible the rehabilitation of those who have such potential and there is some discussion of having Old-Age, Survivors, and Disability Insurance pay for the rehabilitation of its disability cases similar to programs of other countries.

Benefits under Old-Age, Survivors, and Disability Insurance are based on average earnings and range from $40.00 to $127.00 per month for an individual and from $60.00 to $254.00 per month for a family.

## The System Is Contributory

The American system of Old-Age, Survivors, and Disability Insurance has emphasized a principle not found in some of the social insurance programs of other countries. In contradistinction to some social insurance programs that are financed in part by general revenues of the government, the United States program is financed through contributions by employees, their employers, and the self-employed, without any subsidy from the general revenues of the government. Employers and employees each pay the same tax rate; the tax rate for a self-employed person is approximately 1½ times the employee rate. Taxes are paid on the first $4,800.00 of a worker's earnings. This principle of workers' contributions is an important philosophical principle of social insurance. It re-affirms the concept that security for the individual should, to the extent possible, grow out of his own work; under social insurance, the worker earns his future security as he earns his living. His eligibility and the amount of the benefit is related to his earnings, a fact which reinforces the general system of economic incentives.

This contributory principle, which was derived from the original German social insurance program, has been finding increasing support in nations which earlier rejected this principle or had adopted it only partially. For example, in Sweden, it has been the subject of considerable discussion and has been accepted for part of the system. Canada, likewise, has been reviewing it; and in Great Britain, a Royal Commission recently asserted that the contributory principle was "an important measure of social discipline." [22]

## The System Is Soundly Financed

A major goal of the Old-Age, Survivors, and Disability Insurance system is that it shall be soundly financed. The system involves several features:

### A Self-Supporting System

It is agreed that the system shall be self-supporting, that is, that the special social security taxes and interest earnings of the trust funds must be sufficient to finance all expenditures. Contributions received under the schedule described above, when added to income from interest on the trust funds, are expected to be sufficient to meet the cost of benefits indefinitely into the future, as far as can be foreseen.

### Actuarial Soundness

It is generally agreed that the program must be financed on an actuarially sound basis. This does not mean, however, that a government program must establish reserves similar to private life insurance. Actuarial soundness implies that, in the long run, the total income must be sufficient to match total outlay.

### Trust Funds

The Social Security Act creates two trust funds: a "Federal Old-Age and Survivors, Insurance Trust Fund" and a "Federal Disability Insurance Trust Fund." Into these funds are deposited the taxes collected from the employees, employers, and self-employed. A Board of Trustees is established by the act, consisting of the Secretary of the Treasury, who is the "Managing Trustee," the Secretary of Labor, and the Secretary of Health, Education, and Welfare. The Commissioner of Social Security serves as Secretary of the Board of Trustees. The trustees are required to report to congress annually on the actuarial status of the trust funds and on estimated income and disbursements for the ensuing five years. These reports have assumed great importance in view of the fact that the figures and statistics presented therein are relied upon by congressional committees as a basis for congressional action. The monies in the trust funds are invested in government securities, and interest earned is added to the funds. Assets in the funds now total approximately 21 billion dollars.

Although the financing of the program is controversial, the Committees of Congress, students of the problem, and official advisory committees, have all concluded that the program is soundly financed. The major finding of the Advisory Council on Social Security Financing in 1959 (a group established by law) stated:

> The Council finds that the present method of financing the Old-Age, Survivors, and Disability Insurance program is sound, practical, and appropriate for this program. It is our judgment, based on the best available cost estimates, that the contribution schedule enacted into law in the last session of Congress makes adequate provision for financing the program on a sound actuarial basis.[23]

## Participation Is Compulsory

Another feature of the system is that coverage is compulsory, with very few exceptions. This principle has been adhered to since the beginning of the system, in order to protect it from adverse selection of risks as well as to protect the country as a whole against widespread destitution caused by the very risks insured against, namely, old age, disability, and death of the wage earner.

## Benefits Are Wage-Related

Again in contradistinction to some social insurance systems, the social security program in the United States emphasizes the relation of the economic status of the worker to the benefits he receives. For example, a person who has been credited with maximum (average annual) earnings of $4,800.00 or more during his working life will receive the maximum monthly retirement benefit of $127.00; a person who averages only $3,600.00 will receive only $105.00. This accords with a firmly ingrained belief on the part of the American people that a man should receive rewards in accordance with his individual efforts and contributions.

Furthermore, the wage-related principle makes it possible to pay retirement incomes that are related to differing individual levels of living and to diverse economic conditions in different parts of the country. By and large, a person's earnings from work establish his level of living and determine the income he will want to maintain in retirement. If benefits were provided in the same amount for everyone, either the amount would have to be so high for some that it would exceed their earnings, or it would be so low for those who had worked at higher earnings levels that it would not provide meaningful security for them.

## Emphasis Is Placed on the Family

Many children in the United States are in homes where family income is low or only moderate. Rural areas where income levels are low have more than their proportionate share of the nation's children. In many families with young children, the father has not yet reached his full earning power and the mother is needed at home. The parents have had to meet the extra expenses of setting up the home and starting the family, so they often have not been able to save much money.

For these reasons, it is especially important that families with children have some assured means of support when the breadwinner's earnings stop or are greatly reduced. Because of the survivor protection under the federal insurance system, nine out of ten of the mothers and young children in the nation now have the assurance that they can receive monthly benefits if the father of the family dies.

Thus, the Old-Age, Survivors, and Disability Insurance program contributes to strengthening and maintaining family life by providing income upon death of the breadwinner. This reduces the necessity for mothers to place children in foster care in order to be free to accept a job. Most families can now rest assured that death of the breadwinner does not mean a complete cessation of income.

### Benefits Replace Earnings Lost

A basic principle of the Old-Age, Survivors, and Disability Insurance system is that benefits are paid only when earnings cease or become lower because of one of the three risks which are "insured," namely, old age or retirement, death, or disability. Old-Age, Survivors, and Disability Insurance is not generally an annuity system or pension program based upon age, disability, or death alone. Benefits are not generally paid to persons who have suffered no loss of income. This concept is an extremely important one but has given rise to one of the most controversial features in the program, namely, the "work test" or "retirement test."

Simply stated, the retirement test provides a method of determining whether a worker has "retired" from gainful employment as required by law. Since the risk insured against is *loss* of earned income from work because of old age, retirement, or death of the breadwinner, the retirement test establishes a standard to ascertain whether the situation of the worker and his family is such as to warrant the conclusion that the contingency insured against, namely, loss of earned income, has occurred.

Under the present law, a worker who is 72 years of age or over is considered retired regardless of earnings. This recognizes the practical situation that very few persons over age 72 are actively working. Also, without the age 72 provision, people who worked to a very advanced age might never get benefits even though they had paid contributions longer than most other people. When a worker applies for benefits after age 62 and before reaching age 72, the retirement test applies, and it applies to earnings from all types of employment, not merely covered employment. A worker may receive full benefits if he earns $1,200.00 or less in a year. In general, if he earns above $1,200.00, then his benefits may be decreased by $1 for every $2 earned up to $1,700.00; that is, on the next $500.00 of earnings over and above the $1,200.00. For all earnings above $1,700.00, $1 of benefits may be withheld for each dollar earned.

Although controversial, the retirement test supports a basic concept of the program, namely, that the risk insured against is not just old age or death but *loss* of earned income resulting from these factors. To abolish the test would change the character of the program from insurance against earnings loss to an annuity program under which persons who continued to work full time at their regular jobs could receive full benefits at age 65.

Undoubtedly, the retirement test will be the subject of considerable discussion and it will probably be changed from time to time. It appears, however, destined to remain a basic concept of the Old-Age, Survivors, and Disability Insurance program for some time to come.

## PREDICTION OF FUTURE CHANGES IN SOCIAL SECURITY

We have described briefly the Old-Age, Survivors, and Disability Insurance system as it exists today. The present program is the result of many changes since the original act was passed in 1935. The next few years will see many changes also. Prophecy is dangerous, but I venture predictions on the following: (1) Coverage will become more widespread, and will include physicians and others not now included. I do not believe that the physicians of this country will wish to maintain the position that they, members of one of the most affluent professions, should not pay the taxes assessed on all other professions and others gainfully employed. (2) Benefits will be raised. The average benefit of about $77 per month for a retired beneficiary is not enough to provide even a minimum floor of protection. (3) The wage base will be raised.

At present only the first $4,800.00 of a worker's wages are taxed. In 1939, under the $3,000.00 wage base in effect, 97 per cent of all workers had earnings of $3,000.00 or less. Only 3 per cent had earnings in excess of $3,000.00 and 93 per cent of all earnings was taxed. In 1960, the $4,800.00 base results in taxing only 78 per cent of earnings because of the large number of persons earning above the $4,800.00 maximum. (4) The definition of disability will be liberalized. At present persons are eligible only if they cannot engage in any substantially gainful employment and are suffering from disabilities which are total and not likely to improve. (5) Finally, I believe that the social insurance principle will be applied increasingly to meet the costs of medical care and replace income lost by reason of illness or disability.

Let us remember that social insurance in the United States already meets a substantial portion of the wage loss caused by sickness or disability as well as a sizable amount of the medical care bill. One form of social insurance, namely, Workmen's Compensation,[24] has since 1908 replaced earnings lost by reason of work-connected disability or illness. In any one week, approximately 500,000 persons receive workmen's compensation benefits.[25] In addition to cash benefits, all states provide medical treatment. In two-thirds of the states, all necessary medical care is available; in the remainder, certain maximum duration and dollar amounts are imposed. Medical care payments now account for about one-third of total workmen's compensation benefits.

## THE SOCIAL SECURITY SYSTEM AND MEDICAL CARE

The great gap in coverage under the United States social security program is the lack of protection against wage loss resulting from temporary disability or short-term sickness. Although there is no large-scale pressure for such coverage now (medicare for the aged being the current hit theme in the political arena), I believe that future consideration of this problem is inevitable. Throughout the world, the discovery has been made that social insurance is an effective way of insuring against stoppage of income because of illness, and I predict that in the next decade, we shall revive the interest in such sickness and disability programs that was prevalent prior to 1950.

During the 1930's, there was considerable agitation to establish a social insurance program covering wage loss resulting from temporary disability or short-term sickness. The Committee on Economic Security, which was the committee whose studies and recommendations led to the introduction of the Social Security Act, urged that study be given to a program to cover temporary disability and illness. Following the enactment of the Social Security Act without such temporary disability coverage, a number of states considered the establishment of state programs. Four states established such programs under state law: Rhode Island in 1942, California in 1946, New Jersey in 1948, and New York in 1949. These four plans provide weekly payments for temporary disability to several million workers in the four states. The California plan also provides for limited hospital payments.

Although these plans have been successful, they have not spread to other states for many reasons. Perhaps the most important factor is the issue of public versus private insurance. In New York, employers insure with private insurance companies; in Rhode Island, employers must insure with a state fund; in California, employers can insure either with a state fund or private company. Several states which sought to establish such programs found it impossible to reconcile the opposing points of view and therefore did not press for a program. In addition, there were those who felt that a state-operated program was not worthwhile, that the varying state provisions without federal standards would not assure a satisfactory program, and that such a program should be part of Old-Age, Survivors, and Disability Insurance. The growth of voluntary insurance, likewise, eased the pressure for public temporary disability programs. In 1939, less than 8 million persons had voluntary insurance covering temporary sickness. Today, more than 130 million or about three quarters of the population have some type of prepaid insurance protection. However, this insurance covers medical care costs on a limited basis and very little coverage is given to replacing lost income. The estimated loss of income from sickness and disability to wage and salary workers in 1960 was $8.6 billion.[26] Of this loss, approximately $1.0 billion or less than 12 per cent was returned in cash benefits from insurance policies. Although there is still such a huge wage loss because of illness, insurance against the cost of medical care has blunted the move toward public cash payments through social insurance in case of wage loss because of illness. Finally, there was the usual cry of "socialized medicine." I doubt whether anyone can demonstrate that the practice of medicine in New York, California, New Jersey, and Rhode Island, has become more "socialized" than in other states which do not have such programs. But, of course, those who use this argument will assert that such public programs under state governments are better and less "socialized" than a similar program under federal auspices.

Whatever the arguments, it is inevitable that some program must make up for wage loss from illness. On an average day, more than two million workers are absent from work because of temporary disability. It is short-sighted not to insure their income in the same way that we have insured against loss of income because of unemployment, old age, permanent and total disability, and death.

## Medical Care for the Aged

In the meantime, attention is being centered on another problem, namely, medical care for the aged under Social Security. The discussions and debates have been numerous and often violent, resulting in more heat than light.

The controversy arises because of a convergence of several factors: the age of retirement continues to go down; longevity has increased; the income of the aged is very low, and social security payments constitute a major portion of the total income of all persons over 65 years of age; and long stays in the hospital and nursing homes for the aged have not been covered adequately through voluntary insurance. These and other factors combine to make the problem a serious one. As a result, many old people are forced to go on relief solely because of medical expenditures. More than half of the residents in the nursing homes of America are on relief. The new program, Medical Assistance for the Aged, commonly called the Kerr-Mills program, has not assisted materially in solving the problem. As of January 1963 116,000 persons were receiving care under such Medical Assistance for the Aged programs.

For the most part, however, they were persons who had been transferred from Old Age Assistance where they could have received care anyway. More than half of all expenditures were being made in five states. Furthermore, many members of the medical profession are beginning to realize that the Medical Assistance for the Aged program has in it more danger of governmental control than anything being prepared under the late President Kennedy's and now President Johnson's proposals. Under Medical Assistance for the Aged, a state can decide to limit its program in almost any way it wishes; it can prescribe the number of physicians' visits per illness; it can determine the length of hospital stay; it can decide the fees to be paid, and so on. Furthermore, it brings many persons, hitherto self-supporting, into the public welfare office.

There is no need to detail here the arguments for and against the use of the social security mechanism to provide medical care benefits for the aged. These have been set forth in hundreds of articles, in the Congressional Record, and in public utterances by advocates and opponents of the proposal. I predict that some measure will be passed by congress in the next two or three years which will tackle this problem through the use of the social insurance method of financing.

## CONCLUSION

In this discussion, I have tried to outline the past, present status, and next steps in social security, particularly with reference to Old-Age, Survivors, and Disability Insurance, which constitutes the basic program under the Social Security Act, and some of the implications of social insurance for health and medical care services. I have also mentioned two problem areas: the replacement of income lost by reason of temporary disability or illness and medical care for the aged.

\*       \*       \*

A rich country such as ours cannot afford to have millions of its citizens without income because of illness, nor can it afford to deny medical care to its ever-growing number of aged. In the past, men frequently resigned themselves to such a situation. Today, our people have made the discovery that there is a way of insuring against various social risks; namely, through the device of social insurance, a device that is now keeping millions of Americans from the hardships and poverty which would otherwise have come because of unemployment, old age, death of the wage earner, disability, or industrial accidents. These problems, along with the problems of medical care for the aged and replacement of lost income because of illness, are national problems in which all citizens have an interest. We have it in our power to make a contribution to the solution of the financial aspects of these problems through social security. We have demonstrated that the machinery of social insurance through Old-Age, Survivors, and Disability Insurance has been administered soundly, efficiently, and economically. I believe that this demonstration of social security's contribution has established it so securely in the minds and hearts of the American people that it will be extended to those areas where it can make its appropriate contribution and continue to assist in that most important goal of our society, the economic security of the American people.

# MEDICAL EDUCATION IN THE HOSPITAL

Edward D. Churchill, M.D.

THE Report of the Committee of both Houses of the Massachusetts Legislature recommended in 1810 the Act to incorporate The Massachusetts General Hospital and pointed to: "The immense benefits to be derived from a General Hospital, as a school for improvement in surgery and physic" and considered these benefits "too obvious to require illustration." The same report foresaw that "the skill thus acquired, by the increased means of instruction, will be gradually, and constantly diffused, through every section of the Commonwealth," and commented on, "the advantages to be derived to the community from improvement in medical science."

Trustees were chosen on February 2, 1813. On January 9 of the following year they addressed a statement to the public from whom subscriptions were requested. A new almshouse had just been built on Leverett Street and it was thought necessary to clarify the difference between the purpose of the almshouse and the purpose of what was to be the General Hospital. The Report of the Committee of the Legislature had already made this distinction in the stipulation that "it is not to the indigent alone that the advantages of the institution are to be extended."

Three years before the cornerstone of the Bulfinch building was laid and six years before the first patient was admitted, a statement of the trustees was published in the October 14, 1815 issue of the Columbian Centinel, a Boston newspaper, now long extinct. It described how the trustees interpreted their responsibilities to the Commonwealth and to the public. This was the design of the new General Hospital: "The end of the Institution is cure of the disease, whether bodily, or mental, under which they (the patients) labour. To this all its arrangements bend. To this, its whole organization is made subservient. It purposes to afford the best medical aid; the best nurses; the most suitable apartments; all the assistance which sickness requires; and all the comforts, which are subsidiary to convalescence." What an open-end contract to have labored under for 150 years!

My assignment is to present the Hospital's Responsibility to the Community with respect to its serving as "a school for improvement in surgery and physic." I may start, as did the Committee of the Legislature in 1810, with the assumption that the "benefits are too obvious to require illustration." My subject matter will be still further narrowed by considering only the role of the hospital as a "school for improvement in surgery," for while its role in physic (internal medicine) has been equally important and in many aspects has developed in a parallel manner, each has met the problems of change in its own way, and I do not pretend to a competence that would make what I might say about physic worth while or even accurate. Only a few other historic events will be cited when they throw light on the adaptive changes that have taken place in the past thirty years during which time I have been but one of many participants.

## CHANGE AND THE MEDICAL PROFESSION

The phrase *adaptive change* has already been used, and doubtlessly will reappear during my presentation. This phrase has a nineteenth century Darwinian ring and today is commonly heard at the climax of some debate about a proposed innovation. A familiar version is the cliché: "Let us proceed by evolution rather than revolution." With this solemn warning the debate is brought to an end and all agree to maintain the comfortable status quo.

At this point, I wish to comment on this process of so-called adaptive change, rather than make the assumption that it is a permanent, built-in mechanism of free institutions and democratic society. This assumption — that the power of adaptive change is our most treasured secret weapon *vis à vis* more rigid totalitarian societies is open to some question. James Reston had this to say about change:

The "central problem of today is the failure of men and institutions to keep up with events. No matter how men try to meet the revolutionary changes of the time — and most of them are doing their best — they find old attitudes of mind, old laws, old ways of picking and promoting legislators, and old methods of selecting and rewarding executives blocking their progress."

Everyone who has accustomed himself to working in an old institution such as the Massachusetts General Hospital recognizes the slowness of effecting change and is likely to attribute the lag to the strong forces of tradition. But, these forces are not serious hurdles, and one soon becomes accustomed to the slow rate at which changes in attitude and ways of thinking take place. One can always anticipate the acceptance of a change with the rise of a new generation and patiently wait. The blocking action of vested interests and the fear of dispossession gradually fade away as a new generation takes over.

To my mind, Reston's alarm over the "failure of men and institutions to keep up with events" is justified, but stems from a far more serious cause. Our democratic institutions assume that they are flexible and that they possess a built-in mechanism for change, but in fact have lost or are losing the ability to make *significant* change. A large institution becomes an existential society, and its energies are consumed in the very process of existing from day to day. The Red Queen encountered this predicament years ago. We cannot change in a significant way. This thought is disturbing, particularly when we look over our shoulders at societies with ten-year plans and directed futures. So while it is agreed that the hospital has a very real responsibility to the community, it is far from certain that if change is necessary it can be accomplished. Certainly the staff has not presented to the trustees a clear cut design for the future comparable to the one the board was able to present to the community in 1814. Then as now, a Board of Trustees can only seek guidance in professional affairs from the staff to which it has delegated the responsibility of carrying out the professional activities of the hospital; so when I express doubts as to the ability of the hospital to meet its responsibility to the community by significant change if such is needed, I have made it clear in which direction I am pointing.

Let it be clear that I have not implied that significant change is required to meet this hospital's responsibility to the community. Perhaps tightening a bolt here and shoring up there is all that need be done. I have merely brought out into the open the fact that the professions which unite and integrate their activities to form a hospital find themselves singly and in their coordinated endeavors quite powerless to bring about significant change. The reasons are obvious. The professional segments which form a hospital closely intermesh with the larger groups which constitute the professions of the community, and these in turn, with the national professional communities. The term "organized medicine" is but a myth, if in its usage it is implied that the profession has a built-in mechanism for change, or acts as a totalitarian society. Medicine, like other professions, is but a loose association of individual entrepreneurs. A convincing example of the inability of the profession to bring about change from within can be found in the prolonged struggle required to raise the standards of medical education from the low level that prevailed in the last century. The prime reason for the organization of the American Medical Association in 1847 was to elevate the standard of medical education, and one of the first acts was the appointment of a Committee on Medical Education. During the next 57 years, this committee issued pronouncements, resolutions, and recommendations at annual meetings of the association. Of all the resolutions adopted, and there were hundreds of them, not one can be regarded as resulting in any specific good.[1] At the turn of the century organizational changes in the American Medical Association resulted in the formation of the Council of Medical Education in 1905. The council defined as its goal an "ideal standard" and began work toward this end, despite the considerable resentment encountered in the medical colleges. In December 1908 the council saw the light and sought the aid of the Carnegie Foundation for the Advancement of Teaching. What is known as the "Flexner Report" was issued in 1910. The governing boards of colleges and universities throughout the country had turned a deaf ear to the pleadings of the council but were ready to listen when Abraham Flexner spoke from the rostrum of the Carnegie Foundation. It can be said parenthetically that the fiscal aid of this foundation was then of vital assistance in the establishment of a pension system for teachers. The story of the reforms that were introduced at local levels is too well known to repeat. The episode is used to illustrate three points: first, the inability of the profession to achieve significant change from within; second, the importance of the formulation of an "ideal standard" by leaders of the profession as a goal toward which to move; and third, the necessity to apply moral suasion from outside to bring about significant change.

## MEDICAL EDUCATION AT THE MASSACHUSETTS GENERAL HOSPITAL

With these general observations the subject can be brought to the microcosm of the postdoctoral schools of surgery and physics within the walls of the Massachusetts General Hospital. First, however, for those not familiar with the terminology of education in medicine the following definitions may be helpful.

Predoctoral education is under the control of the Faculty of Medicine of a medical college or medical school. A hospital participates by providing the opportunity for clinical instruction to students who come to the hospital each day in considerable number and receive instruction in the care of the sick and injured. The Massachusetts General Hospital is academically associated or "affiliated" with the Harvard Medical School. Harvard University assumes no responsibility for the care of the sick, either financially or managerially. Its buildings on Longwood Avenue in Boston contain the preclinical departments of the medical sciences, administrative offices, and a central medical library. The hospital's responsibility to the community resides in providing clinical opportunities during this four-year predoctoral period. This responsibility is shared by other hospitals associated academically. Instruction is solely the responsibility of the Faculty of Medicine. Nearly every member of the Massachusetts General Hospital staff is likewise a member of this faculty.

Postdoctoral education embraces two major activities: (1) Education of recent medical school graduates through periods of appointment at the hospital as intern and resident. This period in surgery extends into 5 or 6 years. Involving as it does the increasing responsibility for patient care, these doctors are licensed by the State Board of Medicine and engage in intramural practice under the supervision of the permanent or visiting staff. Interns and residents form the house staff and were formerly known as house pupils. Appointment to the house staff is made by the trustees of the hospital, and its members are responsible through the visiting staff to the trustees for their participation in the care of patients. Medical students (predoctoral) are forbidden by law to assume responsibility for the care of the sick either by prescribing medicine or performing operations. (2) Courses for practicing physicians are conducted at the hospital and elsewhere under the Harvard Graduate School of Medicine or other outside agency.

This lecture therefore is focused on the education of recent medical school graduates who, as I have explained, constitute the house staff. The conduct of this program, commonly referred to as *training* is one of the many responsibilities of the hospital to the community.

In September 1939 an eighty-page report entitled "Graduate Training at the Massachusetts General Hospital" was presented to the trustees by the General Executive Committee which is the "medical board" of the hospital. In view of what has been said, a retrospective glance at this document is of interest. It starts with a "Preamble" drawn from the wisdom of President A. Lawrence Lowell.

A design, complete and elastic, is essential, and for want of a better word we may call it a pattern — not an inappropriate expression, for it connotes a picture in the mind with the essential features clearly drawn, the subsidiary ones sketched in, the background well marked, and the foreground or approach indicated.

"Such a pattern is by no means rigid," Mr. Lowell explained, "the final objective is perfectly definite, but the details are fluid and must be kept so throughout." [2]

The Introduction of the report itself defined the objective. The basic tenet of the report was that an institution with the resources of the Massachusetts General Hospital "in accepting the responsibility of caring for the sick assumes a second responsibility to train physicians. This is a responsibility that cannot be taken lightly or passed off as an automatic by-product of caring for patients. The method of training physicians requires independent appraisal of its merits as an intensive program in graduate education. These two functions of the hospital — care of the sick and training of the doctor — then require integration for mutual benefit, without sacrifice of fundamental excellence by either."

In a section entitled "Type of Training" the educational resources of the hospital were carefully appraised. Also, it was stated that "the needs of the community are to be considered in shaping a policy for graduate education." The decision was made that: "The Hospital may best provide the community with family doctors by continuing the excellence of, and further strengthening, its training in internal medicine. It may also serve an equally vital need of American medicine by providing proper training for specialists and by the establishment of higher standards in this training."

Each department was invited to review its educational program and include proposals for change in the report. From here on I shall deal with surgery, and only with salient items. The proposals for significant change in the existing system were hammered out in many staff and committee meetings. It may be recalled that the White building was then in process of construction and provided a tangible basis for a new order.

## The Selection of Candidates

The primary task in an educational endeavor is to determine how many students the resources of an institution can accommodate and what criteria are to be used in selecting them from a larger number of applicants. I shall deal with the latter item first. The process of selection is essentially that of prediction. In selecting men about to obtain their doctorate, a long and objective record of academic achievement is readily available. In addition, an intuitive judgment is made, based on a personal interview in which a considerable number of the active staff participates. Because the quality of the educational experience which an accepted candidate will enjoy in his years at the hospital will depend on the intimate personal relations he develops with the individual members of a sizable staff, I consider it of great importance that they share in the selection process.

Not until 1962 was I aware that we had long been adhering to the common sense terms of a formal statement published by the trustees in 1884.

The object of the Trustees is to appoint as house pupils the best available men. It would be a mistake to suppose that those appointments are offered as prizes to the best scholars or to those who pass the best examination by the staff. Those examinations are not intended to be thorough tests of knowledge. Candidates who have maintained high rank at the Medical School, and who are successful at the examination of the staff have secured important advantages. But, besides good scholarship, other qualifications are to be considered, such as dexterity, good character, good manners, tact, the power of getting on with other men. In short, all the qualities, moral, intellectual, and physical, which go to make the successful physician or surgeon, the Trustees try to obtain in the House Pupils.

This statement admirably expresses the attitude still governing the selection of candidates and goes far to explain why Alan Gregg was in a position to say: "The teaching and supervision given an intern or resident in a teaching hospital involves an intimacy with his teacher that surpasses anything he has experienced in the previous twenty years of his education." [3]

I trust that I have made it clear that the educational endeavor in surgery at the hospital is and always has been a product of the surgical staff as a whole, and not one dominated by one or two surgeons of senior rank. It is inevitable with a total roster of between 50 and 60 men in training and a sizable permanent staff, that the helpful personal attachments between the two groups form naturally in accord with compatible personalities. The important thing is that they form, and without rivalries or so-called apple polishing. After each period of close professional association in the discharge of hospital duties, the staff member is invited to write his appraisal of the trainee's performance. These evaluations are filed as a confidential personnel record.

### The School of Surgery at the Massachusetts General Hospital

The number of younger surgeons that can be accepted by an institution depends on the clinical work load of the institution. In surgery this is measured by the number of patients treated by operation, rather than by the number of beds, many of which may be inactive. The range of surgical therapy conducted is also of great importance, as well as the competence of the allied and supporting services, including nursing.

Intensely motivated men who have completed their predoctoral education in contemporary U.S.A. medical colleges learn rapidly to assume responsibilities as they are delegated to them. It is important, in my opinion, that they should be somewhat overworked while on clinical tasks rather than idle. In writing of the surgical way of life, Dr. Rudolph Matas used the following words: "It has its great joys, its superb and glorious hours; but it has also its tragic hours, its hours of bitterness and desolation. And yet, all love it. They love it in spite of its fatigues, its worries and its emotions because it is also a source of deep satisfaction and lasting joy."

Time for reflection, so vital in creative scientific effort, can lead to brooding and discouragement in those hours of "bitterness and desolation." Ill considered or harsh criticism from above likewise may be a devastating event in the life of a sensitive and conscientious young man; a wiser course is to pursue a careful analysis of the many variable circumstances which surround every endeavor in surgery, followed by a calm and carefully weighed judgment in which colleagues of all ages participate. Thoroughbred horses respond best to a light touch on the reins, and a school of surgery which aspires to be a center of higher learning can neither be a boot camp nor an antechamber to the economy.

I shall now outline more specifically some of the changes which have followed the 1939 Report to the Trustees. This provided a basic design or pattern against which details could be measured as the need for adjustments arose. As I have implied and illustrated, without this guideline or ideal standard in mind, decisions that bring about change might not have taken place, or at the best would have been random ones rather than truly adaptive and evolutionary. The immediately foreseen adjustments required by the opening of the White building had scarcely been introduced before World War II was upon us. Hasty adaptations to the shortened curriculum and urgent needs of the armed forces were carried out. Beginning in 1947, it was possible to reassemble the pieces and make a fresh start.

The major change envisioned was a replacement of the time-honored personal master-apprentice training by the creation of a learning situation in which the trainee worked as a responsible individual under the guidance of the staff as a whole. I have already spoken of the wide range of personalities in a sizable staff; an even more striking wide range of expert skills had been developing among the individuals that comprise the visiting staff. Orthopedic Surgery, Urology, and Neurosurgery had been divorced from General Surgery decades previously and each had erected its own ladder for training specialists in its respective field. General Surgery was rapidly becoming "Residual Surgery." Further fragmentation as the result of the formal segregation of still more areas of expert skills threatened the conversion of surgery into a larger number of watertight compartments. The central need was to encourage the development of expert knowledge and skills for the benefit of the patients, but at the same time preserve the substance of so-called General Surgery for its educational value to the resident staff and predoctoral medical students alike. For many reasons it was considered important to provide a broad and general education in surgery for these young men.

By general staff consensus, a moratorium was declared on the further organizational fragmentation of the residual content of surgery, and in consequence, the Massachusetts General Hospital has no aggregates of patients representing Plastic, Thoracic, Cardiac, or Hand Surgical Services. When the Vincent Memorial joined the Massachusetts General Hospital group, a Department of Gynecology was established as a semidetached service but with close educational bonds with the Department of General Surgery. Despite this policy, expert knowledge and skills representing all of these areas and others have been nourished and developed, and staff members representing these special fields have achieved international reputations. A Department of Child Surgery has recently been established with a dual valence to Children's Medicine and General Surgery.

However ideal such arrangements have proven in establishing a learning situation for students, residents, and staff, it must be frankly admitted that they have created additional burdens for the permanent staff. Hospital work hours are greatly simplified by congregating one's patients in one place under one resident and one head nurse.

The 1939 Report recalled that 20 years previously it had been "customary for" the young surgeon to complete a short (two-year) period of internship and then secure his real technical training as a member of the out-patient staff. In addition, he usually served as assistant to a senior practicing surgeon in the care of his patients, often scattered in a number of outlying hospitals. The report warned that responsibilities were already being given to the house staff that formerly were considered prerogatives of the visiting staff and that these responsibilities would be increased with the establishment of a much longer period of intramural education. The prediction was made, however, that participation in a formally recognized and intensified educational program which preserved the breadth of general surgery would increase the attractiveness of staff association, and I believe this has proven true. The delegation of responsibility in surgery even when supervision is maintained is always a more trying task than plunging in and doing the job oneself. Only the unified, if not always unanimous, support of the visiting staff has made the program a success. Perhaps the most difficult thing for some surgeons to accept is found in the ancient Greek philosophy of teaching — the greatest honor a teacher may achieve is to have his pupils excel him.

The old personal master-apprentice training was excellent in its time, and those of us who grew up that way look back with gratitude to the experience we acquired under it. But it also had its defects and limitations. One still hears its virtues extolled, and many clinical departments in the medical schools of this country bear the earmark of continental influence in their organizational structure with a lone professor standing at the apex of the pyramid. It is said that the young man must spend his formative years "sitting at the feet of a Master."

Ramon y Cajal, the great Spanish neurologist, had this to say of such euphemisms: "How many of keen intellect we know, who have had no greater misfortune than to have been pupils of a great man. Extreme admiration drains the personality and clouds the understanding."

And Maurice Arthus in pondering on the philosophy of scientific investigation wrote:

. . . the young biologist endeavors to imitate his teacher in every respect; he tries to identify himself with him, to merge himself with him. His infinite admiration will deprive him of his intellectual independence and originality.

Honor your teacher, as is fitting, and respect him sincerely. But accept his directions only if they seem justified. Ask questions — argue. Do not accept his words, all his words, without reservation and criticism. Criticize with moderation, of course, and first of all respectfully, but criticize *firmly*.

Preserve your originality. It is this that will give your scientific work its frankness, its grace, its elegance, its warmth and life among so many banal commonplace, cold and corpse-like works, for originality is the colorful bonnet of the girls of Anjou among the banal Parisian hats.

And Thomas Kuhn, an historian of science, has recently said:

Almost always the men who achieve these fundamental inventions have been either very young or very new to the field whose (methods) they change. Obviously these are the men who, being little committed by prior practice to the traditional rules, are particularly likely to see that those rules no longer define a playable game and to conceive another set that can replace them.

But surgery is not an autonomus science — it is the application of many sciences to the diagnosis and treatment of disease and injury in human beings. The assumption of responsibility for human life and health can never be as free as an experiment in the laboratory, and the primary responsibility of a hospital and of all those within its walls remains as stated 150 years ago: "The end of the Institution is cure of the disease, whether bodily, or mental under which they (the patients) labour." Only insofar as this responsibility is discharged can any educational undertaking be successful, for this is what it is our purpose to teach.

The problem of what is called the "socialization" of doctors has been introduced in recent times, referring to the development of an attitude which enables the physician to consider the general welfare of a patient rather than concentrate on the technological problems with myopic vision. I wish briefly to comment on this subject from the standpoint of the surgeon. I shall illustrate by a concrete example. For years I have taught medical students that when a frightened woman appears at the door, she may be one who had screwed up her courage to tell a doctor that she has felt what she thinks is a "lump" in her breast. If so, ask no further questions but take her immediately into the examining room to find out about what has alarmed her. It is not the time for a formally taken history or inquiry about the illnesses of her grandparents or what her relations may be with her husband. Such matters can come later. What she might say under the stress of the situation would be both inaccurate and probably irrelevant to the immediate decisions that must be made.

This direct and *ad hoc* approach often shocks the student, drilled in the formal case-taking methods of physicians or the interview techniques of the psychiatrist. His first reaction is one of hostility to the surgeon and to believe that he is either ignorant or heartlessly preoccupied with the thoughts of the operation which may be required.

Much of surgery requires this direct but far from impersonal approach to tangible and, one may say quite obvious, decision-making. Once a decision is made, tensions and anxieties relax.

In dealing with hundreds of interns and residents I have rarely had misgivings about the doctor-patient relationships they develop within an environment such as this hospital enjoys. Although mistakes are made, they are perhaps no more frequent than occur in the practice of their seniors.

Gloyne attributes the following to the Golden Sayings of Epictetus in defense of philosophers. I offer it in defense of surgeons.

A Philosopher's school is a Surgery; pain, not pleasure, you should have felt therein. For on entering none of you is whole. One has a shoulder out of joint, another an abscess; a third suffers from an issue, a fourth from pains in the head. Am I to sit down and treat you to pretty sentiments and empty flourishes, so that you may applaud me and depart, with neither shoulder, nor head, nor issue, nor abscess a whit better for your visit? [4]

The 1939 Report which has been mentioned was followed in 1950 by a careful study by a staff committee, headed by Dr. Richard Warren. Another committee led by Dr. J. Gordon Scannell in 1959 gave us our bearings by an independent review. During the past two years, Dr. Fred Richardson and his graduate assistants have made an independent study from the viewpoint of a social anthropologist. Much has been learned from these appraisals. The day-by-day administration of the service elements of the program have been assumed by Dr. Francis D. Moore, Dr. J. Gordon Scannell, Dr. Paul S. Russell, and Dr. Hermes C. Grillo, in succession. It has been their task to adjust the ideals of a broad educational program to the stern necessities of the responsibility for continuous 24-hour care of the hospital patients. And above and beyond any individual, there has always been the understanding participation of the surgical staff as a whole, oftentimes as I have said, at the sacrifice of their time and charismatic prestige.

Other salient features that were either projected by the 1939 Report or have developed subsequently are:

When an applicant has been appointed he may confidently expect to be reappointed annually until he has completed the five years required for admission to the examinations of the American Board of Surgery. This was a radical departure from the so-called pyramidal programs in which places for reappointment diminish each year, and men are constantly being eliminated from the roster with less than the required number of years to their credit. This change to what is now called the "rectangular" program rather than "pyramidal" has done away with competition and rivalry for reappointment and promotion. There is no place for competition and rivalry at the bedside of a sick patient, where excellence of care depends on the vigilance of unified teamwork. I can point to no one change that has brought as significant improvement in patient care as this simple expression of confidence in the sustained motivation of selected men.

With due notice so that a replacement can be found, a man may withdraw from the surgical training to pursue other interests. Over the years there has been but a 10 per cent attrition rate from *all* causes, such as transfer to a surgical specialty, sickness, or personal desire to seek an alternative career. When a man desires to give up surgery completely every effort is made to find a place for him here or elsewhere, so that he may take up an alternative course with minimal loss of time. He does not lose face, and the hospital may be as proud of the few men who have left as of those who have completed the full program. A man may leave for active duty with the armed forces and take up his work here again, usually on the day of his discharge.

With six months advance planning, men are released for one or more years to pursue research in scientific laboratories in this country or abroad. They are assisted in obtaining opportunities for such work and fellowship stipends to make it feasible. Again, they return to continue clinical training from where they left off.

It is far easier to identify these specific changes that have been made than it is to describe or appraise the tangible attitudes and qualities of the house staff which have emerged. I am told by the anthropologist that the house staff has taken on the form of an age-peer group with strong in-group membership identification. The use of this term in secondary education frequently carries the meaning of "social adjustment" of the pupil to the norms of the group. This may be far from desirable when stressed to bring about conformity of effort, behavior, and attainment. With mature adults in a postdoctoral school of surgery the only observable conformity has been the common devotion to meet the needs of the patients, an essential attribute of a doctor. In recent years some conscious effort has been exerted to avoid having participation in research undertakings reach the status of becoming something "expected" of every resident. The majority of the house staff remains headed toward the dignified and useful career of surgical practice in some urban community. A great virtue of the rectangular system is that no man feels he must spend a period in the experimental laboratory in order to gain promotion in the clinical training program. Certainly the house staff's loyalty to the hospital and its high purposes has been enhanced. The permanent staff provides a reference group which serves to maintain on-going standards and is a safeguard against retrograde trends.

The members of the visiting staff have by no means lost their influence, as some like to make it appear, but act as informal consultants. By accepting these younger surgeons as adult members of the profession and building on their talents and strengths they are giving the *one* support an older man *can* give a younger man nowadays — the encouragement of self-reliance in a man facing his own world in his own time. The younger men immediately become essential parts of the administration of the hospital and carry on their shoulders a major share of the professional task of providing the best of surgical care.

It sometimes seems to me that doctors are so accustomed to prescribing medicines in milligrams, diets in exact calories and ingredients, and performing operations with meticulous standardized techniques that these habits are carried over into their educational endeavors. By so doing they are likely to miss the point of adult education entirely. The house staff is made up of mature and highly educated men. Our task has been to create for the individual the strongest possibility for personal initiative, competence, and self-reliance.

Ambroise Paré, the great sixteenth century surgeon, was both a devout and deeply religious man and a superb teacher. In the year 1583 on the tenth day of December, Paré was summoned to care for a man in Beauvais and found:

"his legs all ulcered and all the bones cariez'd and rotten; he prayed me for the honor of God to cut off his Legge by reason of the great paine which he could no longer endure. After his body was prepared . . . I caused his Legge to be cut off, fowre fingers below the rotula of the knee, by Daniel Poullet one of my servants, to teach him and to embolden him in such workes; and there he readily tyed the vessels to stay the bleeding, x x x I will not here forget to say that the Lady Princesse of Montpensier knowing that he was poore, and in my hands, gave him money to pay for his chamber and diet. He was well cured, God be praysed, and he was returned home to his house with a wooden Legge.[5]

Whether we call these young surgeons servants, apprentices, assistants, house pupils, or residents, it is the time-honored privilege of older surgeons to "embolden" them to face the grim tasks that must be undertaken and to perform them without the timidity that comes from the fear of inadequacy.

## CONCLUSION

I shall revert to the thesis already developed concerning the introduction of an innovation or change. Whether or no this change in the education of surgeons can be described as significant is not a matter for our judgment at the present time, although I venture to predict that as the nature of what the surgical staff of this hospital has accomplished in the past two decades becomes generally understood, its importance may well transcend the sum total of scientific and technical contributions achieved by its individual members during this same period.

In this instance, the innovation was entirely an intramural one and as such was uninhibited by reference to the profession of the community. It required no force of moral suasion from without. It did, however, depend on the guideline of a design — not a rigid, predrawn blueprint, but a pattern with a definite objective against which details could be measured as specific decisions were required which would lead to adaptive change.

# THE HOSPITAL AND THE CONTINUING
# EDUCATION OF THE PHYSICIAN

Russell A. Nelson, M.D.

THE community hospital is a natural setting, perhaps even an indispensable focal point for the continued education of the physician. I would like to speak of the education of the physician and the relation of the hospital to it in three phases. The first is that of the medical student; second, the intern and resident in specialty training; and third, postgraduate or continuing education of the practicing physician. I hope to show that there is great concern in the medical profession about the inadequacy of the continued education of the physician and that this is a major problem facing not only medical education, but all of American medicine and hospital practice. In the evolving role of the hospital in the education of the physician it should be pointed out that the hospital is emerging as a more influential center for medical care and practice and is becoming even more of an educational institution than in decades past. I hope, also, to show that a change in emphasis by the hospital in its educational role with more attention to the postgraduate area may facilitate a badly needed regional integration of hospital and medical services.


## THE EDUCATION OF THE PHYSICIAN

Among the distinguished professions, medicine is recognized as one which traditionally and strongly assumes responsibility for education of the current members of the profession and the oncoming generations of student physicians. The Oath of Hippocrates features the doctor's responsibility to educate his successors and has led to the continuing interest of the profession in medical education. Since medical practice is and always will be a combination of the application of known medical science and the application of human relations known as the "art of medicine," the education of the physician or student is a combination of formal scientific curriculum, scientific investigation, and an apprentice relationship with seasoned, experienced physicians. As the biological and social sciences affecting man become better understood and more sophisticated in their development, the educational process becomes less apprentice in character. Nevertheless, all thoughtful physicians recognize that even in these days of great scientific advance, medicine is still a very inexact science, and much of the education of the doctor must be based upon an empirical medicine which, in turn, is based upon the experience of the practicing physician. The movement, however, is steadily, although slowly, in the direction of more exact information and a more scientific method of instruction.

Although medical science has thoroughly permeated hospital practice, it remains true that the hospital's basic contribution to the education of the physician is in the preceptor or apprentice phase which we call "Clinical medicine." This concept can be expected to remain for a long, long time and gives to the hospital its unique opportunity in education.

## Predoctoral Medical Education

The medical education of a doctor begins in medical school. Here we find the course of study based increasingly on the solid ground of medical science with standards well established and the affairs of the process well in the hands of the universities and colleges. It was not always so, however. Fifty years ago much of the education of the medical student in the United States was in a disgraceful state, with low standards and inadequate instruction. This situation was remedied with dispatch following Abraham Flexner's study[1] which was conducted under the auspices of the Carnegie Foundation and the American Medical Association. The reform was brought about by a single basic recommendation: the education of the medical student should be in a medical college which should, in turn, be an intimate part of a university, and university standards of education should be applied to the medical school.

Within a few decades the deplorable state of affairs of 1910 was almost entirely corrected, and today we have a medical school system in this country which is probably the best in the world. Of course, there are serious problems of finance, recruitment, and others, but these are not considered to be sufficiently severe to threaten the inherent quality of American medicine.

## Postdoctoral Education — Intern-Resident and Clinical Fellow Training

The second phase in the education of the physician comes during the postdoctoral period where hospital and specialty training in the internship-residency period and, in recent years, the clinical fellowship are found. Here, educational requirements are not so firmly under control as in the undergraduate period and changes have evolved slowly. Fifty years ago relatively few physicians took internships before entering practice. Now, essentially all do. Twenty-five years ago only a few physicians took extra hospital training in one of the medical specialties. Now, nearly all graduates undergo this advanced training. It seems clear to me that we are progressing to a point where all medical graduates will spend two, three, four, and even five years of education and training in clinical and special scientific fields. Thus, the formal if not absolutely required period of medical education won't be just the four years in medical school, but those four years plus three, four, or five more years spent in the graduate period.

The great advance in medical science has been, of course, accompanied by a growth in specialization in clinical medicine; indeed, specialization has fostered that growth. Specialization itself makes this protracted period of graduate education a necessity and stimulates the young graduate to this long and arduous additional task. It is interesting to observe that despite the investment in time and the delay in earning capacity, the young medical graduates of today are to a sharply increasing extent entering internship-residency training. Table 1 shows the increase in the number of young physicians in internship-residency training in American hospitals between 1930 and 1960.[2,3] It shows that the number of interns has increased by nearly double, but that the number of residents in specialty training has increased several hundred per cent, most of

TABLE 1. NUMBER OF INTERNS AND RESIDENTS IN HOSPITALS
APPROVED FOR TRAINING BY THE AMERICAN MEDICAL
ASSOCIATION, 1930–1960

| Year | Interns | Residents | Total |
|------|---------|-----------|-------|
| 1930 | 5,500[a] | 1,500[a] | 7,000[a] |
| 1940 | 7,553 | 3,900[a] | 11,453[a] |
| 1950 | 6,821 | 14,595 | 21,416 |
| 1960 | 9,115 | 28,447 | 37,562 |

[a] Estimated.

this in the period after 1940 and, actually, since the conclusion of World War II. The 37,000 M.D.'s listed in internship-residency training in 1960 represent between 15 and 20 per cent of all active physicians in the United States.

There is another important factor at work in graduate education. It relates to the change in medical practice in hospitals and the increasing need for physicians available on a 24-hour basis to provide medical services for the seriously ill in-patients whose tempo of care in hospitals has been accelerated so much. There is also an enlarging need for physicians in hospitals to meet the needs of patients in the emergency departments and to provide medical services in the expanding out-patient sections. Hospitals and medical staffs have turned to interns and residents to fill this requirement and, as is well known, there are not enough of these individuals to fill the approved positions. This mixture of education and service presents one of the serious problems. Although, according to the American Medical Association,[4] only 21 per cent of hospitals have approved graduate training programs, they are the larger institutions and account for half of all hospital beds.

Table 2 shows the number of intern-resident positions filled in 1950 and 1960[5,6] and illustrates several interesting and important points. The total number of positions offered and approved has increased in that decade from 28,000 to 45,000 or slightly over 60 per cent. This is a measure of the increasing need for these individuals in hospital practice. It also shows that the percentage of the positions offered which are filled by American school graduates had diminished from 67.6 to 61 per cent in this decade. Although the total vacancies remain about the same at 7,700, the gap is partly filled by a five-times increase in the number of positions filled by

TABLE 2. STATUS OF INTERNSHIPS AND RESIDENCY PROGRAMS
APPROVED BY THE AMERICAN MEDICAL ASSOCIATION,
1950 AND 1960

| Year | Number of internships and residencies | | | | |
|------|-----------------|-----------------|-----------------------------|-------------------------------|-----------------|
| | Total offered | Total filled | Filled by U.S. graduates | Filled by foreign graduates | Total vacant |
| 1950 | 28,734 | 21,525 | 19,453 (67.6)[a] | 2,072 | 7,209 |
| 1960 | 45,333 | 37,562 | 27,626 (61.1)[a] | 9,935 | 7,771 |

[a] In per cent of total offered.

foreign medical graduates. The American medical educational system is failing to supply enough physicians to serve as interns and residents in approved hospitals and we have become importers of medical man power.

The foreign medical graduate in American hospitals creates a very special problem which is characterized by great difficulties in language, inadequate educational preparation, and degree of supervision. In some hospitals it has led to a lowering of the quality of medical care. The program very often leads to frustrated foreign guests taking home impressions of American medicine, medical education, and America itself that are not wholesome or in the best interest of our international relations.

The standards for intern-residency training programs are set by the practicing profession through the American Medical Association and the various specialty societies. All programs require approval by the American Medical Association and to have any chance of success a hospital must be so approved. With medical service such a heavy component in the graduate educational process and with the standards set by the practicing profession, it is inevitable that these standards are minimal. This, too, has led to the disparity in number of positions approved as compared to those filled and may, in fact, compound the problem because the available students are distributed in numbers too small to receive effective education or proper supervision. In 1960, the Internship Review Committee of the American Medical Association approved nearly twice as many hospital programs as the committee members felt they could personally recommend to a student.[7]

It seems very likely that the conditions of resident and intern graduate education will not be improved without vigorous action. In many respects, the conditions that exist in graduate education resemble those pertaining to undergraduate medical education at the turn of the century. There is a heavy aspect of service to patients and the standards are largely set by the practicing physicians in the hospitals. A thorough review is overdue and may result from the action of the Council on Medical Education in Hospitals of the American Medical Association in initiating a study[8] by a group headed by President John Millis of Western Reserve University. It is very likely that a single recommendation which would place the responsibilities of this education under sponsorship of the medical schools would go far in solving the problem. This, in fact, might be one of the principal points to come out of an impartial review of the situation.

If a share of the responsibility for intern and resident education is transferred from the hospital as sole sponsor to the medical school, as cosponsor, this would create an educational resource and release energy in many community hospitals which it is hoped could be mobilized for education in the postgraduate period.

## DEVELOPMENT OF CONTINUED EDUCATION OF THE PHYSICIAN

Like other professions, medicine prides itself on its dedication to continued education of the physician. Medical students and house officers are repeatedly exhorted to continue the life of the student throughout their professional life to come. The development of medical societies, both special and general, and the increasing number of medical journals, are all expressions of the attempt of practicing physicians to avail themselves of current knowledge. Despite these urges, they are increasingly frustrated in attempts to keep up. Literature inundates them; there is little time to study and few places to be taught. The problem continues.

In 1955, Vollan[9] of the American Medical Association reported a survey of postgraduate medical education in the United States and classified the methods of education of the practicing physician into five categories: (1) Reading of medical books, monographs, periodicals, and the abundant literature that every physician receives from pharmaceutical firms. (2) Individual professional contacts between the physician and his colleagues, consultants, pharmacists, and the representatives of pharmaceutical firms. (3) Attendance at hospital meetings, such as staff meetings, clinicopathological and radiological conferences, and journal club meetings. (4) Attendance at national, state, and local general or special medical society meetings. (5) Attendance at formal postgraduate courses.

Vollan's studies indicate that hospital staff meetings are considered one of the most ineffective methods of postgraduate education. He points out that most of these staff meetings are felt to be perfunctory and are concerned with current matters of hospital organization and only to a limited extent with the presentation of new medical information. There have been, however, a number of interesting and worthwhile demonstrations in postgraduate education by individual hospitals or groups of hospitals sometimes related to medical schools. One of the most productive is well known to the physicians of New England. It is, of course, the plan of the Bingham Associates[10] so successfully directed by Dr. Samuel Proger of the Pratt Diagnostic Clinic. This plan is based on sending modern laboratory diagnostic aides and members of the house staff of a Boston hospital to smaller hospitals in New England. It has been successful to the limits of its influence. A somewhat similar plan based on the rotation of members of the house staff from the University of Michigan[11] to hospitals in that state has been reported successful. Another example, limited in scope but interesting in its effects, is the relationship of the Hunterdon Medical Center and Hospital in New Jersey with the New York University School of Medicine.[12] Here a small community health center with full-time medical staff and an academic affiliation has had a significant impact on the continued medical education of general practitioners in that region of New Jersey.

Another interesting and successful venture is the association of the Albany Hospital and Medical College with the staffs of hospitals in the surrounding area. This plan is based on luncheon staff conferences at stated times in the outlying hospitals, the teaching being accomplished through the medium of a two-way FM radio with headquarters in the teaching medical center.[13]

Vollan's analysis, based on inquiries made to several thousand physicians, indicated that the majority questioned felt formal courses were the most rewarding of exercises. However, the most significant finding in Vollan's study is the over-all situation which shows that despite gradual improvement fewer than 25 per cent of practicing physicians indulge in any kind of formal or organized postgraduate education.

At the Second World Congress on Medical Education,[14] held in Chicago in 1959, representatives of many foreign countries reported similar inadequate attendance by practicing physicians in any form of continued educational program. In Great Britain serious attempts were made, including reimbursement of general practitioners for time away from their practice, but still only about 10 per cent of such practitioners attended educational exercises.

It is abundantly clear that the need for the continued education of the practicing physician is greater than ever and that it is growing year by year as the sheer bulk of medical knowledge increases under the stimulus of an unprecedented volume of medical research in this country. In recent years there is evidence that the medical profession is increasingly concerned about the inadequacy of some of its members. The stimulus to the physician to improve his knowledge is, in the main, his own conscience and desire to keep abreast. More and more, physicians are becoming trained as specialists and are being certified by specialty boards organized for this purpose. However, once board certification is achieved there is no further examination or checking upon the physician's maintenance of an adequate level of competence. Only the Academy of General Practice has the requirement of a fixed amount of postgraduate education for continued qualification.

Membership on hospital staffs is dependent upon satisfactory compliance with medical standards as set by the Joint Commission on Accreditation of Hospitals, but there is no standard concerning postgraduate education of the physician. Dr. John Leonard[15] of the Hartford Hospital medical staff, a man known for his interest in education in the hospital, suggested in a presentation at the Congress on Medical Education in 1961 that the medical profession and hospital staffs should develop requirements concerning postgraduate education for the maintenance of hospital staff appointments.

The American Medical Association and the Association of

American Medical Colleges are concerned about continuing education. Until recently these associations have done little except urge the development of more and better programs for postgraduate education, make reviews of the over-all situation, and express the belief that something should be done. These two associations and the American Hospital Association sponsored a study titled "Lifetime Learning for Physicians," [16] which was published in June 1962. This study offers a provocative stimulus to the field of medical education. In contrast to other studies, it spends less time analyzing the present situation and more on an imaginative approach to solutions. To indicate the seriousness of the situation two of the report's three assumptions (the third said that the problem is national and requires a national plan) are: (1) "Our first assumption is that the continuing education of physicians is one of the most important problems facing medical education today," and (2) "There is a serious gap between available knowledge and application in medical practice."

In regard to the latter point, the study points up some dramatic illustrations of this serious gap as it relates to the advances in the field of drug therapy. For instance, in the last ten years there have been: an increase of 370 per cent in the drugs known as "anti-obesity" preparations; an increase of 400 per cent in preparations used to treat cardiovascular disease; an increase of 250 per cent in drugs used in the treatment of diabetes; and an increase of nearly 2,000 per cent in the diuretic preparations used in the treatment of heart and kidney disease. The problem of keeping up with names, chemical compositions, and dosages is a substantial one in itself.

I enjoy most, however, the description of the situation ten years ago as given by your own Boston physician, Dr. Laurence B. Ellis, in his "Reflections on Postgraduate Medical Education for Practicing Physicians." [17] Dr. Ellis says:

The continuing professional education of practicing physicians constitutes one of the most important, difficult and neglected problems facing American medicine today. It is unnecessary to labor the point that the complexity and rapidity of developments in all branches of medical knowledge have forced the modern physician to be continually going to school if he is to be considered competent and well trained. It is no longer sufficient for a man to have a background of study in a good medical school and as an intern and resident. Granted, therefore, that the doctor needs retraining, a corollary is that the general practitioner in the country needs this retraining most of all. This is true because of the wide scope of his practice, which often embraces, of necessity, specialties with which the urban practitioner does not concern himself and because of his relative isolation from contacts with his medical fellows. The problem of providing adequate opportunities for medical education of these doctors is the most difficult. Undoubtedly, one of the great deterrents to entering country practice has been this failure to provide proper means for keeping up to date. A solution would go a great way toward maintaining medical practice at a high standard in the rural areas and also in easing maldistribution of physicians between the country and the city.

In view of these facts it is surprising how little attention the problem has received. Neither the proponents of "individual enterprise" nor the advocates of socialized medicine have much to say about this cardinal requirement for providing good medicine. Medical schools, so much bedeviled by their own economics, have, with few exceptions, hesitated to branch into a field that might entail a drain on their overburdened exchequers. Foundations have provided millions for research but have done relatively little about the weak link in the chain between producer and ultimate consumer. Of what use is all the knowledge building up in the laboratories if its practical fruits, the proper technics of application, are not being taught?

Conditions today, ten years later, are much the same, it is sad to observe.

The report "Lifetime Learning for Physicians" [18] could have significant impact on the postgraduate education program. Dr. Bernard Dryer, the Study Director of the Joint Study Committee in Continuing Medical Education, indicates that the problem is national and requires a national plan. He further points out that medicine has not taken full advantage of the modern teaching techniques and instructional aids that have developed in recent years. He refers particularly to the use of electronic equipment as teaching aids and television, which he believes can be a useful teaching device if properly programmed. The report suggests the development of a series of presentations in the various fields of medicine which could be made available as "core" curricula for educational programs in local communities and regions. It is suggested that the universities and medical schools be central forces for the organization of such local and regional programs with the actual instruction occurring in medical societies, health departments, and community hospitals. Dryer refers to this over-all program as a "university without walls" for the continued education of the physician.

It is proposed that there be created a nationwide "university without walls" for continuing medical education. This term implies that the organization should have the function and independence of a university, but need not have the physical plant, resident faculty, and resident student body which a university ordinarily has. Its functions should be those of teaching, research, development, and coordination in continuing medical education.

Three of the objectives as stated in the report are:

Focus should be on the patient, through the physician.

All physicians should have equal opportunity to continue their medical education, in order that all physicians may be lifelong students.

The opportunity for continuing education should be available at a time, place, and pace convenient to each physician.

Although not so clearly stated as the objectives, the report seems to identify the community hospital as a very important focal point for the education. Hospital trustees, administrators, and active staff members, I believe, will all recognize the potential of educating the doctor on some nationally conceived scheme in the community hospital. There are many arguments that can be made in favor of the use of the community hospital but, again, I wish to refer to the words of Dr. Ellis, who vividly describes the inadequacies of the formal course method of education and speaks highly for the hospital.

The character of most instruction also leaves much to be desired. My great uncle attended Harvard Medical School by purchasing a series of course tickets for lectures on pharmacology, materia medica and so forth. Educators shudder at the quality of that type of undergraduate instruction today, when bedside teaching and learning by doing are the order of things. But how does the modern general practitioner get his instruction? — by lectures, usually poorly delivered, at a time of day when both he and the lecturer are nodding with fatigue. Why is the type of instruction that was outmoded fifty years ago for medical students the best for the physician in practice? The answer is that it is not, but that postgraduate education is fifty years behind the times.

At present the best modern physician education is obtained by daily attendance at a large modern teaching hospital with exposure to the stimulus of eager residents and medical students in discussions at the bedside of well studied patients, and by intimate and informal contact with many specialists in various fields at conferences, at the luncheon table, and in the hospital corridors. Those fortunate enough to have this kind of teaching frequently do not appreciate it, it is so much a part of their medical lives. It cannot fully be attained except in limited areas. But this goal can be aimed for everywhere, and it has been demonstrated in many comparatively rural areas that it can be reached.

In the first place, education should be part of the daily life of the physician, not a special event like a holiday. Therefore, it must be brought to him.

Dr. Ellis goes on to say: "The best way of bringing medical teaching to the doctor's own doorstep is to develop in the community hospital an approximation of the teaching hospital." And then he describes how regular visits by residents in training and consultants can create this approximation.

Dr. Ellis recognizes the value of such a teaching program in the community hospital as far as medical care standards and general features are considered. He says:

This type of program has incidental effects that should be of vast benefit to the local medical community. It is a great stimulus to the establishment of the regional hospital as the hub around which the medical practice in each area rotates. This it accomplishes by helping to maintain and even raise medical standards, giving the community a sense of pride and accomplishment and making it a more attractive place in which to settle and practice. When coordinated programs are established between hospitals the neutral ground of these programs brings together groups from different hospitals within the city or between neighboring towns, which are sometimes divided by factional differences.

## THE HOSPITAL AS AN EDUCATIONAL INSTITUTION

Not only are hospitals convenient places for the education of the physician, but hospitals themselves are deeply rooted in education. For many years the large teaching centers have been engaged in extensive and high-quality educational programs in medicine, nursing, dentistry, and other allied health fields. Our hospitals are patterned after the hospitals in Europe, particularly those in Great Britain where education of the student has been a function of the hospital for many centuries. English medicine in particular brought to our hospitals and medical schools the clinical clerkship and bedside teaching of the medical student. The values of this to medical education are now fully accepted.

In Flexner's report on medical education in the United States of the early twentieth century, in addition to the basic recommendation that the responsibility and sponsorship of medical student instruction should be in the universities, he repeatedly pointed out the desirability, if not the necessity, of each medical school having a close and intimate attachment with a good hospital in which the instruction in clinical medicine could be carried out. In the years following the report, leading medical educators were repeatedly emphasizing the need for each school to have such an intimate hospital association. This concept has developed far beyond the expectations of those days, and with the great growth in specialty training, hospitals have not only accepted medical students, interns, and residents, but are now aggressively seeking even a larger educational role.

There have been changes in the setting of medical education in our community hospitals. The decrease in the numbers of charity or ward patients has moved the education of students and house staff into the private patient's room. There are more standards and requirements for education to be met in the hospital and this greater organization and direction of educational efforts require full-time physician members of hospital staffs. In the attempt to improve intern and residency training there has developed a new position in hospital medical organization known as the "Director of Medical Education." Individuals in this position are appointed with the responsibility to organize, direct, and sometimes actually conduct educational programs. Beginning only a few years ago, there are now nearly 1,000 directors of medical education in our hospitals.[19] Although it is true that one of the major reasons for the development of these positions was to recruit interns and residents, the by-products for hospitals which may never qualify for house staff training may be very great. One may be an improved method of staff education itself, one of the most effective forms of postgraduate education of the physician.

## THE CHANGING ROLE OF THE PHYSICIAN IN THE HOSPITAL

There are other reasons which favor the development of postgraduate education of the physician on hospital staffs. In modern medical practice, physicians must have hospital appointments and privileges to care for their patients who are seriously ill. Not too many years ago, a physician could conduct most of his practice in the office or in the home. This is changing and, increasingly, the physician depends upon the facilities and services of the hospital for the proper care of his patients. More physicians are developing practices in groups, and they do so often in close association with a hospital. Hospital medical practice proceeds at a much faster pace than formerly, and standards of quality of physician care in hospital practice are increasing. Physicians on the staff must meet those requirements imposed by the new and rapidly increasing standards. Physicians, being self-governing and self-disciplining as far as quality of medical care is concerned, are finding it increasingly difficult to do this with only a "visiting" or "attending" status on the hospital staff. More and more, the physicians feel the need for better organization of the departments within the hospital, with an increasing number of hospitals developing full-time chiefs-of-service for better operation of the departments. This means that the physician is becoming an intimate partner in the daily operation of the hospital, and methods are being developed to give him more authority in the daily management of the hospital. This will increase the opportunity for the doctor to develop the hospital's teaching program.

At the same time, there is evidence that the physician in his local and state medical society is exposed less to continuing education and more to the physician's socioeconomic and political responsibilities. Thus, it can be argued that the natural shift of the physician's educational opportunity is in some degree from medical society to hospital staff.

## A HOSPITAL PROGRAM FOR THE CONTINUING EDUCATION OF THE PHYSICIAN

These observations on the need for education, changes in medical practices and the hospital's role in them suggest general goals toward which our communities might work.

Each major medical teaching center, that is, a medical school and its affiliated hospital or hospitals, might become the headquarters of an administration and a faculty which could provide the leadership required to generate an educational program to serve the physicians and hospitals lying in the center's natural area of geographic proximity and medical influence. The center would provide from its own resources (and this could be a flexible matter and vary widely) the program for teaching of medical students, some intern-resident training, medical research, and formal postgraduate courses for the region's physicians.

Each center would, in turn, have a primary affiliation with several large community hospitals where staff physicians selected by the center faculty could develop intern-resident education under the direction of the school and organize the regular staff work of the hospital around a postgraduate educational program. There should be substantial staff overlap between the major center and these affiliating teaching hospitals.

Each affiliating teaching hospital would, in its turn, associate with the staffs of several smaller, nonaffiliated community hospitals for regular "work-a-day" postgraduate education. It is believed there are many competent teachers on the staffs of affiliating teaching hospitals who, if given the proper organizational support, would relish the opportunity to give vent to their teaching urges by joining the staffs of smaller hospitals.

A plan such as I propose here, of course, needs over-all organization and support. A national organization might supply materials and some general guide lines, but the compelling force must come from the local teaching center. These schools and hospitals will need facilities, funds, and personnel beyond those now available for their "at home" programs. The center faculties will also need more effective control of the medical staff organization of the community hospitals which affiliate with them. This will be no easy task!

Let me urge that experiments and demonstrations along this line be encouraged. Except for the cost of nationally developed materials, the added costs in the teaching medical center for faculty and staff and the appointment of paid medical officers in affiliating hospitals (which positions could be justified on the basis of medical supervision as well as medical education) are not likely to be too great. The hospital facilities exist now, the physicians in practice

want and can participate in the educational process at the proper
level, and they need not be provided substantial extra compensation
for their educational time.

Demonstrations and experiments will prove the desirability of
developing a standard for the accreditation of hospitals that relates
to such an educational program; and if the system proves effective,
a hospital's full accreditation would ultimately depend in part upon
its ability to participate in such a regional educational program.

This educational program, of course, is reminiscent of the plan
on the integration of hospital services suggested by Mountin, Pennell, and Hoge of the Public Health Service in 1945. Their publication "Health Service Areas: Requirements for General Hospitals and Health Centers," [20] proposes a regional plan for hospital
services for the entire United States, with rural hospitals and health
centers being related to district and regional hospital centers. Progress in the development of a system of this type has been discour-
agingly slow. It still is sound from the standpoint of the efficient
delivery of high-quality hospital services. It fits hand in glove with
a regional system of postgraduate education of the physician.

As the title of this Lowell Lecture series indicates, our hospitals
are community agencies created, supported, and directed by community groups. Hospitals and the medical profession they serve
must change with the changing dimensions of medicine and general
socioeconomic changes. Solo, independent home and office practice
of medicine is *not* now meeting, and *will* not in the future meet,
the needs of modern medicine and society. Medical practice will
be more and more performed by groups working on a team basis
with a merging of many special talents. Likewise, hospitals must
face the challenge of not giving their services on a solo, independent basis, which today means that each hospital attempts to give all
possible services to all members of the community. A group hospital
service mechanism must emerge as the only efficient and progressive method. A regional system of graded hospital services seems
highly desirable. The teaching medical center — a medical school
and affiliated hospitals — is logically the base unit of this type of
integrated hospital service.

As it always has, the education of the physician will be heavily
related to the hospital and hospital services. It seems logical and
exciting to develop postgraduate medical education on such a re-

gional hospital system. Let us hope that some of our communities, and particularly our teaching medical centers, will see this opportunity and make the start into a new and improved system of hospital and medical education.

# MEDICAL EDUCATION AND MEDICAL CARE: AN EXAMINATION OF TRADITIONAL CONCEPTS AND SUGGESTIONS FOR CHANGE

Thomas McKeown, M.D.

THE organization of a modern medical service, concerned with the prevention and treatment of disease as well as with the care of those for whom neither has been wholly successful, is among the most complex tasks facing society. Some of the reasons for the complexity are obvious. There is first the difficulty of defining objectives. Is medicine concerned only with the prevention of disease and the care of the sick — in itself a sufficiently exacting goal — or should it also seek to promote the elusive concept of positive health? Secondly, even if the more limited objective is accepted, the available indexes of achievement are quite inadequate. We have some information about mortality, less about morbidity, and almost none at all about the ability of a doctor or the efficiency of a hospital. Thirdly, there is the formidable problem of assessing priorities within the wide range of resources on which health depends. What priority do the medical services merit in relation to the other competing social services which contribute powerfully to health? And what is the relative importance of medical measures which range from psychotherapy to surgical procedures? Finally there is the costliness of the application of medical knowledge which makes the finance of medical care a source of anxiety even in the wealthiest countries. These are among the problems which must be faced, and there can be no easy solution.

There is however another class of difficulty, less obvious, but not less important. It is that in important respects the traditional pattern of medical service is inappropriate to the major tasks which lie ahead. For while the problems with which medicine is confronted and the methods available for their solution have both changed dramatically during the past hundred years, the pattern of service has tended to remain fixed in a mold determined in quite different circumstances. Let us now examine the grounds for this assertion.

## THE PROBLEM

In relation to health the experience of England and Wales has been fairly typical of that of other developed countries. Until the eighteenth century, over any considerable period there was only a slight excess of births over deaths and the population increased very slowly. It began to increase rapidly about 1770 and the rise has continued to the present time. It is attributed, plausibly before 1838[1] and confidently after that date (when national birth rates and death rates were first recorded), to a decline of mortality. From the public viewpoint there is no more important issue in medical history than the explanation for the reduction of mortality since the eighteenth century. Reasons have been given for the belief that in order of relative importance the main influences before the twentieth century were: a rising standard of living; the hygienic changes introduced by the sanitary reformers; and a favorable trend in the relationship between infectious agent and human host. The effect of therapy was restricted to smallpox and had only a trivial effect on the total reduction of the death rate.[2]

The interpretation of the reasons for the continued decline of mortality during the twentieth century is considerably more complex, because of the introduction since 1900 of the personal health services and the discovery of some effective forms of therapy. But whatever uncertainties there are about the reasons for the decline of mortality there is no serious doubt about its effects. A comparison of mortality according to age at death in 1838–1854 and 1950–1952 indicated that whereas formerly there were substantial numbers of deaths at all periods of life — prenatal, prereproductive, reproductive, and postreproductive — they are now largely restricted to the prenatal and postreproductive periods.[3] The effect on cause of death has been equally dramatic. One hundred years ago, and indeed until well into the twentieth century, infectious disease was everywhere the predominant problem. Today the most important problems confronting medicine in developed countries are: prenatal mortality and malformation; mental defect and mental illness; and the disease and disability associated with aging. This conclusion is also consistent with the admittedly inadequate evidence concerning morbidity.

## THE METHODS

Since control of reproduction has played no significant part in advancement of human health, the effective control of disease has so far depended almost entirely upon control of the environment, and chiefly of the postnatal environment. This has been brought about either by modification of the physical environment in which the individual lives, or by direct interference with the body through such measures as protective inoculations, drug treatment, and surgery.

Until the nineteenth century the scope of all these measures was very restricted. Apart from the rising standard of living which was a by-product of the industrial revolution, the improvement of the physical environment began with sanitary reform in the mid-nineteenth century. Internationally this task is far from complete; indeed in a large part of the world it has scarcely begun. But in developed countries great advances have been made, and if control of the physical environment is still incomplete, we are at least aware of the steps upon which it depends. On the other hand the control of the social environment — the influence of the behavior of human beings upon one another — is merely beginning. It can hardly be doubted that this is one of the most important methods now available for development.

With the single exception of vaccination against smallpox it is doubtful whether specific therapy, protective or curative, had any substantial effect on the course of disease before the present century. Until 1800 surgery was limited to a few procedures — amputation, lithotomy, trephining of the skull, incision of abscess, and operation for cataract — whose results in the absence of anesthesia and knowledge of antisepsis were exceedingly bad. In the light of what we now know, few of the many drugs then in use can have been effective. In the nineteenth century the improvement in understanding of the nature of disease, and particularly of infectious disease, and the discovery of anesthesia and antisepsis, prepared the way for the advance of methods in the twentieth. There are now a considerable number of specific preventive procedures of varying effectiveness, chiefly against infectious disease. And since the discovery of insulin in 1920 the range of useful curative treatment has been considerably enlarged.

From this short review it is clear that useful methods to prevent and treat disease have evolved rapidly in the past. They were almost nonexistent in the early nineteenth century and exist in profusion today. It seems quite certain that methods can be expected to develop even more rapidly in future, possibly on the following lines: an extension of the methods already in use for control of the physical environment; the discovery and application of knowledge concerning the social environment; the elaboration of more effective methods of prevention and treatment of disease in the individual; and the introduction of more satisfactory methods of care of patients who in spite of attempts to prevent and treat disease are left with some degree of residual impairment. This last is a very large, and at present greatly underestimated task.

## THE SERVICES

If methods which are developing rapidly are to be applied to problems which are constantly changing, the services through which they are mobilized must also evolve. Unfortunately the pattern of medical services tends to be relatively inflexible. It owes its character largely to historical circumstances, among which the following were particularly important. (1) The earlier limited concept of public responsibility. In the first half of the nineteenth century society accepted virtually no responsibility for health. In a little over a hundred years its obligations have increased rapidly, and today the only decision is between a large and a complete public commitment. But during the past century multiple interests —

public, religious, voluntary, and private — have become involved in the administration and finance of medical care. This complex framework now prejudices a rational organization of services. (2) A second important influence was the way and the order in which different facets of service came to public attention. The different origins of mental, chronic, and general hospitals has had a profound impact on the present-day hospital services, and the fact that prevention of infectious disease was more urgent than cure largely determined the character of the public health service. (3) Another significant influence was the predominance of infectious disease, particularly in young people, in the period when our concept of service was acquired. When many young patients were suffering from short-term remediable illnesses it was understandable — although on a longer view regrettable — that hospital design and service should be conceived in relation to short-term investigation and treatment. The same premise is quite inappropriate when the predominant problems are mental illness and the diseases associated with aging.

These considerations help us to understand the forces which have shaped the medical services; they also suggest steps which will be necessary if they are to be remolded. In any circumstances the task of assembling medical services appropriate to the needs of the second half of the twentieth century must be difficult; it will be impossible if decisions cannot be taken on their merits. Hitherto services have been improvised to fit into an existing administrative and financial framework; the complexity of the resources on which health depends is such that their potential cannot be realized unless administration and finance are made to accord with the needs of service.

There are many circumstances which restrict the improvement of medical services but three are of outstanding importance. They are: the separation — physical, administrative, and in some countries financial — between mental, chronic, and acute hospitals; the division between institutional and extrainstitutional care; and the separation of preventive from curative medicine imposed by the traditional pattern of public health service. In the present context we shall be concerned chiefly with the first of these themes but reference will also be made to the other two.

## THE SEPARATION OF MENTAL, CHRONIC, AND ACUTE HOSPITALS

Many of the problems which confront the hospital service are rooted in the traditional separation of acute, mental, and chronic hospital services from one another. This subdivision does not correspond to the medical, nursing, and social needs of patients and is wholly attributable to historical circumstances. I shall describe the way in which it developed in the United Kingdom.

### Origins

The divisions of the hospital population are attributable to two reasons. The first is because the various facets of the hospital problem presented to society different problems at different times. Until the nineteenth century the main object of the asylums was protection of the community from the supposed risks of the insane, and the method adopted was a penal one: patients were locked up and chastised. Gradually during the nineteenth century the idea that patients needed care took root. But it was only recently that the possibility of investigation and treatment was seriously considered, and by then a tradition of separate administration of mental hospitals was firmly rooted.

The institutional care of the chronic sick also developed in a different form. Traditionally the problem was inseparable from that of destitution; those who were sick were often poor, and those who were chronically sick were almost invariably so. The important arm of the British hospital system which cared for the sick poor for almost a hundred years came into existence, unplanned, in 1834, when admission to a workhouse was made a condition of public assistance under the Poor Law. It is scarcely surprising that in these circumstances the concept of institutional care for the chronic sick was that of a bare minimum, wholly divorced from the investigation and treatment which from the late nineteenth century became the predominant interest in general hospitals.

The second reason for the present division of the hospital system was the need to provide for certain classes of patients at public expense. Had the mentally ill and chronic sick not been accepted as a public responsibility, they would not have been cared for at all. But a very substantial part of hospital practice was under voluntary auspices in Great Britain until 1948. It was inevitable that the different methods of administration and finance should be reflected in separate hospital systems.

### Disadvantages

The disadvantages of the isolation of the major classes of hospitals from one another may be summarized as follows: (1) The traditional segregation does not provide at each hospital center patients homogeneous in respect of their medical and social needs. Patients in mental and chronic hospitals may exhibit the full range of mental and physical illness, and some of them are indistinguishable clinically from others admitted to general hospitals. Even in general hospitals the population is by no means homogeneous, a fact to which the recent concept of progressive patient care gives welcome recognition. (2) The distinction between the major classes of hospitals gives the erroneous impression that patients fall naturally into acute and chronic classes. If services were adequate there would undoubtedly be some bimodality in the distribution of duration of hospital care, but the sharply bimodal distribution is an artifact attributable to deficient services at mental and chronic hospitals and to the reluctance of general hospitals to retain patients for more than short periods. The need for acute care may be prolonged and some short-term patients do not need the services of a general hospital. (3) The difficulty of staffing mental and chronic hospitals, which, with an aging population, can only become more serious, is largely caused by their isolation. Doctors and nurses who work in them must isolate themselves from the main streams of medical interest. (4) Segregation of hospitals has also removed from the view, and hence from the interest, of research workers some of the most important medical problems. It can hardly be doubted that progress in understanding of mental deficiency and schizophrenia would have been more rapid if those affected were seen more often at general, and particularly at teaching, hospitals. (5) When they are isolated from one another hospitals cannot achieve economies by pooling resources and by relating facilities to patients' needs. The concept of hospitals as single, more or less self-contained units was an inevitable consequence of their isolation. The range of services which patients require is so wide that it should be reflected in variation in design, equipment, and staffing. The single building provides only limited scope for this adaptation of design to function. (6) The traditional hospital building, which is in large part the product of the system of segregation, is inherently inflexible. Having regard to the rapidity and unpredictability of change in medical problems and methods, the hospital should be capable of growth and change. The scope for both is greatly restricted in the contemporary hospital.

*Proposals*

In order to avoid these and some other disadvantages it was suggested that in future hospitals should be planned with the following features: subject to a reservation in the case of teaching hospitals, all types of patients should be accommodated at the center in approximately the proportions in which they occur in the whole hospital population; patients should be classified strictly according to their medical, nursing, and other needs and placed in the facilities most suitable for their care; the hospital community should consist of a number of buildings, of varied size and permanence of structure, each designed, equipped, and staffed according to the needs of the patients to be admitted; medical and nursing services should be provided by a common staff; and the relationship of the hospital center to the community around it should be much more intimate than hitherto.

The most significant effect of implementation of the first two proposals would be elimination of the traditional divisions between the physically and mentally ill, and between old and younger patients. The third proposal would change the hospital from a single building providing a full range of services for selected patients to a group of buildings providing complementary services for all classes of patients. A common staff would mean that all doctors and nurses would make a contribution to the care of all types of patients. The last proposal would remove the barrier which now separates the services in hospitals from those provided by general practitioners and local health authorities.

*A Balanced Hospital Community*

A hospital center incorporating the features suggested above was referred to as a balanced hospital community.[4] Its adoption would affect in greater or less degree almost all hospital services, but its greatest impact would be on psychiatric and geriatric care, which have suffered most from past deficiencies.

The decision to eliminate the mental hospital would indeed be a large one requiring substantial justification. The central reason is that it is only by ending the different sites of mental and other hospitals that we can hope to shift the different attitudes to mental and other illness. On the common site and with a common staff it should also be possible to raise the standard of care for the mentally ill to a level long regarded as obligatory in the general hospital. Similar considerations apply to the geriatric patients, who in Great Britain today have inherited the facilities in chronic hospitals provided formerly by the Poor Law Authority for the destitute sick. Under the National Health Service there has been a considerable improvement in standards of care in these hospitals, but they still suffer from the deficiencies inherent in their isolation.

The assembly of all institutional medical care at the same site will provide the opportunity to establish, and to use efficiently, the full range of services related to patients' needs. The education of a mental defective, the retraining of a psychotic, speech therapy for the hemiplegic, basic nursing of a bed-fast invalid, the delivery of a normal infant, and investigation of a congenital cardiac abnormality are all part of the medical task. Yet they are entirely different activities requiring different space, equipment, and staff. The grounds for separating them in different facilities are as strong as for separating arts, biology, and engineering on the university campus, or for not requiring the shopper to walk past or through a public library in the same building to get to the butcher's store. But while multiple buildings are essential so too is the integration of services. It is imperative that elderly patients who become seriously confused should be admitted quickly to psychiatric care, and that patients under psychiatric supervision who no longer require it should be transferred. It is the structural interrelation of buildings and functional integration of services which distinguishes the balanced hospital community from the concept of the hospital center which was current during the 1930's.

## THE DIVISION BETWEEN INSTITUTIONAL AND EXTRA-INSTITUTIONAL CARE

It is evident that the size and character of the task confronting hospitals is greatly influenced by the services which exist outside them. Even if our concern is mainly with hospital services some attention must be given to the three questions: What services, if any, should be provided in patients' homes? Where should the ambulant patient normally see his doctor? What relationship should exist between hospital and other services? The variation in the answers being provided in different countries and even within the same country indicates that these questions need more critical examination than they have so far received.

### Home Services

In some countries, including the United States, it is becoming increasingly difficult to maintain medical services in patients' homes, and there are some people who doubt whether it is desirable to do so. In Great Britain, where home services are a traditional feature, a valiant attempt is being made to encourage and support the general practitioner who provides them.

If economical use of the doctor's time were the only consideration there can be little doubt where the balance of advantage would lie. Nevertheless there are reasons why home care is desirable. It may be more economical, if the alternative is to admit the patient to hospital. It facilitates, if it is not certainly essential for, the provision of personal medical care (under which each patient has his own doctor). And it enables the doctor to know and to manipulate the patient's social and physical environment. These considerations may be particularly important in the care of psychiatric and geriatric patients who will call so heavily on medical services in future.

## Ambulatory Care

Although not the central issue related to domiciliary care, the site at which the ambulant patient normally sees his doctor is important. There are three possibilities: the doctor's surgery or office; the hospital; or some neutral center such as a polyclinic or health center. The variations in nomenclature in current use for these facilities need not detain us.

The center for ambulatory care should have three requirements. It should be capable of accommodating a group of doctors and ancillary workers. It should be equipped with facilities for investigation and some forms of treatment. And it should be reasonably accessible to the homes of patients who use it. The first two requirements rule out the independent doctor's office as the ideal site, and the third, in some countries at least, usually rules out the hospital. Hence there is probably a place for some intermediate facility between home and hospital, less well equipped than the hospital out-patient department, but better equipped and staffed than is usually feasible in the independent office or surgery.

## The Relationship Between Hospital and Other Medical Care

So far we have envisaged the care of the sick patient at home and of the ambulant patient at health centers unless the services needed are of a kind best provided in hospital. We must now consider the relationship which should exist between home and hospital services. Clearly if there are to be no home services this issue does not arise. But if home services are offered we must consider the role, if any, of the domiciliary doctor in hospital and his relationship to the hospital-based specialist.

In Great Britain the National Health Service does not require the doctor providing home services to work in hospital, although it allows him to do so as a clinical assistant. There are two reasons, however, why hospital appointment of the domiciliary doctor should be an essential feature of a medical service. First, it is only in this way that he can keep abreast of the rapid advance of medical knowledge. And second, the free movement of patients — particularly the mentally ill and aged sick — between the wide range of extra-institutional and institutional facilities require that a change of site should not involve a change of doctor.

The relationship of the domiciliary doctor working in hospital to the hospital-based specialist is a complex matter and considerable thought and experience will be necessary in order to shape it. It has been suggested [5] that the concept of family practice stands in the way of this development, and that it would be better to base domiciliary care on the work of four doctors — obstetrician, pediatrician, general physician, and geriatrician. Each would function as a personal doctor and would be responsible for hospital as well as home care. They would be supported in the hospital by specialists who would provide services involving complex techniques as well as those of a simpler technical character in which referred work is a necessary condition of expert practice. Under these arrangements personal care would be based on broad age groups with relatively homogeneous medical and related social problems and referred work would be restricted to techniques and diseases to which it is appropriate.

### The Separation of Preventive from Curative Medicine

The third of the three major problems referred to at the outset has less direct bearing in the planning of hospital services. Yet it is an essential element in the medical scene and deserves at least brief consideration in any comprehensive discussion of medical services.

In most developed countries the public medical services are little more than a hundred years old. For about the first half of this period they were restricted to the control of the physical environment, and it was inevitable that they should have been administered by local health authorities. Early in the twentieth century it was decided to extend public responsibility into the field of personal care, but the form of this extension was a matter of prolonged and bitter dispute. In the end the compromise arrived at was that the new personal health services should be concerned exclusively with preventive measures. Almost inevitably, from the outset they were linked administratively with the existing environmental services under local authorities. This history determined the character of the traditional public health service based on the premise that the prevention of disease was a public matter and its treatment was private. This principle was ignored only in relation to mental illness, the destitute sick, and infectious disease, where the public commitment for medical care was inescapable.

The long-term significance of this decision is of course that the grouping of preventive personal care with environmental services separated them from the main body of medical work both outside and inside the hospital. Moreover this division is not restricted to countries where treatment of disease is still largely under private finance. It has been retained in Great Britain and elsewhere whether the public obligation for curative services is extensive or complete.

It is unnecessary to labor the disadvantages of this tradition which has been widely criticized in recent years. The anomaly of antenatal care divorced from other obstetric services, and of separation of responsibility for the well and for the sick child, has been recognized. It remains to be decided how best to realign the preventive personal health services but there can be little dispute about the necessity to do so.

## MEDICAL EDUCATION AND MEDICAL CARE

In the foregoing discussion it has been suggested that the problem of organizing the services through which medical knowledge is applied is immensely complex, and some of the restrictions which make it even more difficult have been referred to. It should be stressed that removal of these restrictions will not of itself provide a solution; it will merely create the framework within which a solution can be sought. Moreover since the tasks confronting medicine and the methods at our disposal for solving them are constantly changing, the pattern of service cannot be expected to reach final form but must also continue to evolve. The contribution of the teaching center to this evolution is of crucial importance. A medical service can be no more enlightened than the minds of the doctors who provide it and the intellectual shutters are never again so widely open as during the period of training.

It is for this reason that the traditional restriction of the interests of teaching hospitals is so regrettable. To a considerable extent they have isolated themselves from problems around them. In the developed countries it is possible to graduate with little knowledge or concern about mental illness, and in developing countries it is notorious that doctors cannot be attracted away from the large towns. Their interests are an inevitable reflection of the interests of the teaching center and it will be futile to attempt to change the one without changing the other.

If the interests of teaching hospitals are to be enlarged it is essential to understand why hitherto they have been restricted. The main reason is historical. They inherited the tradition of the voluntary hospitals which from the beginning was highly selective. Their concern was with short-term illness; and the intractable problems of mental illness, sickness associated with destitution, and infectious disease were left mainly to public authorities. However, there are some who believe that even if the selectiveness of teaching centers is historical in origin there is contemporary justification for it. They argue, reasonably, that teaching centers should be the focus of medical research, and conclude, unreasonably, that this justifies limiting their work mainly to patients in respect of whom knowledge is advancing.

The objections to this argument are threefold. In the first place, while some kinds of advance unquestionably require concentration of selected patients, there are other kinds which are prohibited by it. The problems surrounding the etiology of essential hypertension will not be solved by exclusive attention to those affected, and without knowledge of the behavior of blood pressure in the related population. More obvious, even the most able research worker can make no headway with problems he never sees, and reference has already been made to the way in which isolation has retarded advance of understanding of mental deficiency and schizophrenia.

A second objection to the restrictive work of teaching centers is that it does not provide a sufficient preparation for the practice of medicine. It seems unnecessary to stress that at the completion of training the doctor should have a reasonable grasp of the problems confronting medicine in his country at the time, and of the best means within the resources available for solving them. More than this, his view of the contemporary challenge should be such that he will want to make his contribution to meeting it. This will not happen so long as the role of the teaching hospital is restricted to short-term institutional care of a selected group of patients.

The third objection to complacency about the usual organization of teaching centers is that they are prevented from making much contribution to thought about the way in which medical knowledge is applied. Some people consider that while the acquisition of knowledge about health and disease is a matter of profound interest and importance, its application is a humdrum affair which can be left to the administrator. This viewpoint is reflected in the contemporary organization of research which finds little place for concern with services. Thus investigation of the biochemistry of schizophrenia is regarded as a proper subject for scientific enquiry; investigation of services for the schizophrenic is not. In reply it should be necessary only to stress that, on the contrary, the problems raised by the application of medical knowledge in a complex world are at least as formidable as those associated with its acquisition. They are unlikely to be solved unless they are taken seriously at teaching centers.

Indeed it is important to recognize that the need for a fresh approach to the planning of medical services arises on intellectual as well as on humanitarian grounds, and it is interesting to reflect on the reasons why so exacting a task should ever have appeared pedestrian. It was not so in the nineteenth century, when some of the best minds were concerned with the association between social conditions and ill health, and with the public action needed to effect improvement. We owe to their efforts the most important specific measures ever introduced, the control of the physical environment. Unfortunately, by the turn of the century, what had begun as a great adventure had taken the form of a routine service: efficient and essential; but not stimulating or challenging. And subsequent controversy concerning medical services has been overlaid by political, financial, and other considerations which have obscured the essential complexity and interest of the task.

Modern medical services are expensive and have to be paid for and it is probable that the only issue is whether public responsibility for them shall be large or complete. But the provision of a workable financial and administrative framework bears the same relationship to the satisfactory design of a medical service as the release of the first rocket bears to the exploration of outer space. It is no more than a beginning.

## SUMMARY

During the past century the problems confronting medicine have been transformed, essentially from the infectious diseases to those arising before birth or to mental illness and the disease and disability associated with aging. Similarly the methods available for the solution of these problems have evolved rapidly and continue to do so. Unfortunately the services by means of which the methods are mobilized have tended to remain static in a mold determined in earlier and very different circumstances.

Hitherto medical services have been improvised to fit into an existing administrative and financial framework. The complexity of the resources on which health depends is such that their potential cannot be realized unless administration and finance are made to accord with the needs of services. Specifically this requires the removal of traditional barriers: between the major classes of hospitals — acute, mental, and chronic; between institutional and extra-institutional services; and between preventive and curative medicine. The country which first achieves this rationalization of services will have achieved a break-through — to use the conventional phrase — at least as significant as any in the understanding or treatment of disease.

In bringing about this transformation of the medical scene the medical school and teaching hospital have a crucial place. It is widely believed that while the acquisition of knowledge of disease is a matter of profound interest and importance, its application is a humdrum affair which can be left to the administrator. Thus investigation of the biochemistry of schizophrenia is regarded as a proper subject for scientific inquiry; investigation of the organization of services for the schizophrenic is not. To a considerable extent this viewpoint is attributable to the fact that teaching centers have isolated themselves from the problems around them. They have never been prepared to contribute to thought about the organization of services because of the mistaken idea that to do so would threaten the standards and values to which they have aspired. If progress is not to be jeopardized this viewpoint must be changed. And the reason for this change is that the problems raised by the application of medical knowledge in a complex world are at least as formidable as those associated with its acquisition. Their solution will require, and will tax, the best minds that can be brought to them.

# THE HEALTH NEEDS OF COMMUNITIES

Erich Lindemann, M.D.

THERE has been a revolution in the orientation of psychiatrists. During the last decade the segregation of the mentally sick into secluded hospitals has slowly been yielding to the new point of view that mental illness deserves the same services and care as does physical illness. Custodial care has been replaced by chemotherapy and psychotherapy. Special programs for night care and day care as well as half-way houses have been developed to serve better at various stages of the recuperative process.

In general hospitals, also, there has been a gradual increase in psychiatric facilities and, what is more important, a gradual transformation of the professional role of the psychiatrist. Psychiatric services in the general hospital were originally designed for the short-term care of the occasional person with mental disease who might be discovered on hospital wards. Psychiatrists working in the environment of the general hospital would refer these persons to mental hospitals for care. They centered their own services on the psychoneurotic patients, who had no organic pathological condition. However, the needs of the hospital community for psychological understanding of *the patient as a person* in a special situation, insofar as he has to cooperate with a complex program of examinations and medical procedures, gradually led to a vast expansion of a program of consultation on other services.

A dramatic climax of this type of participation in medical and surgical services occurred in 1942 when Dr. E. D. Churchill, Chief of the Surgical Services at the Massachusetts General Hospital, decided to include the psychiatrists in the medical team that was caring for the victims of the Cocoanut Grove fire. It then became obvious that more important than the diagnosis of neurosis was the proper appraisal of the emotional reaction of the patient to life crisis. It was clear that the nature of his illness, and even more, his capacity to cooperate with the physician and surgeon, are markedly affected by his repertoire of coping mechanisms and emotional defenses against overwhelming stress. Suggestions as to his psychological management may make a significant difference in the outcome of his physical care. It became necessary to find a scientific basis for dealing with reactions to emotional crises. A substantial body of information was needed to predict and control pathological behavior patterns. This naturally led to a keen interest in possible preventive measures, based on better understanding of the reactions to stressful life situations in the community.

Preventive practice means widening the horizon of activities in medical care, deliberately including explicit attention not only to those who are sick but also to those who are exposed to the danger of becoming sick in the future.

Certain aspects of preventive medicine are practiced by the physician and pediatrician as a matter of course. The series of inoculations and injections which are administered at proper times to a child in order to protect him from noxious agents in the environment are well standardized and based on a sound immunological investigation. However, when we deal with the behavior and experience of adults, and especially of children, with their personality growth and their proper integration into their cultural and social orbit, we seem to lack such a foundation. Indeed, it would be presumptuous to claim that at the present time we have a solid scientific basis for preventive endeavors in psychiatry. We have more challenge for further research than established knowledge, and more call for imaginative participation by the psychiatrist in new types of programs to secure this knowledge than validated preventive practice. We must face the very large task ahead for joint efforts among psychiatrists, between different professional disciplines, and across national boundaries, both in investigation and in the experimental usage of preventive procedures.

## THE BEHAVIORAL AND SOCIAL SCIENCES AND HUMAN DEVELOPMENT

Let me review with you briefly some of the small, but nevertheless useful advances in the behavioral and social sciences which have changed our perception of human growth and development and have perhaps served to suggest preventive intervention at particular stages of the life cycle.

First of all, what do we mean by prevention in our field? Any action which serves to intervene in a sequence of events starting with hazards to an individual's health and personality development and ending with a disturbed state should, in contrast to remedial work, be thought of as preventive intervention. In prevention, therefore, we deal with hazardous situations, with populations at risk, with the removal of noxious agents or the erection of barriers against such agents, with strengthening the health resources of child and family, and with recognizing those constellations of circumstances in time and space in which preventive intervention is possible and desirable.

For purposes of *secondary prevention* we try to develop resources for early treatment and case finding in order to arrest a disease process. This may do much to obviate the hazard of a more serious outcome which might otherwise prevail. Even rehabilitation by retraining and educating those suffering from the aftereffects of uncured diseases may still be thought of as preventive insofar as it lessens the evil by-products of malfunctioning and deficiency. Secondary prevention is at least a small element in every clinical encounter, whether we teach a feeble-minded child so that he may function better and be less apt to be a social misfit, or treat an enuretic child to avoid psychoneurotic complications, or educate a delinquent child to prevent later criminality. However, our special challenge is that of population-wide measures to forestall the development of neuroses, behavior disorders, psychoses, and emotional impairment before they ever become established: namely, with *primary prevention.*

In some facets of our medical practice, this has become possible. The indirect effects of poliomyelitis and the large apparatus for the rehabilitation of the victims of this disease have become obsolete since the population has been immunized by the proper vaccine. Certain forms of cerebral palsy are now identified and can be controlled by better obstetrical care. Certain inherited genetic defects, such as the abnormality responsible for the improper metabolism of amino acids leading to the development of phenylpyruvic acid with its destructive consequences such as mental retardation, have been recognized and can be controlled by proper dietary measures. Once the specific enzyme is found, its particular function in the organism can be identified and corrected. Many other specific illnesses are awaiting control in this manner. But the very large number of children and adults who have personality difficulties or are impaired in their social and intellectual functioning in a less specific way present a perplexing problem. It is in connection with this whole range of disorders that I would like to cite some recent observations on factors determining normal and abnormal growth and development in order to stimulate your interest in the more detailed discussions which are to follow.

## The Behavioral Sciences

First of all, the *concept of disease* as it refers to disturbances in the growing organism has undergone considerable change. There are only a few clearly defined disease entities in which a predictable sequence of disturbed behavior can be diagnosed and a prognosis made. While this is true of mongolism and a series of other fairly well circumscribed changes in morphology and behavior, by far the majority of conditions about which we are concerned represent unspecific impairments of function. In these conditions, we are not looking for one "cause" but for a multiplicity of contributing factors which are interrelated in "transactional" ways (to borrow a term from general systems theory). While it is clear that somatic events in the individual affect social behavior and that social events affect somatic behavior, the critical details of these transactions are very complex and require painstaking study.

If we look more closely at these conditions, which demand the attention of the physician, we find *failure to perform* or to achieve up to the expectations of society; we have *deviance* from the code of conduct; and we find *disorganization* of function either in the area of mentation or in bodily functioning: all interrelated, and interdependent, and demanding at any moment the proper correlation by the scientist of biological and social components of disease.

The central concern in this field must be with the processes of growth and development, with expectable stages of maturation, and with those factors in the environment which facilitate or impede the inborn evolution which has been prescribed for this organism by the combination of its genes. It is just here that there has been a revolution of thinking. We know a great deal more about genetic units, about chromosome morphology, and about the way in which the information contained in genes is transmitted to the new being. Most important is the fact that this information also prescribes series of developmental events over time and implies certain stages which are more vulnerable than others.

A number of studies[1] concerned with prenatal, natal, and postnatal environmental events go far beyond problems of mechanical danger and proper biological inputs. They are concerned with the way in which the growth of the organism is determined by the effect of early experiences on its inborn learning potential. We now begin to understand that the newborn brings along for each species not only the well-known structurally inherited patterns of rage, fear, fight, flight, and feeding and elimination, but also a number of responses more complex than those necessary for survival and, at later stages, for procreation. These are laid down in a rather specific way within the central nervous system, and the proper evoking of these potential responses by the appropriate stimuli in the environment is of crucial importance.

I do not have to remind this audience of the variety of studies of very early experiences of animals: the so-called *imprinting* which has to take place at quite specific moments of postnatal existence and which strikingly determines the infantile responses to nurturing objects. Numerous studies demonstrate the enduring effects on subsequent development of early *sensory deprivation*, of absence of a nurturing object, and particularly, of the mother. Pleasurable experiences and the early stages of learning are profoundly bound to the appropriate responses of a maternal object. Liddell[2] has shown a dramatic reduction in the capacity for survival of goats who were deprived of their mother, for hours only, during early infancy.

Harlow[3,4] has given us a great deal of systematic insight concerning the crippling of exploratory behavior of chimpanzee infants brought up in the presence of a mechanical mother surrogate. Nurture in the narrower sense, namely providing warm milk, is not the significant factor. Rather, the opportunity for clinging and contact responses is the major prerequisite for normal growth. One of the most important implications of these studies is that the lack of proper nurturing and exploratory situations for the monkey infant both in respect to the maternal object and to other monkey infants will show its deleterious consequences later, in adulthood, more than during the actual growing stages of the organism. The adult monkey who in infancy was deprived of opportunities for normal interaction with a live mother will be severely handicapped both in procreative activities and in her capacity for mothering her own babies.

Numerous studies[5] which have been carried on in various countries in the last two decades on human infants with respect to orphanhood, maternal deprivation, and variations in the early social context all agree that the evil consequences of damaging separation may not show up until many years later.

Recently we have become familiar with the details of the behavior of human infants when they are separated from their mothers in hospitals. Films which show their responses to the mother's return have brought us face to face with the sequence of separation responses in children. John Benjamin's[6] work suggests a striking periodicity during the first few months in the readiness to display massive emotions and elucidates the beginning of early coping mechanisms in response to excessive stimulation as well as to sensory deprivation.

While some of these observations relating to critical periods in emotional development seem to be fairly constant throughout the species, we are also beginning to see a marked degree of individual differences of response even in the newborn. Peter Wolff[7] and Sibylle Escalona[8] have shown that quite early in life the rates of activity and the readiness to respond will vary considerably from child to child, and that the mother's empathic or objecting responses to the given child's particular style of behavior may determine her own pattern of reactions, which, in turn will become important in connection with early imprinting, learning, and the development of affectionate patterns of behavior.

Indeed, the mother's responses to the newborn are likely to have precursors in her attitude and responses to the pregnancy. Gerald Caplan has studied the marked "regressive" concerns of pregnant women with their own early experiences as they anticipated motherhood; and he has also shown the particular challenging impediments to positive responses which occur at the time of a premature birth.[9-11] Grete Bibring[12] has just finished a series of observations on imagery in coping with the arrival of a new human being in the confines of the mother's own existence.

With these observations, we are clearly in the field of studies concerning *social context*. They leave no doubt that developmental sequences are profoundly altered by the nature of the social context in which they occur. While naturally most emphasis has been placed on the mother, quite recently we are learning about the importance of the father for the newborn, particularly in his power to support or impede the maternal behavior of the mother and in his capacity to relate his role and hers properly. One might well ask whether the absence of the mother (maternal deprivation) indeed is more damaging than that of the father. This question was answered in the affirmative by Barry and Lindemann,[13] and their findings have been recently confirmed by Hilgard,[14] who shows a striking statistical excess of maternal loss before the age of five in the antecedents of both adult neuroses and psychoses. This was more damaging to girls than to boys, but only in boys is there a special age of vulnerability to paternal loss which is the period of prepuberty rather than infancy.

## The Social Sciences

If the integrity of the social environment is important for the growing child, then our attention will be called to the *effect of transitions from one environment* to the other, both as these are demanded by the child's own growth and achievement drive and as they are prescribed by the cultural expectations of the society around him.

It is here that *community studies* and the convergent information from a whole variety of anthropological studies become relevant. The social sciences have provided us in the last several decades with conceptual tools to describe action sequences in an individual and to relate them to the behavior of others. We speak now about the different *roles* which are assigned to a child at different age levels, which comprise the legitimate expectations which others can have about him, and which are complementary to the roles which the other significant persons in his human environment play.

Childhood growth comprises a series of more or less stationary periods in which roles can be elaborated and consolidated. These change abruptly to new situations in which the old roles are obsolete and new ways of doing things and coping have to be learned.

Moments of role transition such as entrance into kindergarten, or such as leaving school to go into professional training, the transition from life as a single person into the marriage state, and finally, the state of bereavement when a significant partner has been lost — all these events in the life cycle which we have become accustomed to speak of as *"situational crises"* constitute a special challenge to the organism. Existing coping mechanisms must be reviewed, many of them must be discarded, and new patterns of behavior must be developed.

Finally, new knowledge has become available about the striking variations in different societies and in different social classes with respect to the demands made upon children at specific points of the developmental curve with respect to achievement, conformity, control of aggression, control of sexual impulses, and finally, with respect to independence and autonomy. The work of Erik Erikson[15,16] and of many anthropologists, particularly John Whiting,[17] has shown that "normal" behavior for a typical child at a given age may vary tremendously from culture to culture.

The studies of Redlich and Hollingshead,[18] as well as of John Spiegel,[19] have shown that the working class and the upper classes in many societies differ sharply in their expectations concerning the behavior of the growing child, that the patterns of sanctions and reinforcements demanding compliance from the child differ, that deviant behavior is defined differently, and that the conditions under which help is sought from various professional resources are equally varied.

## THE COMMUNITY HEALTH MATRIX

A host of new considerations not belonging to the traditional image of medical care has forced itself upon us. Instead of dealing with sick organ systems only, we have to consider our patients as persons in crisis whose life has become affected by social changes, by conflicting demands, and who can get the help that they seek only if we learn to understand the community matrix in which they have to function.

There are in every social system networks of opportunities and obligations, of high status and low status, of roles as challenges and commitments; and there are a series of professionalized institutions in each community to help individuals at critical periods. The medical profession and the hospital with its arrangements for the practice of medical care is only one such institution. If we take the community matrix seriously and try to deal with it with a quest for new knowledge or for the application of existing knowledge, we are invading a complex system and are affecting it by our presence. The division of labor within the community, the distribution of power and decision-making, the rights and prerogatives of certain citizens in contrast to others, the access to land and to the basic supplies of food, shelter, security, as well as opportunities for education and occupation are all contained in a complex network of institutions. Medical and health concerns have to be defined and defended in the interplay of forces. The boundary between sickness and crime, between therapy and education, between secular treatment and salvation is unstable and changes over time. It is important for the practitioners of the health professions to become acquainted with the details of this interplay in different types of communities and to become self-conscious participants in the gradual evolution of the services which these people consider as essential for their needs (see Figure 1). Asking for health needs as separate from the concerns of welfare, education, and justice will require a considerable intimacy and acquaintance with the details of community functioning at various levels of our society.

During the last decade, efforts were made by the Psychiatric Service of the Massachusetts General Hospital in two different communities; a middle class suburb and an area described as "slum" and subjected to relocation. Our first community study was the so-called Wellesley Project.

### The Wellesley Project

We chose Wellesley, a suburb of Boston, to develop a *community agency* to serve the needs of training and research in the

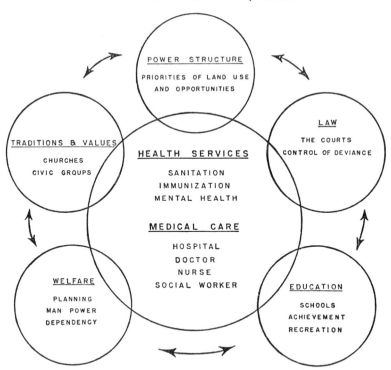

*Figure 1. The essential human needs in community life which are reflected in institutional and professional organizations. The definition of health needs and the provision for their care is determined by the interaction of these segments of the community.*

field of mental health. It was hoped that the services of such an agency could be made acceptable to the community in a five-year pilot period with the expectation that the citizens would support them from then on. This has indeed been the case. Wellesley was chosen because of its willingness to cooperate, and because it presents a typical suburban community in a metropolitan center with a large middle-class population. In 1948, it had approximately 20,000 inhabitants, or 8,000 families, and has since grown to 27,-000 persons.

The services of a mental health agency were conceived as five-fold: First, a referral resource for emergency situations involving emotional disturbances of one or several members of the community. Second, efforts to detect incipient emotional disorders, and the development of methods of preventive care. Third, to ascertain the distribution of emotional disorders within the community and to develop methods of following fluctuations in this distribution through time. Fourth, to ascertain the types of activities of various professional and social agencies which have either remedial or preventive implications in the field of mental health, and to serve as consultants for the further development of these activities. Fifth, participation in community planning in the fields of housing, medical care, education, recreation, and welfare to bring to bear the influence of mental health principles.

It was expected that an agency to execute these services would provide a field station for the training of individuals in social science and public health, as well as psychiatrists and psychologists. Further, it was hoped that this agency would make accessible a normal population for the purpose of studying the relationship of emotional disturbances to the structure and functions of the social environment.

An interdisciplinary team was assembled combining the traditional clinical combination of psychiatrist, psychologist, and psychiatric social worker with a research group consisting of social psychologist, sociologist, and anthropologist. A steering committee consisting of Dr. Walter Bauer of the Massachusetts General Hospital, Dr. Hugh R. Leavell of the Harvard School of Public Health, Dr. Samuel Stouffer of the Harvard Laboratory of Social Relations, and Francis Keppel, former Dean of the Harvard Graduate School of Education, reflected the interdisciplinary nature of the program.

An "action research" model was adopted; this involved the citizens in planning for services and research through a series of lay committees which used the staff members as resource people. This type of organization had some influence on the choice of research problems since the citizens objected to certain approaches, but it has the advantage of facilitating work in other areas through their active cooperation.

It is obvious that the clear definition of a problem often constitutes the better part of its solution. The Wellesley Project compounded the difficult task of delimiting manageable aims within the general area of "mental health" by trying to combine two types of activities: that of establishing a first-aid service within the community; and that of extending clinically relevant knowledge. Both tasks, moreover, are aspects of a third effort: the increasingly explicit and rigorous formulation of a frame of reference in terms of which one can think more systematically about varieties of "health" and "illness" of designated individuals and the nature of the process by which they become "ill" and "cured."

The concepts on which research planning was based were those of "the emotionally relevant human environment," "frequency and duration of social interactions," "role distribution within the social system," and the "equilibrium and disequilibrium at times of crises." Central assumptions were as follows: Given a crisis leading to disequilibrium of a social system, either in a family or other social organization, readaptation will be required from the members of the group. These responses may be adaptive or maladaptive. Responses which appear adaptive at first, may on closer study be found to represent precursors of later disturbances.

The starting point for these studies was a review of reactions to severe bereavement in which it was possible to distinguish a variety of reactions: on the one hand, "normal," effective grief work; and on the other, morbid types of adjustment including psychotic, psychosomatic, and psychoneurotic reaction types; but also certain forms of personality change which merely reduced the survivor's scope of functioning.

It seemed important to find other situations of crisis or transition which would make it possible to study the reactions of individuals with different personality structures and their ways of mastering the attendant problems. One such crisis was repeatedly referred to our clinical service: namely, the return to the family of a mental hospital patient. This situation provided a model for clinical investigation in a community according to which not the referred individual, but the group of which he is a member, becomes the object of service and study. Service records were developed to collect data on the conditions of the social system, the emotionally relevant environment of the ex-patient. Study of the "normal" members of these families led in the direction of a typology of pathological forms of family organization and of hypotheses concerning external pressures which result in the transmission of emotional disturbances from one member to another.

In order, however, to do systematic research on large groups of the population, it was necessary to develop methods of motivating various segments of the community to cooperate. It was possible to win a high percentage of a group of families with nursery school age children and a large percentage of families with children entering kindergarten to agree to help promote understanding of varieties of adjustment to social stress.

The nursery school studies were designed by the social scientists on the team to explore aspects of American middle-class family life which may be relevant for mental health and for the way in which individual families or family members respond to crisis situations. Naegele's study of Hostility and Aggression in Middle Class American Families[20,21] elicited from mothers of nursery-school age children information as to how they typically defined and managed aggression and hostility in themselves, their children, and their husbands and related this information to other data on the social structure of these families. The range of attitudes relative to aggression and hostility in particular and relative to various broader aspects of the maternal role in general was distinctly narrower than the range of personalities represented among them. For that reason, the threefold involvement of these mothers in general American culture, the middle-class version of it, and the small, isolated conjugal family are of relevance in understanding the range of their attitudes. A similar study of the fathers of these same families made by Aberle[22] contributed to understanding the way in which the nursery school age boy becomes the focus of paternal concern relative to his eventual occupational success while his sister remains relatively free of such concern.

Studies of children and their families at the transition point of entry into kindergarten focused on the adaptation required of family members when the child leaves home and goes to school, as well as on the child's own patterns of coping with a new life experience. As in the case of the bereavement studies, it was possible through a series of group meetings with parents to delineate a typical course of anticipation, upset or disequilibrium, followed by readjustment experienced by these families. A free "Pre-School Check-Up" offered to the community and carried out at the Human Relations Center has afforded an opportunity each year for interviewing mothers individually and seeing the child in a play situation, in an attempt to ascertain from a relatively brief contact what type of emotional adjustment prevails within the family orbit and what situations the child is probably going to meet successfully, in contrast with those in which he is probably going to fail. It is hoped that experience gained over a number of years in this type of voluntary preschool assessment will eventually lead to population-wide surveys which can identify and bring preventive services to bear on children who are vulnerable to difficulties in school or to later breakdown.

A similar cross-sectional study of transition was made in the School of Nursing of the Newton-Wellesley Hospital and showed the hazards encountered by first-year nursing students as they attempted to embrace a professional role. The drop-out rate of the first-year class was significantly lowered by providing mental health assistance to the students in the form of group seminars at which they were free to discuss their concerns.

The development of longitudinal studies in which children can be followed from the preschool period or earlier all the way through high school and beyond has been a goal of our community work, but has proved to be difficult to achieve. As a first step, we have instituted follow-up surveys of children who attended the preschool check-up and have made use of teacher and parent observations in order to check on our staff's predictions regarding their ability to adapt successfully to the school environment.

Another method of observing the relation of emotional disturbance to social structure is to study the distribution of emotional disorders within the community. The assumption was made that there exists in every community a manifest caseload known to the professional agencies, and also a hidden caseload of emotionally disturbed individuals who are known only to themselves, their families, or outside institutions. There was also the assumption that the distribution of disturbances was to be understood in terms of differential strain in various geographical areas corresponding to various regions of the social structure. Richardson and Lewis[23] developed a method of subdividing the town into a number of homogeneous residential areas, using criteria readily available from public records, such as date of building construction, assessed valuation, external appearance, and ethnic characteristics. A refinement of this early study has been developed by Baldwin, Simmons, and their co-workers,[24] which makes it possible to identify subdivisions of the larger areas and eventually to study types of neighborhood interaction within these units.

A second phase of this work involved becoming thoroughly acquainted with the modes of operation of the medical profession, the clergy, and the social agencies; particularly with their stereotypes concerning emotional disorders and with their reliability as casefinders. It has only recently become possible to make prudent use of their reporting in terms of a set of diagnostic criteria acceptable to all groups.

In contrast to the nonhospitalized sick population, those individuals who were in mental institutions during the last fifteen years were easily ascertained. The incidence of these disorders in the subsections of this town is, of course, small in absolute numbers. It appeared more promising to contrast the total number of hospitalized individuals for the whole community with that of a comparable segment of the population in another area of metropolitan Boston which differs markedly in socioeconomic status and in most of the criteria enumerated above. Here, as in our other studies, our interest focused on differences in the patterns of affiliation, especially on the changes in affiliation which go with upward and downward mobility in the social system and with mobility from one residential area to the other.

The Wellesley Project, then, represents a mental health agency in the process of development. The research program, rather than being a unitary project, consists of a series of individual projects which developed in response to the challenge of problems arising in connection with the development of service activities. Over a fifteen-year period, about 2000 families have become known to the service. Emotional disorders referred for service have ranged from frank psychoses to psychoneuroses, to delinquency, and to psychosomatic conditions. In addition to direct clinical service, on a short-range basis, to individuals and families, an elaborate program of consultation is carried out with both the Wellesley and Weston public school systems, as well as with clergy, medical practitioners, social agencies, and law-enforcing personnel. The agency is a field station for a training program in community mental health or graduate students in psychiatry, psychology, and social work, supported by grants from the National Institute of Mental Health to the Massachusetts General Hospital.

Tracing and understanding the needs of the community, we have been helpful in creating a mental health agency which fitted

well with the expectations and concerns of the citizens of this suburban middle-class community. These were the advancement and
success of their children, the control of deviance and failure, and
the early discovery of possible impairment of health. They were
able to plan cooperatively and to develop their own program using
us as resource persons.

### The West End Project[25]

Most of the Wellesley citizens receive private medical care, but
what about the population whose members are cared for on general
hospital wards? It is they who present many problems because of
lack of cooperation, lack of understanding of medical procedures,
and excessive dependency on hospital and physician. Could we
develop a similar program for a working class area? We were quite
aware of the fact that members of the working class, particularly
slum inhabitants, are not likely to tell much about their life because
they are afraid of strangers, especially of investigators, no matter
how helpful they wish to be. They are accustomed to collectors of
bad debts and to police investigators. In order to become well
acquainted with such a population, we had to wait for a crisis in
community life. The forced relocation of the population of the
West End in Boston under the Urban Renewal Act presented such
a crisis. Using the representatives of the hospital as a potential resource and possible source of assistance, the inhabitants of this
neighborhood might be willing to share with us information about
their way of life and aspirations, their relationships to each other,
and their notions about ill health, failure, and conflict.

We were able to win the cooperation of the citizens for a
lengthy interview and for visits to their homes, many of which
were very well kept in spite of their poor external appearance.
Many of the dwelling units had been condemned and were considered unsanitary. They had been neglected by the owners and were
becoming less suitable as homes in spite of the efforts of the low-
income inhabitants.

We worked closely with the relocation authorities offering to
this agency services for the severely disturbed or impaired persons.
We also obtained permission from them and the support of com-

munity leaders to whom they introduced us for our plan of visiting and interviewing the families included in our sample.

We found 83 per cent compliance in responding to the interview. There was a pervading sense of loss and resentment about the fact that the region was destined for apartment houses for the well-to-do, that they were losing not only their houses but also their elaborate recreational facilities just across the street, and that they would be deprived of many of their intimate relationships. Again we completed interviews on 86 per cent of the sample after the relocation in their new habitat and were able to relate their adaptation to basic ethnic and cultural factors.

Some of our findings were as follows. This was a working class community. Their average income was not much above four or five thousand a year. They are skilled, semiskilled, unskilled people in their work situation. College education reaches only 10 per cent of this group. The ethnic composition shows predominantly Italians, while others are of Polish, Slavic, Jewish, Irish origin. As many as 72 per cent of the Italians and a similar high percentage of other ethnic groups had arrived in their generation from abroad. This shows that the area was an immigrant platform and presented to its inhabitants the problem of acculturation from the European territory into the American life.

Instead of the kind of small family which we encountered in Wellesley, the so-called "nuclear family" consisting of husband, wife, and children, we found here kinship systems of large numbers of families interlaced and dependent on each other for material and moral support.

Most of the people to whom they turned for support were living in the West End and not outside. There was a sense of intimate human relationships within a bounded area, and there was a much higher rate of communication inside than across the boundary. The concept of "who belongs to us" and "where do we belong" was quite explicitly defined for the West End. The strangers are suspect. It takes a long time to give confidence. Once this confidence is established, one feels free to make demands on him as though he belonged to the family.

Clearly, the problems and concerns which the families in the West End reported were not of the same order as those in Wellesley. They could be classed as medical, social, and legal as defined by the community agency involved, rather than as "achievement problems," "conformity problems," problems of discomfort or disease as seen by middle-class citizens.

Our follow-up study is not completed, but we are collecting data on the following questions: In terms of mental health, we wonder are the people in their new habitat sicker than they were? Are they achieving less than they were? Are they more unhappy than they were? Are they less conforming, and was there more evidence of court records and delinquency than before? City planners concerned with other areas are interested in our findings in planning their program for future urban renewal. One of the most important impressions so far has been that the West End population experienced itself as a target of administrative procedures without responsible participation in the planning for their own future. The opportunity for citizen participation in future relocations is now becoming mandatory. This provision may well become a preventive factor in the adjustment of families involved in a forced change of their habitat.

## HOSPITAL STUDIES

Trying to investigate the health needs of communities we had to learn how to get along with the citizens as participant observers and interviewers. We found ways to communicate with all these persons of different social class and began to be more comfortable with people even if they complained unduly or had strange manners and values. We began to wonder if our own hospital populations have community aspects also. An opportunity to test our capacity to appraise cultural and social variables came when the Emergency Ward changed dramatically its role in the Massachusetts General Hospital. Some years ago the administration had decided to open the doors of the hospital to all the people in the neighborhood who needed care, including alcoholics. The "alcoholic" has attributes which many doctors find objectionable. We became interested in these individuals as representatives of an especially dependent segment of the population with many attributes of a slum population.

It seemed that a "crisis" approach to their calamity might make a difference in terms of their motivation to accept treatment and to continue with it. Our Alcoholism Clinic at that time received just about 1 per cent of the people who were seen in the Emergency Ward with alcoholism. We decided to communicate with these patients not in terms of alcoholism but in terms of life crises which in their opinion had led to conflict, failure, and finally to the alcoholism which brought them to the hospital. A series of studies has demonstrated that after having been interviewed in this manner a much larger percentage of these patients use the Alcoholism Clinic for a sustained program of care than could be expected after a "traditional" clinical referral (Chafetz, et al.).[26]

We further found that with this new attitude, not looking for mental disease only but appraising "health needs" and unsolved life crises, psychiatrists were more and more in demand. Patients were beginning to come to the Emergency Ward for help with unresolved emotional crises. There has been a substantial increase in all Emergency Ward patients. In the last ten years they have doubled in number from about 22,000 to 44,000; however, the number of psychiatric patients has grown much more. They have increased tenfold, from 300 to 3,000 a year, requiring a considerable increase in psychiatric staff. A change has occurred in psychiatric clinical practice in the direction of mental health operations (see Figure 2).

The life crises in which these patients seek help are the kind of predicaments which we encountered both in Wellesley and in the West End: the loss of another person, a bereavement response, a transition problem. If the psychiatrist is content to diagnose such a condition as depression or "alcoholic addiction," he is inclined to dispose of the patient. The need to have assistance with a life crisis is brushed over and not recognized. But, if he is alert to the life crisis behind this presenting symptom, he is motivated to form a team of psychiatrists and social workers to tackle this problem and to reach out for further agency assistance in the community.

In all this activity, the mental health worker is only one component of the medical and surgical team. The orientation to life crises as a legitimate health need begins to influence other staff members, physicians, and administrators alike.

All through the hospital it is now appreciated that the emotional and social needs of the patients must be studied with scientific

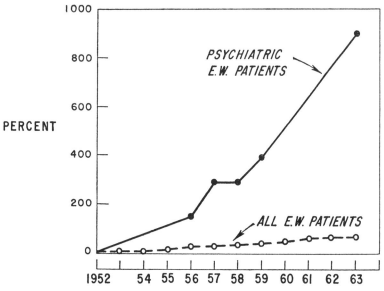

*Figure 2. The increase in the number of referrals for psychiatric "crisis-oriented" consultation in the Emergency Ward over a ten-year period (1952–1963). From Morris E. Chafetz and Howard Blane.*

competence and thoroughness. Dr. Nathan Talbot's program in Pediatrics clearly makes studies of life crises an integral part of the care of sick children and what is even more important, of the preventive care for families with young children. Studies of psychological provisions for healthy growth and adjustment, of patterns of parental behavior and competence are beginning to affect the daily activities in clinic and ward. The evidence being accumulated by his research team shows striking differences in the "psychological nutrition" of healthy and sick children.[27]

In the Medical Clinic, also, social science studies have become a daily preoccupation. The very high percentage of medical patients with significant emotional-social crisis problems is as evident there as in the Emergency Ward. The medical students are taught to identify these crises and to lend appropriate assistance in problem-solving. A careful study by Dr. Stoeckle[28] has shown that persons of different cultural backgrounds decide to define themselves as sick and to see the doctor under quite different life circumstances. *Detailed* knowledge is as important here as in molecular biology!

As the use of the psychological and social sciences advances in medicine, the hospital is more and more able to meet the problems of human crises and, perhaps as a consequence, there appears before us a subtle but definite change in hospital functioning in the direction of community responsibility and community care. The psychiatric service is now sharing in the planning for a large hospital to be built by the Commonwealth of Massachusetts adjacent to the Massachusetts General Hospital. This will give us a large number of beds for severely sick mental patients, but primarily will carry on those functions enumerated today, namely, dealing with a defined population in their respective communities, ascertaining and anticipating life crises and their consequences, providing short-term care in the hospital, and extending programs of assistance into the community. This new pattern of health care which is so urgently needed in the field of psychiatry is clearly interwoven with the new image of a general hospital as a potent resource for community health.

## SUMMARY

The health needs of communities are a matter of high complexity. Needs are at least of two kinds. First there are those seen by research as necessary provisions for normal growth and development and for a satisfying life in a social orbit.

This means provision of proper stimulation and companionship at the right time. It means the provision of special attention and care at critical periods of growth of the child, and it means assistance through all ages at the time of inevitable life crises whether they be developmental or situational in nature. The mental health worker with a secure basis in biology, as well as in social medicine, will join hands with the other care-taking and care-giving institutions and professions in the community to add his advice and counsel.

There is a second type of need with which the health worker must be familiar. The patient may define emotional or social needs as constituting sickness rather than other types of want. Even though such a need may not be of a medical nature in the narrower sense, it may point to conditions in the community which urgently need remedy lest they constitute a mental health hazard. What constitutes a recognized state of need and helplessness varies from community to community. Differences exist within the class structures and within different cultural groups. Differences also are found from institution to institution.

The most difficult task before us is to anticipate and deal successfully with crises of human organizations, such as urban renewal, which affect the well being of many persons involved. This type of consultation requires flexibility and sound footing in a conceptual framework of social science. Only the barest beginning has been made in empirical studies and much work lies ahead.

# AT THE TURN OF THE NEXT CENTURY

David D. Rutstein, M.D.

Dᴜʀɪɴɢ the first half of the twentieth century the hospital changed from a custodial institution to a complex workshop. By the turn of the next century, it will incorporate all preventive and curative personnel and services and will become the center for community health. But the new hospital center will no longer be self-centered. It will be carefully interrelated in a community-wide and regional hospital system to meet the total medical care needs of the individual and the community.

The hospital is already the focal point for medical care. This is fortunate. By examining the assets and liabilities for medical care within the hospital, we can see with our own eyes the essential characteristics of our entire medical care system. There are many examples. The haphazard state of medical care in the United States is illustrated by the lack of coordination among our many different kinds of hospitals and the detached independent operation of the individual hospital. Our general hospitals devoted mainly to the care of acute short-term illness are symptomatic of the episodic nature and lack of continuity which pervades our medical care. Moreover, the discharge of chronically ill patients from the general hospital to the miserably inadequate care in nursing homes re-emphasizes our lack of real concern for the chronically ill and the aged. Separate custodial institutions, euphemistically called hospitals for the mentally ill, document the isolation of psychiatry from the main stream of medicine. Our teaching hospitals with their super-specialists, exquisite techniques, and elaborate equipment amaze us with the complexity and accomplishments of modern medical science. They also verify the diminishing status of the general physician. The contrasts between voluntary and municipal hospitals punctuate the differences in medical care by economic level. The gradual decrease in the number of proprietary hospitals, that is, privately owned hospitals run like a business for a profit, augurs well for an improvement in the quality of medical care. But recent attempts to develop chains of profit-making hospitals (a contradiction in terms) epitomize the threat to life and health if profit-making becomes the primary objective of hospital operation. Most important of all, those individual hospitals scattered throughout our country that have a long tradition of the practice of the best medicine primarily for the benefit of the patient stand out as beacons to guide us to the medical care of the future.

We may go one step further. If we reorganize and strengthen our hospitals, total medical care must improve. This is not to say that reorganization can be done entirely within the walls of the hospital. Each change will reverberate in our communities and affect professional, social, and economic relationships in medical care. But the hospital is the logical place to start. As we tidy up in-patient and out-patient hospital care, community medical care problems will be uncovered. In turn, improving community medical care will place increasing demands on the hospital.

## FORCES AFFECTING HOSPITAL EVOLUTION

Many of the major trends now affecting the future evolution of our hospitals fortunately reinforce each other in a direction favoring better medical care. And the tide is so strong it will not be stayed even by the inertia of our present unplanned approach and lack of system. The forces impelling change include the expansion of medical knowledge, growing specialization, automation, the soaring costs of medical care, and the expectations of the public. All of these will tend toward the centralization, coordination, and more systematic use of hospital services.

### Expanding Medical Knowledge and Increasing Specialization

Constant medical advance depends upon the continued growth of medical knowledge. Application of our rapidly expanding store of knowledge for the benefit of the patient demands a gradually increasing number of narrow specialties and the education of many more specialists. But, this is not to say that every existing general hospital will have to be staffed by every kind of specialist and equipped with all facilities and laboratory aids to perform any procedure conceivably beneficial to the patient. It would be both impossible and undesirable.

Specialists are scarce, and the growing demand for highly qualified specialists is not limited to medicine. It is symptomatic of the increasing complexity of our entire society. There is a real danger that our whole social structure will collapse because its complexities will outrun the supply of those needed to hold it together. In every field — professional, administrative, business, and government — there is an increasing deficit of those needed to fill high-level positions. This is understandable. In our population there is but a limited number of individuals with the combination of intelligence, originality, judgment, motivation, and wisdom necessary to leadership. Moreover, specialization with its inherent rigidity has accentuated the deficit. The flexible adaptability of the natural scientist has been lost. Atomic scientists even in a grave emergency cannot take the place of the neurosurgeon. Every field must be manned with leaders and replacements.

To be sure, we can increase the supply of competent individuals by broadening our educational base and providing the financial support necessary so that every citizen may be educated in accordance with his ability. This problem is now being sharply focused in the congressional debates on aid to education and civil rights. But is is unlikely that by broadening the base we will keep pace with society's growing complexity.

We must husband our resources by strategic location of super-specialist services. In medicine, Sweden has already pointed the way by centralization of such highly specialized procedures as the radium treatment of cancer. Moreover, in the United States in some aspects of care, the concept is already established that every general hospital cannot provide every service to every patient. For example, highly specialized life-saving equipment such as the artificial kidney, needed only by an occasional patient, is available in relatively few hospitals. It has also been clear for a very long time that the laboratories of every hospital cannot perform all required tests. Complicated, unusual, and dangerous laboratory tests are farmed out to laboratories in other hospitals, in state health departments, or to such highly specialized laboratories as that of the Communicable Disease Center of the United States Public Health Service in Atlanta, Georgia. In grave emergencies, hospital resources have been centralized for their most effective use. Thus, in the polio epidemic in Massachusetts in 1955, three hospitals were selected to treat all the patients in the metropolitan Boston area under the supervision of a few highly qualified specialists. The patients received superb care.

In contrast, our wasteful duplication of specialist resources is documented by the almost endless proliferation of highly specialized services, for example, heart surgery, in some of our large cities. We also see, only too often, a superspecialist in a suburban hospital using special equipment purchased at great expense by the local community, attempting to carry out an unusual procedure which can be more safely and effectively performed in the nearby urban medical center. Local pride and individual initiative are laudable virtues, but they must not cost the life or health of the patient. A superspecialist may provide irreplaceable life-saving care. But a relatively few patients will need his help. He must serve a large population if his knowledge is to continue to grow and his skills be kept at peak efficiency. We see that staffing every hospital with a complete roster of superspecialists could be harmful.

We are thus faced with a dilemma. Not every general hospital can provide, but every patient should have, whatever a properly equipped specialist needs to bring a patient the maximum benefits of medical knowledge. There is only one solution. There must be one completely staffed medical center in each hospital district. Other hospitals will as satellites have their services interrelated with those of the major center. Patients will be transferred to the major center for care not available in the satellite community hospital. Many of the major centers will be affiliated with medical schools responsible for undergraduate medical education. Every regional hospital system should also be responsible for the continuing postgraduate education of local physicians under the direction of the most accessible medical school.

All hospitals unaffiliated with the regional system, because of inadequate plant or staff or out-of-the-way location, will have to be closed if patients are to receive satisfactory care in an era of rapidly expanding knowledge and increasing specialization. The implications of these conclusions are enormous because the United

States is a country of small general hospitals, most of which operate independently of each other.

## *Automation*

Automation will have effects both good and bad on the hospital of the future. Labor-saving devices in the kitchen, laboratory, and housekeeping services, automatic analyzers in the routine laboratory, and automatic x-ray film processing are current examples of the benefits. In the near future, we may also look forward to the development of medical machinery such as physiological monitoring and feedback systems. Critically ill patients will require less constant supervision as precise systems are developed for periodic measurement of such vital signs as temperature, pulse, blood pressure, and respiration and for relating these to the treatment of the patient. As an example, patients in shock with low blood pressure would no longer require repeated blood pressure measurements by a physician or a nurse. The level of the blood pressure would be better maintained by continuous automatic measurement in a feedback system. Whenever the pressure fell below a preset critical level, intravenous drug administration to raise the blood pressure would automatically be increased. If the apparatus failed or the patient did not respond, a warning signal would alert the physician or the nurse. Automation systems, by taking over routine duties, will thus permit more efficient use of scarce highly educated and trained personnel.

Analogous are the time and labor-saving effects of computer application to hospital, administrative, and medical research. Accounting procedures, and calculation of administrative statistics, such as the number of admissions, length of stay, bed occupancy, and cost indexes can now be performed automatically. Inventory control in the pharmacy, blood bank, and of hospital supplies and in food purchasing can decrease capital investment and prevent waste.

The computer will be particularly effective as a research tool in hospital medicine when large amounts of data or many variables are involved, but only when the quality of the data justifies its use. Thus the computer analysis of routine hospital records assembled in the usual way is likely to be worthless.

The computer will also be very useful in the application of operations research theory and techniques to the solution of hospital administrative and medical problems. Studies instead of guesses can be made of the optimal size of individual hospital units, for example, the number of beds in a ward, or space allocation in the out-patient department. Such measurements can be related to present and future estimates of hospital use, and to each other. The most efficient combination of individual units and total hospital size may then be related to community needs.

Medical procedures can also be evaluated. From preliminary observation in a study of diagnostic models we have already learned that in emergency care it is not efficient to review the patient's illness in the order of the standard history, physical examination, and routine and special tests. Actually, interns and residents on emergency service demonstrate this as they bypass standard methods and collect their data in what appears to them to be the most efficient order in a particular patient. This process can be made more objective and systematic. Study of chief complaints reveals that there are key questions, examination procedures, and selected tests which will lead more rapidly to diagnosis and to emergency treatment. Other medical procedures are also susceptible to this same kind of analysis.

In the practice of medicine, the computer will be useful in certain delimited areas. For example, numerical results of certain laboratory tests will in the near future be interrelated and interpreted in terms of diagnosis and prognosis. The electrocardiogram and other electronically recorded records will be read and interpreted automatically. On the other hand, the unwary should not be seduced by claims that the computer will replace the physician in the diagnosis of disease. It will be a long time before the computer will look at the patient and say, "He looks sick." Claims that the computer will replace the physician reflect a lack of understanding of the diagnostic process, neglect the simplest principles of data collection analysis and interpretation, and betray a lack of understanding of the computer.

In contrast to its many benefits, automation will bring serious problems in its wake because it cannot make the hospital as efficient as the production line of an industrial plant. A shortened work week can only be tolerated by industry if the increased productivity of labor from automation compensates by yielding the required number of units at a competitive profit-making price. Moreover, a night shift is added in industry only when it will yield significant additional income. In contrast, the hospital has no choice but to operate 24 hours per day and meet increased demands at any hour of the day or night. Certain hospital personnel, particularly physicians, nurses, and maintenance workers, have to be employed or be on call around the clock. And most important of all, many hospital services are highly personal and cannot and often should not be automated.

As industry and labor struggle to minimize technological unemployment from automation, the work week in industry will continue to shorten. Although hospital labor practices have lagged behind those of industry, they must eventually follow the same trend of the shortened work week. The total number of hospital employees will accordingly increase. Labor costs, already 70 per cent of the hospital budget, will continue to rise.

The increase in the hospital budget from automation will demand more efficient operation and will force the hospital to adopt a full seven-day work week. Now in spite of all efforts, there is a distinct letdown in the intensity of hospital activity on weekends and holidays, and during vacation periods. The letdown is greater than can be measured by decrease in bed occupancy. The beds may be occupied by patients, but essential procedures are often postponed because of the absence of certain key personnel. This is understandable because physicians, nurses, and technicians need rest and recreation.

The increase in the number of hospital personnel resulting from the shortened work week will present one advantage. The larger number of staff members and employees could more appropriately be scheduled so as to operate the hospital more effectively seven days per week. In effect, there will be duplicating personnel who can cover for each other. Physicians, nurses, and other hospital workers will thus have periods of recreation while the hospital continues to function at a constantly high level.

As the work week shortens, our concepts of week day and weekend will change. We will think in terms of time on and off duty. This concept of different periods of time on and off for different people during the week will be furthered by increased population pressure. It will have some obvious benefits — in leveling off peaks of highway traffic and commuter crowding, in more effective use of our limited recreational facilities, and in a diminished need for commercial rental space in offices, stores, and shopping centers.

Most careful studies are needed now of factors limiting maximal hospital use throughout the week. All kinds of factors may be relevant. The absence of key personnel has already been mentioned. Others include the diagnosis and average length of stay, the day of the week when a patient is admitted or when certain procedures, examinations, and other tests are performed. Regrouping of beds into larger and fewer units may make seven days per week operation more feasible and cut down the total number of needed beds in the community. Community-wide hospital studies are also needed to estimate the number of "wasted" hospital beds and determine the reasons therefor.

Automation will thus increase the efficiency of many hospital functions and make for seven-day-a-week hospital use, but its total effect over all will increase hospital costs.

### Rising Hospital Costs

A prediction of continued increase in hospital costs in the future is serious indeed. The Consumers' Price Index already shows that for the years 1939 to 1960 the cost of medical care has increased more than that of any other service, and of all items of care hospital costs have risen most sharply. These increased costs are already responsible for the growing demand for more complete medical care insurance coverage, particularly among those most vulnerable to disease — the very young and the very old — and among those whose incomes do not allow for the unpredictable and sometimes very large cost of severe illness.

The increased cost of medical care is reflected in repeated increases in voluntary health insurance premiums. Programs which provide "total care," for example, the Kaiser Plan, or reimburse the total cost of certain services, for example, Blue Cross, must immediately reflect rising medical care costs in their premiums. Private insurance company plans which pay a stipulated amount of money, that is, a fixed indemnity whether or not it covers the cost of necessary services, are less vulnerable. But, in the long run, as costs continue to rise, the public will become dissatisfied with incomplete coverage. A clear example is the recently proposed "over 65 policy" whose relatively small premiums cannot possibly reimburse for, and do not cover the large costs of, medical care of the aged. Any insurance plan which attempts to meet most of the costs of needed medical care must charge a large premium because the cost of medical care is high and is going higher all the time.

Insurance plans are partially responsible for increasing hospital costs. For example, Blue Cross and many other insurance plans specify that reimbursement for diagnostic studies be made only if the seriousness of the patient's illness justifies hospital admission. This limitation on reimbursement is considered necessary for actuarial reasons. Diagnostic tests on ambulatory patients particularly in a doctor's office are deemed unpredictable, difficult to administer, and open to abuse. Actually this limitation unnecessarily forces patients into a hospital for diagnostic studies which could be done as effectively and more cheaply on an ambulatory basis. Patients needing expensive diagnostic tests place irresistible pressure on their physicians to admit them to the hospital where the costs of the tests will be reimbursed. This single limitation in insurance contracts unnecessarily increases hospital admissions, hospital costs, the size of the insurance premium, the total number of hospital beds in the community, and does not improve medical care. Indeed, the opposite is the case. This actuarial restriction may prevent the conscientious physician from diagnosing the early stages of serious illness before the patient develops severe symptoms. This serious and costly limitation to good medical care can be resolved by the development of hospital-affiliated prepayment group practice units.

Costs have been increased also by the haphazard location of most of our hospitals and the lack of cooperation among them. Eventually, rising costs will in themselves force more careful planning of new hospital construction and make for more cooperative hospital operation. Rising costs stress the need for action now while there is yet time. Only too often in medicine, needed changes are postponed until a catastrophe occurs when hurried reorganization is likely to be poorly done. The recent "thalidomide incident" has initiated long-needed reform in drug testing, but the atmosphere of crisis has not been conducive to the evolution of a sound program. Hospitals are vulnerable because most of our present system of hospital insurance depends on full employment. A sharp economic depression will interrupt the smooth flow of payment of insurance premiums. Hospitals will then be faced with caring for a large uninsured population. With constantly rising costs, sudden governmental intervention would be the only solution. Let us not wait for a war, economic collapse, or other national emergency to initiate needed hospital reorganization and financing.

## Increasing Public Expectations

The public's image of the hospital has changed. People used to go to the hospital when they were too sick to be cared for at home. Or, they would not go because it was "the place you went to die." With the impact of science on daily life and the development of "miracle drugs" and dramatic operations, people now go to the hospital to receive the benefits of the technology of medicine. The science and technology of medicine have greatly expanded and this has been reflected in the public's attitude. On television, for example, the hospital scene is furnished in glass, chromium, and stainless steel, and decorated with festoons of plastic tubing and the flashing lights of electronic equipment.

Aided and abetted by sensational articles in the popular press and in the annual fund-raising drives of national health agencies, and by the promises of medical spokesmen of imminent solution of our major medical problems, the public has begun to expect far too much from the hospital and from medicine. Patients are often not satisfied with less than their version of the latest treatment. Physicians now spend a great deal of time reassuring patients, attempting to undo false hopes engendered by careless public statements. This public attitude has and will continue to place great pressure on the individual hospital to do the impossible, that is, to try to provide the public's concept of medical care. This tendency is constantly reflected in unnecessary additions to the hospital budget.

In the future, carefully designed health education programs will be needed to give the public the information they require to make the most effective use of the hospital and of all medical care facilities. The public should also be reassured by the development of regional hospital systems which should make available complete and up-to-date medical care.

## HOSPITAL OF THE FUTURE — CENTER OF COMMUNITY HEALTH

Within the regional system, the present-day general hospital with its in-patient care and its ambulatory services will be the core of the hospital of the future — the center of community health. Affiliated with the general hospital and located within its walls will be specialty hospitals, facilities for the care of the broad spectrum of chronic illnesses including mental disease, a group practice unit, a clinical preventive medical service, the local health department, and voluntary health agencies providing direct services to patients.

### Specialty Hospitals

Although some specialty hospitals have been operating for a long time in close relationship with general hospitals, many of them (mental disease, tuberculosis, maternity, children's, eye and ear, cancer, and orthopedic hospitals) were built as separate institutions in both urban and in isolated rural areas. Urban specialty hospitals were established as voluntary institutions when a small influential group of physicians and laymen were successful in raising funds to meet a community need. Isolated specialty hospitals were set up under governmental auspices for the long-term care of patients when their disease was a threat to their family or neighbors, for example, tuberculosis, or it disturbed the smooth flow of community life, for example, mental disease. The isolation of these hospitals were favored by the belief that country air had healing properties and by lower land values. These reasons have diminished in importance as modern medical care has become more complicated.

As Professor McKeown pointed out in an earlier Lowell Lecture, there are many economic and administrative reasons for bringing the specialty hospital into the general hospital center. There are also medical facts which make this relationship imperative if adequate care is to be provided. Patients in specialty hospitals deserve as good care as those in general hospitals. Treatment limited entirely to the specialty of the hospital is by definition incomplete. The patient in the specialty hospital must be guided by a general physician and have access to whichever specialist may be needed at the moment. In the absence of these, complete medical care is impossible in the unaffiliated and particularly in the isolated specialty hospital. Moreover, many specialty hospitals, particularly those without medical school affiliation, now have difficulty in recruiting interns and residents. Finally, the quality of the practice of the specialist must deteriorate if he separates himself from others in his own field and isolates himself from the main stream of medicine.

The individual specialty hospital is already rapidly disappearing. Hospitals caring for patients with tuberculosis or rheumatic fever are being liquidated or converted to other uses as these diseases decrease in importance. Other specialty hospitals, particularly eye and ear, orthopedic, maternity, children's, and cancer hospitals, are being affiliated with general hospitals as in the Massachusetts General Hospital, the New York Hospital complex, and the new medical center to be built adjacent to the Harvard Medical School. The adjacent geographic location and the affiliation of the specialty and the general hospital will do more than provide good medical care for its patients. It will promote the development of regional hospital systems so that highly specialized services will become more widely available. In teaching hospitals, it will influence the evolution of the medical curriculum to the end that medical schools may once again educate all of the kinds of physicians needed to provide complete medical care.

### Mental Disease Hospitals

Among the isolated specialty hospitals, the sad plight of the mental disease hospitals is most striking. Most of them no longer deserve the name of hospital; they are for the most part institutions providing only custodial care to enormous numbers of sick patients. They lack, among other things, a resident staff, an active roster of general physicians, specialists, nurses, and above all psychiatrists. Most newly fledged psychiatrists prefer to be concerned with a very few patients with relatively minor psychiatric illness rather than devote themselves to the care of a large number with serious mental disease. To be sure, remote custodial institutions do not attract professional personnel. Mental institutions will continue to provide primitive care as long as they remain isolated from the main stream of medicine. To obtain adequate professional staff, they will have to be affiliated directly with general hospitals. But, improvement in medical care for the mentally ill will also require a change in the attitude of the psychiatrist toward fuller integration of psychiatric services in urban, general hospitals.

In other countries, particularly in Scandinavia and in the United Kingdom, serious attempts are being made to do away with the isolated mental disease hospital. Depending upon the needs of the individual patient, a series of graded services is being developed, extending all the way from care in the patient's own home through intermittent ambulatory treatment to part- and to full-time hospital care. New units are being built adjacent to general hospitals so that they will be accessible to the patient, their families, and their physicians. The patient receives medical as well as psychiatric care. In such programs, some patients previously incorrectly classified as hopeless have been rehabilitated. Better medical care assures more precise classification. Moreover, one might wonder whether in some patients hopelessness might not derive in part from treatment in custodial nonmedical institutions isolated from family, community, and from physicians.

In the United States, modern medical care for the mental disease patients will demand an extensive building program of hospital units attached or adjacent to the general hospital. This need was recognized in the legislation proposed to congress by the late President Kennedy. Both in-patient and out-patient facilities are needed to cover the entire range of mental disease. Admission of patients to the new affiliated hospitals cannot be limited to those with the best prognosis or to those of interest to the staff. These tendencies in the past have sharply divided mental patients into two groups to the great disadvantage of those referred to custodial care. During the long interval of time required for the rebuilding of our mental disease hospitals, this gap must be obliterated. A random sample of all patients must be admitted and treated in affiliated hospital units. Experience with the total spectrum of mental illness will assure the development of sound policies on the selection of the kinds of patients to be treated at home, given ambulatory care, or admitted to the hospital for part or full-time treatment.

The juxtaposition of the mental disease hospital and the general hospital will have other important advantages. It will bring the patient with mental disease in contact with scientifically trained physicians and with modern medical research. The patient will be seen through the eyes of a physician in addition to those of a psychiatrist. Research workers may by closer contact become aware of mental disease problems susceptible to solution.

Finally, affiliation with a general hospital will facilitate the recruitment of resident staff. Nurses will also be attracted to general hospital centers in urban areas where normal social life is possible. In hospitals affiliated with medical schools, medical students will see and learn about the whole range of mental illness. Hopefully, in this environment psychiatrists of the future may accept their social responsibilities and develop an interest in and practice among those with major psychiatric disease.

### Institutional Care of Chronic Illness

Chronic disease care is the shame of modern medicine. General hospitals do not provide long-term care except for an occasional wealthy patient who can afford the large per diem costs in the private pavilion. General hospitals welcome chronically ill patients only for the treatment of acute episodes and for important complications. After the emergency is over, general hospitals accept little or no responsibility for those needing continued institutional care. Since most clinical teaching in medical schools is given in general hospitals, emphasis on acute care is reflected in the medical curriculum. Indeed, the present system of medical education in the United States is now almost completely indifferent to the social need for physicians to provide institutional care for those with long-term chronic illness.

A few modern hospitals are built for the care of the chronically ill, e.g., the Lemuel Shattuck Hospital in Massachusetts. But admission is usually limited to patients with better prognoses and only for relatively short periods of time for diagnosis or for establishing a regimen of treatment. These are worthy activities but they do not meet the problem of the care of chronic illness. Because the patients are so many, the beds so few, and the budgets so small, chronic disease hospitals usually make no pretense at long-term continuous institutional care.

There are, however, a few hospitals, for example, the Montefiore Hospital in New York City as already described in an earlier Lowell Lecture by Dr. Cherkasky, which have done a magnificent job of long-term care for relatively few chronically ill patients who are fortunate to have suitable homes and interested, cooperative, and intelligent families. But with the exception of hospitals where research is conducted on the care of the chronically ill or on a particular chronic disease, there are very few hospitals in the United States providing for long-term continuous care of chronic illness. Moreover, as the proportion of those most susceptible to chronic disease, the aged, continues to increase, the problem becomes ever larger.

In the United States, chronically ill patients who are either too sick to be cared for at home or who have unsatisfactory home conditions, must be cared for in institutions. Practically all such patients, regardless of income level, will receive unsatisfactory medical care either in custodial governmental institutions or in nursing homes. Patients on the welfare rolls or in the next higher marginal income group may receive chronic disease care in custodial institutions growing out of the local county home. Such care is usually hopelessly inadequate because essential specialists, equipment, and laboratory services are generally unavailable. Care usually is limited to visits by one or a few general physicians and to a few simple laboratory tests. The physician in such an institution is likely to be on a full-time governmental salary — one of the few real examples of socialized medicine for civilians in the United States.

Practically all chronically ill patients who can afford institutional care and those medically indigent who receive direct governmental payments will be treated in nursing homes. Most nursing homes are located in renovated large residences not designed as medical facilities. According to the National Nursing Home Survey of 1957, about 40 per cent of all licensed nursing homes, in spite of the name, had no professional or practical nurses on the staff. Practically none had an attending physician. Half of the patients in nursing homes had been seen by a physician at least once during the previous month. But one-fifth of all nursing home patients had not been visited once by a physician for at least 6 months, and one out of 6 had not received medical attention for at least a year.

In short, local governmental hospitals and nursing homes are marginal medical institutions filling the gap between hospital and home care for the chronically ill. They provide such a sharp contrast with facilities for patients with acute illnesses that future historians could well compare their care with that given by primitive tribes that send their aged and chronically ill out of the village to fend for themselves.

The Scandinavian countries have pointed the way to the future with some of their experiments in the care of the chronically ill. Special experimental housing units with housekeeping assistance permit home care by a personal physician for many who would otherwise have to be placed in an institution. A few special units in hospitals are set aside for those who need institutional care, but not the intensive treatment of the acute hospital.

In the United States, when we really decide to apply our scientific medical knowledge to the care of the chronically ill, we will first have to do controlled experiments on large population groups. Studies will have to be done in chronic disease hospitals affiliated with general hospitals having good rehabilitation and medical social services. The hospital complex must be functionally related to new housing projects, some units of which, as in Sweden, would be designed for and allocated to the chronically ill and the aged. The chronic disease unit must provide all gradations of care from ambulatory home care to full-time institutional therapy. The experiments will be costly. But, our present custodial system is both wasteful and expensive and it does not provide medical care. Costs and accomplishments in affiliated hospital chronic disease units must be compared with those in the large number of haphazardly located nursing homes needed to care for a control group of the same number of patients.

I fear it will be a long time before we bring scientific medicine to the chronically ill. It is likely that during the next few decades we will continue to delude ourselves that by pouring hundreds of millions of dollars of federal funds into nursing homes, they will suddenly change into permanent well established medical institutions. Congress, with the support of the American Medical Association, has already embarked upon such a course. Nursing homes should, of course, be made as comfortable and as safe as possible until a real medical care program is evolved to care for the chronically sick. State licensing and nursing home standards may prevent the inmates from being burned to death in a fire, but they cannot replace professional leadership or medical and nursing staff. Without professional leadership and staff, adequate and decent medical care for the chronically ill is simply impossible.

Short of a catastrophe or a public scandal we could only hope that the establishment of a regional hospital system will lead to a medical care program for the chronically ill. The public may eventually see the sharpening contrasts between the treatment of acute and that of chronic disease. In the former, at present the benefits of scientific advance are likely to be incorporated into medical care in a general hospital. In existing chronic disease institutions, except for an occasional visit by a physician, care is essentially nonmedical. These differences will become greater as time goes on.

Physicians may eventually tire of travel among many small scattered nursing homes. They must also become dissatisfied with their inability to provide the essentials of professional care without appropriate facilities or supporting staff. Indeed, these factors are already in part responsible for the infrequent medical visits to patients in nursing homes. Even the American Medical Association may eventually stop the promotion of a nonmedical solution for a medical problem. But the time remaining between now and the turn of the next century may not be long enough to bring scientific medicine to the chronically ill.

## The Group Practice Unit

In the hospital of the future, all of the physicians on the staff will comprise a group practice unit located in a building within the hospital grounds. In the major centers, the group practice unit would consist of a complete roster of specialists, all of the general physicians practicing in the immediate area, and ancillary medical personnel. In the satellite centers the roster would include the more commonly consulted specialists and all of the general physicians. The location on hospital grounds will conserve the time of the physician as he provides ambulatory care in his office and in-patient treatment on the hospital wards. Ambulatory care will benefit also from the proximity of the extensive armamentarium of equipment, personnel, and other facilities of the in-patient service.

Each person will have free choice of his own general physician from among those affiliated with the hospital center serving his community. The general physician will be primarily responsible for the patient and for providing continuity of care at all times. The general physician will no longer "lose" his patient on admission to the hospital. Instead, as a member of the hospital staff, the patient's personal physician will carry the same responsibility within the hospital as he does now when his patient is referred to a specialist for ambulatory care. The general physician will thus pilot his patient in and out of the hospital, from one service to another within the hospital, and outside of the hospital to whatever specialist, laboratory, or ancillary service may be needed at any time.

With the creation of group practice units and under the pressure of the increasing complexity and soaring costs of care, the wasteful duplication of facilities in individual physician offices throughout the community will no longer need to exist. Their disappearance will require the creation of a mobile emergency service, an occasional substation for emergency care in a high risk area, for example, adjacent to an industrial plant, and for an efficient transportation system for ambulatory and critically ill patients. Transportation will have to be provided between the community and the hospital and among the hospitals in the regional system.

Except for emergencies and a rare handicapped patient, physicians will no longer make home visits. The visiting nurse, specially trained, will become the emissary of the physician. She will interpret the physician's instructions within the practical limitations of the patient's environment; reinforce health education of immediate applicability; administer prescribed injections or collect specimens for laboratory examination; identify new health and medical care problems; supply personal attention, reassurance, and comfort to the patient; and relay information back to the patient's physician.

By the turn of the century, it is likely that every member of the community served by the hospital center and its group practice unit will be insured against all major costs of medical care not otherwise covered (for example, Workmen's Compensation). It would be desirable that the patient pay a token amount for every service rendered, similar to the present practice in Sweden and unlike that in England. Without any significant financial barrier, the patient could then be freely referred within the regional system to any physician or specialist for any laboratory or other test, or to ancillary medical personnel needed for his care.

This proposed plan of hospital care for the future assumes that our society will continue to expect that everything possible will be done for every patient. The time may indeed come when a conscious decision may be made not to provide certain medical services or procedures because of excessive cost or lack of qualified specialists, other personnel, or essential equipment. In my own view, a modern civilized society must place a high enough premium on good medical care so that any scientific knowledge, professional skill, or resource which can preserve life or prevent or cure disease will be available to every citizen. But, arbitrary limitations on medical benefits for the aged, based on the amount of funds appropriated by the legislature rather than on medical need, have already been established in certain states (Colorado and New Mexico). If and when a conscious decision is made to limit medical care, it is to be hoped that priorities, based on objective medical standards, will be established as to the most effective use of available funds and personnel in the preservation of life and in the prevention and treatment of disease.

## Preventive Medicine in the Hospital

Thus far we have been concerned only with those services required for the treatment of disease. But at the turn of the next century, prevention will be a major function of the hospital as it evolves into a center for community health. Modern preventive medicine is concerned not only with the prevention of disease, but also with the prevention of disability and the postponement of untimely death. Preventive medicine, for many years a tool of the public health officer, is now an integral part of clinical medicine for the individual patient. Moreover, the science of epidemiology

— the study of all the factors that affect the occurrence and course of illness — can now be helpful in diagnosis as it has been in the prevention of the spread of disease in the past.

Accumulating medical knowledge has blurred and is now obliterating the line between preventive and curative medicine. The biochemist is identifying the predisposing chemical basis of more and more illnesses. Prevention can now be applied to noninfectious diseases. Individual medical procedures override both prevention and treatment. There are many examples: the search for phenylketonuria in all newborn babies to prevent mental deficiency, preventive advice to a patient planning to travel to an underdeveloped country, and the complete medical care of a patient with chronic disease to include prevention of complications, of deformity or disability, and vocational guidance and rehabilitation.

At the turn of the next century when you or your children are seen by a physician, you will be evaluated simultaneously for prevention and for treatment. Pediatricians are already spending more time on prevention than on treatment, particularly when they care for small babies. Medical care in all fields will be concerned increasingly with prevention to conform with the trends in our accumulating knowledge, and to anticipate your medical needs.

The major hospital centers of the future will include a consultation and research unit in preventive and social medicine. The staff of the preventive medical service would consist of specialists in preventive and social medicine, epidemiologists, and statisticians. A consultant in preventive medicine in each satellite hospital in the regional system will provide care and will be affiliated with a unit in the central hospital. Consultation on the individual patient by the specialist in preventive medicine might concern such questions as the desirability of immunization under special conditions of exposure and risk, for example, polio immunization for a pregnant woman or for a member of the hospital staff. Or, he may be asked to interpret epidemiologic data as it may affect the management of a case, for example, diet in a patient with coronary disease. He would also advise on procedures to be adopted by the staff to protect vulnerable patients, for example, the prophylaxis of a hospitalized rheumatic fever patient against the high risk of streptococcal infection which might trigger another attack of his disease.

The preventive medical service will be responsible for advising the staff on control of spread of illness from the community into the hospital, within the hospital to other patients and to staff, and from the hospital to the community. There are many examples; but this responsibility is most vividly delineated by our present epidemics of staphylococcal infection. The usual story begins with a physician or nurse carrying a virulent staphylococcus in his nose infecting the skin of a newborn infant in the hospital nursery. The disease may then spread to other infants in the nursery or to other members of the staff. After discharge, an infant may start an epidemic in his family and in the community. His mother may come down with a breast abscess. Other children in the family may develop skin infections from the infant or their mother. The children then spread the infection to their playmates in their neighborhood and in the local school. Then the epidemic goes round and round as patients with the infection are brought back to the hospital for treatment. Without epidemiologic control, some of our hospitals now act as foci for community epidemics of virulent strains of the staphylococcus. The consultant in preventive medicine will have direct responsibility for control of the hospital aspects of such epidemics and for working with the Health Department in control of the community epidemic.

The specialist in preventive medicine, aided by the wealth of information continually accumulating on environmental and genetic etiologic factors will also be concerned with controlling the spread of noninfectious disease. After consulting, for example, on a case of man-made disease caused by a toxic chemical in the air of an industrial plant, in smog, in a food additive, or in an insecticide spray, the specialist in preventive medicine will initiate a series of steps to protect the patient against further exposure and to prevent the development of additional cases. He will, with the assistance of the local health department and other appropriate agencies, seek out the source of the responsible toxic substance or other environmental factor. Such epidemiologic investigation is usually successful, because in contrast to naturally occurring illnesses it is relatively easy to identify the etiologic factor of man-made diseases. In cases of disease where genetic factors are most prominent, the situation is more difficult but the specialist in preventive medicine, as the facts justify it, will give eugenic advice.

In major hospital centers, the preventive medicine staff will conduct research in preventive and social medicine, medical economics, and epidemiology, and provide research consultation in biostatistics and biomathematics to other investigators. Collaborative research would be conducted with the clinical departments on studies which demand investigation of the population from which the hospital patients are selected, for example, the role of environmental factors in the increasing incidence of leukemia, or the relation of previous drug treatment to the etiology of lupus erythematosis and other connective tissue diseases.

## Local Health Department Within the Hospital

Traditionally, the local health department has been geographically separated and functionally isolated from the hospital and from therapeutic medical care. In their early beginnings, health departments were mostly concerned with engineering and sanitation, and in the environmental control of water, milk, and food supplies. With the advent of immunization, tuberculosis control, and preventive programs for maternity and infancy, the functions of the health department turned toward clinical medicine. Now, the rapid mushrooming of man-made diseases has imposed new responsibilities on the health department in environmental disease control. Man-made hazards from radiation, antibiotic-resistant germs, accidents, toxic chemicals, and new drugs demand a close working relationship between health department and clinician. Moreover, many of the newer health department programs on chronic illness demand active clinical participation.

The continued geographic and functional isolation of the official health service from clinical medicine, regardless of its effect on community health, became a firm tenet of organized medicine in order to "keep politics out of medicine." In England, in 1948 when the National Health Service was begun, on insistence of the British Medical Association the official health authority was set up in an administrative pyramid completely separate from those of the hospitals and specialists and the general physician services. The shortsightedness of this policy in England is now being recognized. The policy has not been of any real advantage to the physician, and has fragmented and increased the cost of medical care.

In the light of the recent Porritt Report, it is doubtful whether the British Medical Association would make the same recommendations today. In the United States at the present time, even if we wanted to, we could not interrelate health department and hospital functions and bring them together in the same geographic area. The independent operation and unplanned distribution of hospitals in most of our communities would make it impossible to select a single appropriate location.

The evolution of the regional hospital system will open the way for an effective unification of preventive and curative services. The health department will be transferred from its political surroundings in City Hall to the professional environment of the hospital center. The function of the health department will be interrelated with that of the therapeutic service through the preventive medical service in such activities as community-wide immunization against diseases (for example, polio and measles), interrelating school health services to total medical care as is done so well in Denmark, in the prevention and treatment of man-made diseases and in using community facilities in the total care of chronic illness. Both the hospital and the health department should benefit from the influence of the other. The standards of the health department would be improved by its location within the medical center, and by the exposure of the health department staff to the practice of scientific clinical medicine. At the same time, the hospital staff would become more aware of the relationship of its activities to community health. With strong professional leadership, there would be no question of bringing politics into medicine. Rather, the close relationship between the two agencies would bring a high standard of scientific medicine into our official health services and make the clinician more aware of his preventive responsibilities.

A firm link between the hospital and the health department can best be forged by having both under the same administrator. As hospital administrator, and health officer, he must have had education and experience in both fields so as to direct a unified health and medical care program for the community. The administrative task will be facilitated as hospital functions and medical care continue to take on a combined preventive and therapeutic character.

## *Voluntary Health Agencies*

Provision also must be made to bring voluntary health agencies within the functional scope of the center. Those providing direct services, for example, the Visiting Nurse Association, should be housed in the center. If the visiting nurse is to act under the supervision of the physician in establishing liaison between home and hospital care, she must be close by. With regard to the many voluntary health agencies not providing direct services, it is likely that society will tire of the continuing proliferation of individual health agencies each devoted to a single disease or organ system. Hopefully, at the turn of the next century there will be a single strong voluntary organization in the hospital center composed of many subunits, each channeling the interest of its supporters toward the conquest of its own health problem.

## SUMMARY AND CONCLUSIONS

At the turn of the next century, there could evolve from our present hospitals a regional system of community health centers for all aspects of preventive and curative medicine. The mechanism, although difficult to implement, is easy to visualize. But, would the patient in such a complicated medical environment, receive good medical care? The answer is "yes" if two additional factors are present. First, the practice of medicine must keep pace with continuously improving formal standards of care incorporating all available scientific knowledge.[1]

And most important of all, soundly based scientific medical care is impossible unless there exists a spirit of dedication to the principle that the health and the welfare of the patient come first. This spirit of dedication has permeated the Massachusetts General Hospital these many years and has in no small measure contributed to its fame. Without it a hospital will become a hollow shell. You may build your towers of glass, you may fill laboratories with the most advanced equipment, you may rebuild wards with the most modern conveniences, you may man hospitals with famous investigators and the most skillful clinicians. Yes, you may evolve the most elaborate system of regional health services, but without this sense of dedication you will not provide good medical care. In my view, your greatest responsibility is to preserve your tradition of dedication to the patient and then build your medical center of the future — your center of community health — around that principle.

NOTES

INDEX

# NOTES

### KNOWLES: THE TEACHING HOSPITAL

[1] R. M. Titmuss, *Essays on the Welfare State* (New Haven, Yale University Press, 1959), p. 135.

[2] A. G. L. Ives, *British Hospitals* (London, Collins, 1948), p. 17.

[3] G. Rosen, *A History of Public Health* (New York, MD Publications, 1958), p. 151.

[4] R. H. Shryock, *Medicine and Society in America, 1660–1860* (New York, New York University Press), p. 9.

[5] L. Shattuck, *Census of Boston for the Year 1845* (City of Boston, 1846), p. 5.

[6] O. Handlin, *Boston's Immigrants* (Cambridge, Mass., Harvard University Press, 1959), p. 239.

[7] *Ibid.*, p. 11.

[8] Shattuck, *Census of Boston*, p. 113.

[9] Handlin, *Boston's Immigrants*, p. 12.

[10] J. B. Blake, *Public Health in the Town of Boston, 1630–1822* (Cambridge, Mass., Harvard University Press, 1959), p. 33.

[11] R.. M. Lawrence, *Old Park Street and its Vicinity* (Boston, Houghton Mifflin, 1922), pp. 33–35.

[12] R. W. Kelso, *The History of Public Poor Relief in Massachusetts* (Boston, Houghton Mifflin, 1922), p. 112.

[13] W. R. Lawrence, *History of the Boston Dispensary* (Boston, 1859), p. 14.

[14] M. D. David and A. R. Warner, *Dispensaries: Their Management and Development* (New York, Macmillan, 1918), p. 6.

[15] J. W. Trask, *The United States Marine Hospital, Port of Boston* (U.S. Public Health Service, 1940), pp. 11–12.

[16] Shryock, *Medicine and Society in America*, pp. 7–9.

[17] H. R. Viets, *A Brief History of Medicine in Massachusetts* (Boston, Houghton Mifflin, 1930), p. 42.

[18] T. E. Moore, The early years of the Harvard Medical School. *Bulletin of the history of Medicine*, 27:530–561 (see p. 535), Nov.–Dec. 1953.

[19] *Ibid.*, p. 555.

[20] T. F. Harrington, *The Harvard Medical School: A History, Narrative and Documentary* (New York, 1905), pp. 274–278.

[21] L. K. Eaton, *New England Hospitals: 1790–1833* (Ann Arbor, University of Michigan Press, 1957), pp. 34–36.

[22] As quoted in J. E. Garland, *Every Man Our Neighbor* (Boston, Little, Brown, 1961), p. 5.

[23] N. I. Bowditch, *History of the Massachusetts General Hospital* (Boston, 1851), p. 55.

[24] *Address of the Trustees of the Massachusetts General Hospital to the Subscribers and to the Public* (Boston, 1822), p. 16.

[25] M.G.H. Annual Report, 1849, p. 5.

[26] Eaton, *New England Hospitals*, p. 105.

[27] R. H. Shryock, in *One Hundred Years of American Psychiatry*. J. K. Hall, ed. (New York, Columbia University Press, 1944), p. 15.

[28] F. A. Washburn, *The Massachusetts General Hospital: Its Development, 1900–1935* (Boston, Houghton Mifflin, 1939), p. 268.

[29] A. Deutsch, *The Mentally Ill in America*, 2d ed. (New York, Columbia University Press, 1949), pp. 158–185, 197–198.

[30] Washburn, *Massachusetts General Hospital*, p. 459.

[31] *Ibid.*, p. 467.

[32] M.G.H. Annual Report, 1914, pp. 61–62.

[33] Washburn, *Massachusetts General Hospital*, pp. 249–250.

[34] M.G.H. Annual Report, 1850, pp. 13–14.

[35] C. S. Burwell, "The evolution of medical education in 19th century America," *J. Med. Educ.* 37:1163 (November 1962).

[36] N. W. Faxon, *The Massachusetts General Hospital: 1935–1955* (Cambridge, Mass.: Harvard University Press, 1959), p. 239.

[37] Blue Cross Report to the Nation, 1962.

[38] Source Book of Health Insurance Data, 1963, N.Y., Health Insurance Institute.

### KNOWLES: THE BALANCED BIOLOGY OF THE TEACHING HOSPITAL

[1] K. L. White, T. F. Williams, and B. G. Greenberg, "Ecology of medical care," *New Eng. J. Med.*, 265:885–892 (November 2, 1961).

[2] E. Freidson, *Patient's Views of Medical Practice* (New York, Russell Sage Foundation, 1961), pp. 142–151, 180.

[3] E. C. Shortliffe, T. S. Hamilton, and E. H. Noroian, "Emergency room and changing pattern of medical care," *New Eng. J. Med.*, 258:20–25 (January 2, 1958).

[4] H. D. Lederer, "How the sick view their world," *J. Social Issues*, 8:4–15 (1962).

[5] United States Bureau of the Census, Current Population Reports, Consumer Income, Series P-60, Nos. 9 and 36.

[6] D. MacDonald, "Our invisible poor," *The New Yorker*, 38:82–132 (January 19, 1963).

[7] Freidson, *Patient's Views*, p. 230.

[8] H. J. Werner, "Premedical trends (communication)," *J. Med. Educ.*, 36:1327–1328 (October 1961).

[9] L. Trilling, "Commitment to the modern," *Harvard Alumni Bulletin*, 64:739 (July 1962).

[10] *The President's Report*, Harvard University, 1961–1962, p. 21.

[11] E. K. Russell, "Medicine as a social instrument: nursing," *New Eng. J. Med.*, 244:439–445 (March 22, 1951).

[12] *Ibid.*, pp. 443, 444.

[13] The Committee on the Function of Nursing, *A Program for the Nursing Profession* (New York, Macmillan, 1948), p. 101.

[14] S. Schulman, "Basic functional roles in nursing: mother surrogate and healer," in: *Patients, Physicians and Illness: Sourcebook in Behavioral Science and Medicine*, E. G. Jaco, ed. (Glencoe, Ill., The Free Press, 1958), pp. 528–537.

[15] A. L. Lowell, *What a University President Has Learned* (New York, Macmillan, 1938).

[16] E. Ashby, "Administrator: bottleneck or pump?" *Daedalus*, 91:264–278 (Spring 1962).

[17] *Ibid.*, p. 271.

[18] *Ibid.*, p. 272.

[19] H. Laski, "Limitation of the expert," in *The Intellectuals*, G. B. de Huszar, ed. (Glencoe, Ill., The Free Press, 1960), pp. 168, 171, 172.

[20] A. Bestor, "Education and its proper relationship to forces of American society," *Daedalus*, 88:75 (Winter 1959).

[21] A. Flexner, *Medical Education in the United States and Canada* (New York, Carnegie Foundation, 1910).

[22] Freidson, *Patient's Views*, p. 230.

[23] T. McKeown, "Responsibility of medical education in initiating change," *J. Med. Educ.*, 36:150–159 (December 1961).

[24] J. de S. Derek Price, *Science Since Babylon* (New Haven, Yale University Press, 1961), pp. 107, 108.

[25] President's Science Advisory Committee Report, "Strengthening the Behavioral Sciences," *Science*, 136:233–241 (April 20, 1962).

READER: CONTRIBUTION OF THE BEHAVIORAL SCIENCES

[1] Robert K. Merton, George G. Reader, and Patricia L. Kendall, *The Student Physician* (Cambridge, Mass., Harvard University Press, 1957), pp. 81–90.

[2] *Ibid.*, pp. 287–293.

[3] *Ibid.*, pp. 90–101.

[4] *Ibid.*

[5] Robert K. Merton, Samuel Bloom, and Natalie Rogoff, "Studies in the Sociology of Medical Education," *J. Med. Educ.*, 31:556 (August 1956).

[6] *The Ecology of the Medical Student*, a reprint of the Fifth Teaching Institute, 1958, Association of American Medical Colleges, Evanston, Ill.

[7] Gene N. Levine, Natalie Rogoff, and David Caplovitz, "Diversities in Role Conceptions," Bureau of Applied Social Research, Columbia University, 1955 (mimeographed, 65pp), Confidential Report.

[8] David Caplovitz, "Student-Faculty Relations in Medical School," unpub. diss., Columbia University, 1961.

[9] Patricia L. Kendall, James A. Jones, and Candace Rogers, "The Effects of the Cornell Comprehensive Care and Teaching Program on the Attitudes and Values of Fourth-Year Medical Students," Bureau of Applied Social Research, Columbia University, 1960 (mimeographed, 203pp), Confidential Report.

[10] *Ibid.*, p. 61.

[11] *Ibid.*, pp. 84–85.

[12] *Ibid.*, p. 130.

[13] M. E. W. Goss, "Role of the Full-time Staff in the Clinic for Compre-

hensive Care and Teaching," CC&TP Research Memorandum No. 6, series A, 1956 (mimeographed, 6pp).

[14] M. E. W. Goss, "Change in the Cornell Comprehensive Care and Teaching Program" in Merton, *et al.*, *The Student Physician*, pp. 249–270.

[15] M. E. W. Goss, "Influence and Authority Among Physicians in an Outpatient Clinic," *Amer. Soc. Rev.*, 26:39–50 (February 1961).

[16] *Ibid.*, p. 50.

[17] M. E. W. Goss, "Administration and the Physician," *Amer. J. Public Health*, 52:183–191 (February 1962).

[18] Margaret Olendzki, "Chart Study of a Sample of General Medical Clinic Patients," CC&TP Research Memorandum, No. 3, series D, 1955 (mimeographed, 30pp).

[19] Margaret Olendzki and George G. Reader, "Appointment-Breaking in a General Medical Clinic," paper presented to Medical Care Section, American Public Health Association, October 19, 1959.

[20] Margaret Olendzki, "Statistical Trends since the Establishment of the Comprehensive Care Program," CC&TP Research Memorandum, no. 2, series C, 1956 (mimeographed, 17pp).

[21] *Ibid.*, p. 13.

[22] Lois Pratt, Margaret Mudd, and George Reader, "Clinic Patient's Expectations of Medical Care," Paper presented at Medical Care Section, American Public Health Association, November 14, 1956.

[23] Arthur W. Seligmann, Niva E. McGrath, and Lois Pratt, "Level of Medical Information Among Clinic Patients," *J. Chron. Dis.*, 6:492–509 (November 1957).

[24] Lois Pratt, Arthur Seligmann, and George Reader, "Physicians Views on the Level of Medical Information Among Patients," *Amer. J. Public Health*, 47:1277–1283 (October 1957).

[25] Lois Pratt, "Communication in the Doctor-Patient Relationship: Doctor's Views on Patients' Information about Disease," unpublished, 1956 (mimeographed, 10pp), p. 8.

[26] Alice Ullmann and Gene G. Kassebaum, *Soc. Serv. Rev.* 35:258–267 (September 1961).

[27] Doris Schwartz, Barbara Henley, and Leonard Zietz, *The Plight of the Elderly Ill* (Maximillan, New York, in press).

[28] Doris Schwartz, Mamie Wang, Leonard Zeitz, and M. E. W. Goss, "Medication Errors Made by Elderly, Chronically Ill Patients," *American Journal of Public Health*, 52:2018–2029 (December 1962).

[29] *Ibid.*, p. 2028.

[30] M. E. W. Goss and George G. Reader, "Collaboration Between Sociologist and Physician," *Social Problems*, 4:82–89 (1956).

### CHERKASKY: THE HOSPITAL AS A SOCIAL INSTRUMENT

[1] E. M. Bluestone, *et al.*, "Home Care — an Extra Morale Hospital Function," *Survey*, April 1948.

[2] Martin Cherkasky, "Hospital Service Goes Home," *The Modern Hospital* (May 1947).

[3] Isidore Rossman, "The Reduction of Anxiety in a Home Care Setting," *J. of Chron. Dis.*, 4:527–534 (November 1956).

[4] David Littauer, I. Jerome Flance, and Albert Wessen, *Home Care*,

American Hospital Association, Chicago 1961 — Hospital Monograph no. 9.

[5] Hospital Research and Educational Trust, *Guide to Organized Home Care* (Chicago, 1961).

[6] U.S. Public Health Service, *A Study of Selected Home Care Programs*, Washington, D.C., U.S. Government Printing Office, 1955 (P.H.S. Publication No. 447).

[7] U.S. Bureau of the Census, *Statistical Abstract of the United States: 1962*, 83d ed., Washington, D.C., 1962, p. 348.

[8] E. Richard Weinerman, "Medical Care in Prepaid Group Practice," *Archives of Environmental Health*, 5:561–573 (December 1962).

[9] George Silver, Martin Cherkasky, and Joseph Axelrod, "An Experience with Group Practice — The Montefiore Medical Group 1948–1956," *New Eng. J. Med.*, 256:785–791 (April 25, 1957).

[10] Joseph Axelrod, "Group Practice of Medicine and Surgery," *Resident Physician* (September 1956), vol. 2.

[11] Paul Densen, E. Balamuth, and Sam Schapiro, *Prepaid Medical Care and Hospital Utilization*, American Hospital Association, Chicago 1958 — Hospital Monograph Series no. 3, p. 34.

[12] Martin Cherkasky: *Family Health Maintenance Demonstration*, Research in Public Health, Papers presented at the 1951 Annual Conference, Milbank Memorial Fund (New York, 1952).

[13] Milbank Memorial Fund, *The Family Health Maintenance Demonstration* (New York, 1954)

[14] G. A. Silver, *Family Medical Care* (Cambridge, Mass., Harvard University Press, 1963).

[15] Committee on Labor and Public Welfare, United States Senate, *The Condition of American Nursing Homes*, Washington, D.C., U.S. Government Printing Office, 1960, p. 7.

[16] Harold Baumgarten and Ray E. Trussell, "Teamsters Plan Next Step in Health Care," *The Modern Hospital*, 98:79, 180 (May 1962).

[17] Teamsters Joint Council No. 16 and Management Hospitalization Trust Fund: *Meeting the Challenge of Health Care Today* (New York, 1962).

[18] Martin Cherkasky, "Medical Care," *Amer. J. Public Health*, 52:767–772 (May 1962).

[19] N. W. Faxon, ed., *The Hospital in Contemporary Life* (Cambridge, Mass., Harvard University Press, 1949), p. 62.

TRUSSELL: MAINTAINING QUALITY IN HOSPITALS

[1] R. E. Trussell, "The Municipal Hospital in Transition," *Bull. N.Y. Acad. Sc.*, 38:221–236 (April 1962).

MASUR: GOVERNMENT AND HOSPITALS

[1] J. Pollack, "The Union Health Movement as Voluntarism" (MS), presented at the Twenty-first Eastern States Health Education Conference (New York Academy of Medicine, April 27–28, 1961).

[2] *The Advancement of Medical Research and Education Through the Department of Health, Education and Welfare*. Final Report of the Secretary's Consultants on Medical Research and Education, Stanhope Bayne-

Jones, M.D., Chairman (Washington, D.C., Government Printing Office, June 1958).

[3] *Building America's Health*, A Report to the President by the President's Commission on the Health Needs of the Nation, 5 vols. (Washington, D.C., Government Printing Office, 1952).

[4] *Federal Medical Services*, A Report to the Congress by the Commission on Organization of the Executive Branch of the Government (Washington, D.C., Government Printing Office, February 1955).

[5] *Federal Support of Medical Research*, Report of the Committee of Consultants on Medical Research to the Subcommittee on Departments of Labor and Health, Education and Welfare to the Senate Committee on Appropriations, 86th Congress, Second Session, Boisfeuillet Jones, Chairman (Washington, D.C., Government Printing Office, 1960).

[6] *Medical Care in the United States — The Role of the Public Health Service*, A Report to the Surgeon General from the National Advisory Health Council (Washington, D.C., Government Printing Office, 1961).

[7] *Medical School Grants and Financing*, Report of the Surgeon General's Committee on Medical School Grants and Finances (Washington, D.C., Government Printing Office, 1951).

[8] *Physicians for a Growing America*, Report of the Surgeon General's Consultant Group on Medical Education, Frank Bane, Chairman (Washington, D.C., Government Printing Office, 1959).

[9] *Reorganization of Federal Medical Activities*, A Report to the Congress by the Commission on Organization of the Executive Branch of the Government (Washington, D.C., Government Printing Office, 1949).

[10] F. Goldmann, *Public Medical Care Principles and Problems* (New York, Columbia University Press, 1945).

[11] *The Voluntary Hospital System*, Statement of Board of Trustees (Chicago, American Hospital Association, 1961).

[12] "The Saskatchewan Story: A Review and Prospect" — (1) M. S. Acker, "Saskatchewan's Health Services in Prospective," (2) R. F. Badgley, "The Public and Medical Care in Saskatchewan," (3) A. F. W. Peart, "The Medical Viewpoint," (4) J. G. Clarkson, "The Saskatoon Agreement and Amending Legislation Developments in the Post-Agreement," (5) S. Wolfe, "The Saskatchewan Medical Care Insurance Act, 1961, and the Impasse with the Medical Profession," *Amer. J. Public Health*, 53:717–735 (May 1963).

[13] Section 635 of the Public Health Service Act as amended, 42 USC 291m.

[14] G. A. Harrison, *Government Controls and the Voluntary Non-profit Hospital* (Chicago, American Hospital Association, 1961).

[15] A. W. Willcox, "Hospitals and Government in the Decade Ahead," *Trustee*, 14:1–5 (September 1961).

[16] A. H. Raskin, "Our Economy: Mixed and Mixed-up," *The Reporter*, 27:27–31 (October 11, 1962).

[17] L. Carroll, "Sylvie and Bruno," *Complete Works of Lewis Carroll* (Modern Library Giants, no. 28).

[18] N. W. Faxon, *The Hospital in Contemporary Life* (Cambridge, Mass., Harvard University Press, 1949).

[19] *Ibid.*, pp. 61–62.

[20] C. V. Kidd, *American Universities and Federal Research* (Cambridge, Mass., Belknap Press of Harvard University Press, 1959).
[21] *The Washington Post*, Editorial, June 7, 1962.

PETERSON: MEDICAL CARE RESEARCH

[1] I. C. Merriman, "Social Welfare Expenditures, 1960–1961," *Social Security Bulletin*, November 1962.
[2] O. W. Anderson and J. J. Feldman, *Family Medical Costs and Voluntary Health Insurance: A Nationwide Survey* (New York, 1956).
[3] *Health Statistics from the U.S. National Health Survey*, U.S. Dept. of Health, Education and Welfare, U.S.P.H.S. series B., no. 30, November 1961.
[4] E. Balamuth, P. M. Densen, and S. Shapiro, *Prepaid Medical Care and Hospital Utilization*, Hospital Monograph Series no. 3, American Hospital Association, 1958.
[5] O. W. Anderson and P. B. Sheatsley, "Comprehensive Medical Insurance: A Study of Costs, Use and Attitudes Under Two Plans," Health Information Foundation Research Series no. 9, 1959.
[6] I. Baldinger, P. M. Densen, E. W. Jones, and S. Shapiro, "Prepaid Medical Care and Hospital Utilization," *Hospitals*, 36:62–68, 138 (November 1962).
[7] *Special Study on the Medical Care Program for Steelworkers and Their Families*, A Report by the Insurance, Pension and Unemployment Benefits Department, United Steelworkers of America, Atlantic City, September 1960.
[8] G. Forsyth and R. F. L. Logan, "The Demand for Medical Care," Nuffield Provincial Hospitals Trust (Oxford University Press, 1960).
[9] C. R. Lowe and T. McKeown, "The Care of the Chronic Sick: I — Medical and Nursing Requirements" *Br. J. Soc. Med.*, 3:110–126 (July 1949).
[10] Forsyth and Logan, "The Demand for Medical Care."
[11] D. L. Crombie and K. W. Cross, "Serious Illness in Hospital and at Home" (*The Medical Press*, October 14, 1959), p. 316–322.
[12] F. N. Garratt, J. M. MacKintosh, and T. McKeown, "An Examination of the Need for Hospital Admission," *Lancet*, 1:815–818 (April 15, 1961).
[13] Forsyth and Logan, "The Demand for Medical Care."
[14] H. F. Becker, "Controlling Use and Misuse of Hospital Care," *Hospitals*, 28:61–64 (December 1954).
[15] E. A. Codman, "The Product of a Hospital," *Surg., Gynec. & Obst.*, 18:491–496 (April 1914).
[16] G. G. Ward, "The Value and Need of More Attention to End-Results and Follow-up in Hospitals Today" (read at the Annual Hospital Conference of the American College of Surgeons, Chicago, October 22–23, 1923).
[17] P. M. Densen, S. Shapiro, and L. Weiner, "Comparison of Prematurity and Perinatal Mortality in a General Population and in the Population of a Prepaid Group Practice, Medical Care Plan," *Am. J. Public Health*, 48:170–187 (February 1958).
[18] J. A. H. Lee, J. N. Morris, and S. L. Morrison. "Fatality from Three

Common Surgical Conditions in Teaching and Non-teaching Hospitals," *Lancet*, 2:785–791 (October 19, 1957).

[19] J. A. H. Lee, J. N. Morris, and S. L. Morrison, "Case-Fatality in Teaching and Non-teaching Hospitals," *Lancet*, 1:170–171 (January 1960).

[20] L. P. Andrews, B. G. Greenberg, O. L. Peterson, and R. S. Spain, "An Analytical Study of North Carolina General Practice, 1953–1954," *J. Med. Educ.*, 31:1–165 (December 1956).

[21] K. F. Clute, *The General Practitioner, A Study of Medical Education and Practice in Ontario and Nova Scotia*, University of Toronto Press, 1963.

[22] C. Jungfer, "General Practice in Australia: A report on a Survey" (MS), Adelaide S., Australia.

[23] R. A. Nelson, "The Hospital and Education," *Hospitals*, 36:48–50, 174 (August 16, 1962) and 36:50–55 (September 1, 1962).

POLLACK: THE VOICE OF THE CONSUMER

[1] Adam Smith, *An Inquiry Into the Nature and Causes of the Wealth of Nations* (New York, Random House, 1937), p. 625.

[2] Henry E. Sigerist, *A History of Medicine*, Vol. II: *Early Greek, Hindu, and Persian Medicine* (New York, Oxford, 1961).

[3] G. R. Driver and John C. Miles, *The Babylonian Laws* (Oxford, 1960).

[4] *The Dialogues of Plato*, tr. B. Jowett (New York, Random House), II, 603.

[5] James Harvey Young, *The Toadstool Millionaires* (Princeton, 1961), p. 247.

[6] New Medical Material, vol. 5, no. 4, p. 18.

[7] *Attitudes Toward Co-operation in a Health Examination Survey*, Health Statistics, U.S. Dept. of Health, Education and Welfare, series D, no. 6.

[8] Pierce Williams, *The Purchase of Medical Care Through Fixed Periodic Payment*, National Bureau of Economic Research, 1932.

[9] American Medical Association, *Report of Commission on Medical Care Plans*, part II, 1958.

[10] *In the Public Mind*, the *Fortune* Survey, vol. 26, no. 1, July 1942.

[11] *Digest of Official Actions*, 1846–1958, American Medical Association (Chicago, 1959), p. 317.

[12] *Medical Care Financing and Utilization*, Health Economics Series no. 1, U.S. Department of Health, Education and Welfare, Public Health Service (Washington, 1962).

[13] Alfred M. Skolnick, *Growth of Employee-Benefit Plans, 1954–61*, Social Security Bulletin, vol. 26, no. 4, April 1963, pp. 4–11.

[14] Louis S. Reed and Dorothy P. Rice, *Private Medical Care Expenditures and Voluntary Health Insurance, 1948–61*, Social Security Bulletin, vol. 25, no. 12, December 1962, pp. 3–13.

[15] *Ibid.*

[16] Warren F. Draper, *The Medical Care Program of the United Mineworkers of America Welfare Retirement Fund*, presented at the New England Assembly, Hotel Hilton, Boston, Massachusetts, March 25, 1958, unpublished paper.

[17] Ray E. Trussell and Frank Van Dyke, *Prepayment for Hospital Care*

*in New York State*: A Report on the Eight Blue Cross Plans Serving New York Residents, School of Public Health and Administrative Medicine (New York, Columbia University, 1960).

[18] Ray E. Trussell and Frank Van Dyke, *Prepayment for Medical and Dental Care*: A Report on the Seven Blue Shield and Other Plans Serving New York Residents, School of Public Health and Administrative Medicine (New York, Columbia University, 1962).

[19] Carl Binger, "The Change in Education," in A. E. Corcoran, *A Mirror Up to Medicine* (Philadelphia, Lippincott, 1961), pp. 171–172.

SOMERS: PRIVATE HEALTH INSURANCE: PROGRESS AND PROBLEMS

[1] H. M. Somers and A. R. Somers, *Doctors, Patients and Health Insurance* (Washington, D.C., The Brookings Institution, 1961), pp. 534 (with appendix).

SCHOTTLAND: THE SOCIAL SECURITY SYSTEM AND MEDICAL CARE

[1] International Labor Office, *Social Security: A Worker's Education Manual* (Geneva, 1958), pp. 2–7.

[2] Social Security Board, *Social Security in America* (Washington, D.C., U.S. Government Printing Office, 1937), p. 470.

[3] I. M. Rubinow, *Social Insurance* (New York, Henry Holt, 1913), p. iii.

[4] United States Social Security Act: 49 Stat. 620 (1935); 42 USCA 7 (1940).

[5] International Labor Office, *Social Security*, p. 12.

[6] United States Congressional Record, vol. 79, pt. 6, 74th Congress, 1st sess., 1935, p. 5858.

[7] A. M. Schlesinger, Jr., *The Coming of the New Deal* (Boston, Houghton-Mifflin, 1959), p. 312.

[8] Congressional Record, vol. 79, pt. 6, 74th Congress, 1st sess., 1935, p. 5875.

[9] *Ibid.*, p. 6051.

[10] *Ibid.*, pt. 9, p. 9285.

[11] *Ibid.*, p. 9440.

[12] *Ibid.*, pt. 6, p. 6054.

[13] Schlesinger, *The Coming of the New Deal*, p. 311.

[14] Congressional Record, vol. 79, pt. 6, 74th Congress, 1st sess., 1935, p. 6063.

[15] *Ibid.*, p. 6054.

[16] J. D. Richardson, comp., *A Compilation of the Messages and Papers of the Presidents* (New York, Bureau of National Literature, 1897 II, 5142 [Special Messages, February 16, 1887]).

[17] Helvering v. Davis, 301 United States 619, 81L, ed. 1307, 57 Sup. Ct. 904 (1937).

[18] Schlesinger, *The Coming of the New Deal*, p. 315.

[19] A. M. David, "Old-Age, Survivors and Disability Insurance: Twenty-five Years of Progress," *Industrial and Labor Relations Review*, 14:12 (October 1960).

[20] *Ibid.*, p. 13.

[21] Ewing v. Gardner, 185 F.2d, 781, 784, 1950.

[22] *Great Britain Parliament Papers*, Committee on the Economic and Financial Problems of the Provision for Old Age, Report. Cmd. no. 9333, sec. 167, 1954.

[23] *Financing Old-Age, Survivors, and Disability Insurance*, A Report of the Advisory Council on Social Security Financing. 1959 (Washington, D.C.: Government Printing Office, United States Department of Health, Education, and Welfare, sec. II), p. 3

[24] E. E. Witte, "The Theory of Workmen's Compensation," *American Labor Legislation Review*, 20:411–418 (December 1930).

[25] H. M. Somers and A. R. Somers, *Workmen's Compensation* (New York, John Wiley, 1954), p. 59.

[26] A. M. Skolnik, "Income Loss Protection Against Short-Term Sickness, 1948–1960," *Social Security Bulletin*, 25:5 (January 1962).

### CHURCHILL: MEDICAL EDUCATION IN THE HOSPITAL

[1] American Medical Association, *A History of the Council on Medical Education and Hospitals of the A.M.A.* (1904–1959) (Chicago, 1959).

[2] A. Lawrence Lowell, *What a University President Has Learned* (New York, Macmillan, 1938).

[3] Alan Gregg, "Horizons at Half Century," *Bulletin of the American College of Surgeons*, 40:65–72 (March–April 1955).

[4] S. Roodhouse Gloyne, *John Hunter* (Edinburgh, 1950), p. 83.

[5] Geoffrey Keynes, ed., *The Apologie and Treatise of Ambroise Paré* (Chicago, University of Chicago Press, 1952), p. 10.

### NELSON: THE HOSPITAL AND THE CONTINUING EDUCATION OF THE PHYSICIAN

[1] Abraham Flexner, *Medical Education in the United States and Canada*, Bulletin no. 4 (Boston, Merrymount, 1910).

[2] A History of the Council on Medical Education and Hospitals of the American Medical Association, 1959.

[3] "Medical Education in the United States, 1961–62," *Journal of the American Medical Association*, 182:735–808 (November 17, 1962).

[4] *Ibid.*

[5] History of the Council on Medical Education.

[6] "Medical Education in the U.S."

[7] Russell A. Nelson, Accreditation of Internship Programs, Proceedings of the 58th Annual Congress on Medical Education, Council on Medical Education and Hospitals, American Medical Association, February 1962.

[8] "Medical Education in the U.S."

[9] Douglas D. Vollan, Postgraduate Medical Education in the United States: A Report of the Survey of Postgraduate Medical Education Carried Out by the Council on Medical Education and Hospitals of the American Medical Association, 1952–1955 (Chicago, American Medical Association, 1955).

[10] Joseph E. Garland, Jr., *An Experiment in Medicine: The First Twenty Years of the Pratt Clinic and the New England Center Hospital of Boston* (Cambridge, Riverside, 1960).

[11] Harry A. Towsley, "University of Michigan Plan for Postgraduate

Medical Education: An Example of the Potentialities of Regional Hospital-Medical School Affiliation," *JAMA*, 164:377–380 (May 25, 1957).

[12] Charles F. Wilkinson, Jr., "New York University Plan: An Example Showing the Potentialities of Regional Hospital-Medical School Affiliation," *JAMA*, 164:381–383 (May 25, 1957).

[13] Frank M. Woolsey, Jr., "Two Years of Experience with Two-Way Radio Conferences for Postgraduate Medical Education," *J. Med. Educ.*, 33:474–482 (June 1958).

[14] Medicine: A Lifelong Study, Proceedings of the Second World Congress on Medical Education, Chicago, 1959 (World Medical Association, 1961).

[15] John C. Leonard, Proposed Accreditation of Continuing Education Programs, Proceedings of the 58th Annual Congress on Medical Education. Council on Medical Education and Hospitals, American Medical Association, February 1962.

[16] Bernard V. Dryer, "Lifetime Learning for Physicians," *J. Med. Educ.*, 37:89–90 (June 1962).

[17] Laurence B. Ellis, "Reflections on Postgraduate Medical Education for Practicing Physicians," *New Eng. J. Med.*, 250:243–245 (February 11, 1954).

[18] Dryer, *Lifetime Learning*.

[19] "Medical Education in the U.S."

[20] Joseph W. Mountin, Elliott N. Pennell, and Vane M. Hoge, Health Service Areas: Requirements for General Hospitals and Health Centers, Public Health Bulletin no. 292, United States Public Health Service, 1945.

### MC KEOWN: MEDICAL EDUCATION AND MEDICAL CARE

[1] T. McKeown and R. G. Brown, "Medical Evidence Related to English Population Changes in the Eighteenth Century," *Population Studies*, 9:119–141 (November 1955).

[2] T. McKeown and R. G. Record, "Reasons for the Decline of Mortality in England and Wales During the Nineteenth Century," *Population Studies*, 16:94–122 (November 1962).

[3] T. McKeown, "Priorities in Preventive Medicine," *New Eng. J. Med.*, 264:594–599 (March 23, 1961).

[4] T. McKeown, "The Concept of a Balanced Hospital Community," *Lancet* 1:701–704 (April 5, 1958).

[5] T. McKeown, "The Future of Medical Practice Outside the Hospital," *Lancet*, 1:923–928 (May 5, 1962).

### LINDEMANN: THE HEALTH NEEDS OF COMMUNITIES

[1] B. Pasamanick, ed., *Epidemiology of Mental Disorder* (Washington, D.C.) American Association for the Advancement of Science, Pub. 60, 1959; J. Hirsch, "Recent development in behavior genetics and differential psychology," Diseases of the Nervous System. (mongr. suppl.) 19:17–24 (1958); and E. H. Hess, "Imprinting," *Science*, 130:133–141 (July 1959).

[2] H. S. Liddell, "Experimental neuroses in animals," in: *Stress and Psychiatric Disorder*, J. M. Tanner, ed., (Oxford, Blackwell Scientific Publications, 1960) pp. 59–64.

[3] H. F. Harlow and R. R. Zimmermann, "Affectional responses in the infant monkey," *Science*, 130:421–432 (August 1959).

[4] H. F. Harlow, "Development in affection in primates," in: *Roots of Behavior*, E. L. Bliss, ed., (New York, Harpers, 1962) pp. 157–166.

[5] J. Bowlby, "Separation anxiety," *Int. J. Psycho-Anal.*, 41:89–113 (March–June 1960); J. Bowlby, "The nature of the child's tie to his mother," *Int. J. Psycho-Anal.*, 39:350–373 (September–October 1958); G. L. Engle, "Homeostasis, behavioral adjustment and the concept of health and disease," in: *Mid-Century Psychiatry*, R. Grinker, ed., (Springfield, Ill., Thomas, 1953) p. 33–59; G. L. Engle, *Psychological Development in Health and Disease* (Philadelphia, Pa., Saunders, 1962); and R. A. Spitz, "Hospitalism: an inquiry into the genesis of psychiatric conditions in early childhood," in: *The Psychoanalytic Study of the Child* (New York, International Universities Press, 1945), I, 53–74.

[6] John Benjamin . . . (personal communication).

[7] P. Wolff, "Observation on newborn infants," *Psychosomatic Medicine*, 21:110–118 (March–April 1959).

[8] S. K. Escalona and G. M. Heider, *Prediction and Outcome* (New York, Basic Books, 1959); and S. K. Escalona, M. Leitsh, *et al.*, "Early phases of personality development," Monographs of Society for Research in Child Development, Inc., vol. XVII, 1952.

[9] G. Caplan, "Psychological aspects of maternity care," *Amer. J. Public Health*, 47:25–31 (January 1957).

[10] G. Caplan, "Concepts of mental health and consultation," (Washington, D.C., Children's Bureau, U.S. Dept. of Health, Education and Welfare, Publication no. 373, 1959), pp. 185–187

[11] G. Caplan, ed., *Prevention of Mental Disorders in Children: Initial Explorations* (New York, Basic Books, 1961).

[12] G. L. Bibring, "Some considerations of the psychological processes in pregnancy," in: *The Psychoanalytic Study of the Child* (New York, International Universities Press, 1959) XIV, 113–121.

[13] H. J. Barry and E. Lindemann, "Critical ages for maternal bereavement in psychoneuroses," *Psychosomatic Medicine*, 22:166–181 (May–June 1960).

[14] J. Hilgard, "Maternal bereavement in psychoneuroses and alcoholism," presented at Annual Meeting of the American Orthopsychiatric Association (Los Angeles, 1962); and J. R. Hilgard, M. F. Newman, and F. Fisk, "Strength of adult ego following childhood bereavement," *Amer. J. Orthopsych.*, 30:788–798 (October 1960).

[15] E. H. Erikson, "Growth and crises of the 'healthy personality,'" in: *Problems of Infancy and Childhood*, M. Sean, ed., (New York, Josiah Macy, Jr. Foundation, 1950).

[16] Idem, *Identity and the Life Cycle* (New York, International Universities Press, 1959).

[17] J. W. M. Whiting and I. L. Child, *Child Training and Personality: A Cross-Cultural Study* (New Haven, Yale University Press, 1953).

[18] A. B. Hollingshead and F. C. Redlich, *Social Class and Mental Illness: A Community Study* (New York, John Wiley, 1958).

[19] J. P. Spiegel, "The resolution of role conflict within the family," *Psychiatry*, 20:1–16 (February 1957).

[20] K. Naegele, "A mental health project in a Boston suburb," in: *Health, Culture, and Community*, B. D. Paul, ed., (New York, Russell Sage Foundation, 1955).

[21] Idem, "Some problems in the study of hostility and aggression in middle-class American families," *Canad. J. Econ. and Pol. Sc.*, 17:65–75 (February 1951).

[22] D. Aberle and K. Naegele, "Middle class fathers' occupation role and attitudes towards children," *Amer. J. Orthopsych.*, 22:366–378 (April 1952).

[23] G. Lewis, "A technique in social geography for the delimitation of urban residential subregions," unpub. diss., Harvard University, 1956.

[24] E. Lindemann, "The Wellesley project for the study of certain problems in community mental health," in: *Interrelations between the Social Environment and Psychiatric Disorders* (New York, Milbank Memorial Fund, 1953), pp. 167–186.

[25] H. J. Gans, *The Urban Villagers* (Illinois, The Free Press of Glencoe, 1962); M. Fried, "Grieving for a lost home," in: *The Urban Condition*, L. J. Duhl, ed., (New York, Basic Books, 1963), pp. 184–200; and M. Fried and E. Lindemann, "Sociocultural factors in mental health and illness," *Amer. J. Orthopsych.*, 31:87–101 (January 1961).

[26] M. E. Chafetz, *et al.*, "Establishing treatment relations with alcoholics," *J. Nerv. and Ment. Dis.*, 134:395–409 (May 1962).

[27] N. B. Talbot, "Has psychologic malnutrition taken the place of rickets and scurvy in contemporary pediatric practice?" Borden Award Address, *Pediatrics*, 31:909–918 (June 1963).

[28] J. D. Stoeckle, I. K. Zola, and G. E. Davidson. "On going to see the doctor; the contributions of the patient to the decision to seek medical aid," *J. Chron. Dis.*, 16:975–989 (September 1963).

RUTSTEIN: AT THE TURN OF THE NEXT CENTURY

[1] D. D. Rutstein, "Better Health for Americans: The need for standards of medical care," *Transactions & Studies of the College of Physicians of Philadelphia*, 4 ser., vol. 29, no. 4, April 1962.

# INDEX

Administration: of clinics, 79–81; function of, 34; hospital health department, 315

Admission rates, *see* Utilization

Aged, 201–220; community center, 104; financing care, 183; health insurance, 151, 193; hospital population, 26; medical care, 218; mental illness in, 262; Old-Age, Survivors, and Disability Insurance, 207–215

Alcoholism, 288

Ambulatory services, 64–92; faculty attitudes, 69–74; and the hospital, 65, 264; hospital costs, 101; need for physicians, 240; and social science studies, 290; student attitudes, 74–79

American Hospital Association, 133; and continuing education, 245

American Medical Association (AMA): commission on medical care plans, 181; council on medical education and hospitals, 114, 224; intern-residency training, 241; survey of postgraduate medical education, 242

Anderson, Odin, 149

Association of American Medical Colleges, 244–245

Automation, in hospitals, 297–300

Becker, Harry, 157

Behavioral (social) sciences, 64–92, 271–292; medical curricula, 45–46; out-patient studies, 65, 290; patient care, 87–90; psychological development, 274; social environment, 277–278

Bingham Associates, 243

Blue Cross: Massachusetts, 20; New York, 115; per cent of expenditures, 187; reimbursement for diagnostic services, 301; utilization, 154

Blue Shield: government relationship, 116; Health Insurance Plan of Greater New York, 153; per cent of private expenditures, 187

Canadian Medical Association, 135

Change, and medical profession, 222–224

Chronic disease, and institutional care, 306–308

Cocoanut Grove Fire, 271

Codman, E. A., 158

Community center, 104–105

Community health, 271–292, 303–317. *See also* 254–270

Consumers, organized, 167–186; Teamsters' Union, 107–109, 197

Cornell Comprehensive Care and Teaching Program, 67; faculty attitudes, 69–74; student attitudes, 74–79

Costs, medical care: charges in *1930*, 16; contemporary, 26–27; distribution by families, 149; and family income, 150; financing, 172–177; hospital and prepaid group practice (HIP), 101; hospital utilization, 101; increasing, 114–116, 195, 300–302; and local government, 114; organization of medical services, 198–199; and public health department, 314

Director of Medical Education, 249

Dryer, Bernard, 246

Ellis, Laurence B., 245

Emergency Ward: increasing use of, 25; and mental illness, 289; need for physicians, 240

"Family Health Maintenance Demonstration, A," 102–103

Fatality rates, *see* Mortality rates

Flexner, A., 238, 248

Foreign medical graduates, 241

General practitioner: Academy of General Practice, 244; performance studies, 161–163

Group Health Insurance of New York (GHI), 153

Group practice, *see* Medical group practice

Harlow, H. F., 275

Harvard Medical School, 9–11, 179–180

Health insurance, 187–200; comprehensive coverage, 191; demographic factors, 189; financing of medical care, 172–178; HIP of Greater New York, 100, 153; Medical Care Insurance Act (Saskatchewan), 135; per cent coverage as related to age, 151; and semi-private location, 25

Health Insurance Plan of Greater New York (HIP), 100, 152; and perinatal mortality, 158–159

Hill-Burton program, 129, 137–140

History of teaching hospitals, 1–21; of nursing profession, 32–34, 51

Home care: Great Britain, 263; relation to hospital, 96–99

Hospitals: administrator, 34–37; balanced function, 37, 43–45; balanced hospital community, 262; changing role of physician, 249; charges paid by insurance, 151; and the chronically ill, 94; government, 128; government-voluntary collaboration, 137–140; guiding philosophy, 47, 62–63; and home care, 96–99, 264; Massachusetts General, 1–46, 221–236; Montefiore, 93–110; professional staff, 119–120; proprietary, 118, 120; public utility concept, 142; restrictions of teaching, 266–268; role as educational institution, 248–249; separation of mental, chronic, and acute types, 259; seven-day work week, 299; specialty, 303; teaching function, 226–227, 237–253; trustee, 37; types of, 113; utilization, 101; and voluntarism, 133; voluntary, relationship to government, 132

Hospital Survey and Construction Act, 1946, see Hill-Burton program

Human Relations Center, see Wellesley Project

Hunterdon Medical Center, 243

Interns, see Medical education

Joint Commission on Accreditation of Hospitals, 113, 117–118, 244

Kaiser Foundation Health Plan, 155

Labor-Management Hospitalization Trust Fund, 107–108; and Montefiore Hospital, 121

Leonard, John, 244

Medical care, quality of, see Quality of care

Medical Care Insurance Act (Saskatchewan), 135

Medical care research, 147–166. See also Physician; Costs, medical care; Medical research; Quality of care

Medical education, 221–236, 237–253, 254–270; Bingham Associates, 243; continuing education in hospital, 250–253; Cornell Comprehensive Care and Teaching Program, 67; expansion of knowledge, 294; faculty attitudes, 69–74; field of practice by class rank, 164; future curricula, 45–46; hospital (post-graduate), 39–41, 225, 239; post-doctoral, 239–242; AMA survey, 242; pre-doctoral, 238; restrictions of teaching hospitals, 266–268; student attitudes, 74–79; student development, 28–32; types of, 225, 237

Medical group practice, 99–103; and Health Insurance Plan of Greater New York, 100, 152; in the hospital, 309–311; pre-paid, 101

Medical research: government, 144; as hospital function, 65; medical care, 46, 147–166; patient care, 87–90; social problems, 42

Medical Social Service, see Social service

Mental illness: care of the aged in hospitals, 262; community health (Wellesley Project), 279; emergency ward, 289; history of institutions for treatment of, 13–20; hospitals for, 304–306; origins of hospitals for, 259. See also Psychiatry

Millis, John, 242

Mortality rates: decline of, 158–159, 255; in teaching and non-teaching hospitals, 159–160

National Health Service (Great Britain), 262; and British Medical Association, 314; role of the doctor, 264

National Nursing Home Survey, 307

Nurses: care by in the clinic, 87; and doctors, 57–58; history of education of, 32–34; and patient classification, 261; student, 284

Nursing home: and chronic disease, 307–308; Montefiore's Loeb Center, 104–106

Nursing service: and family structure, 49–50, 52; history of, 51; of today, 53

Patient, 22–46; behavior of, 26, 55–56; care of, 38, 89–90; cost of care and Gross National Product, 147; and chronic disease, 306–308; evaluation of care of, 81–86; increasing expectations of, 302; needs of, 169–170

Physicians, 221–236, 237–253; and change, 222–224; and changing role in the hospital, 249–250; and clinic administration, 79–81; educational development of, 28–32; field of practice by class rank, 164; future role of, 45–46; and hospital utilization, 197; hospital education of, 39–41, 237; and National Health Service, 264; organization of medical practice, 180–181; performance of general practitioner, 161; relationship to nurses, 57–58; specialization, 294; striking (the Saskatchewan Medical Care Insurance Act), 135; training, 69–79

Prevention of disease, 257; in children, 290; in the hospital, 311; primary and secondary, 273; and psychiatry, 272; separation from curative medicine, 265

Preventive medicine, 311–314

Psychiatry, 254–292 passim

Public health department, in the hospital, 314

Quality of care: and behavioral sciences, 87–90; evaluation of, 81–86; in municipal hospitals, 121–123; and organized consumer, 178; and Teamsters, 107. See also Medical care research

Regional planning, 117; Hill-Burton program, 137–140; hospital-medical school, 296; and rising costs, 301

Rehabilitation, 104–106

Residents, see Medical education

Rubinow, I. M., 205

Saskatchewan episode, 135

Social medicine, 254–317 passim

Social responsibility, 1–21, 48

Social security, 201–220; Old-Age, Survivors, and Disability Insurance, 207–215

Social service: and family health maintenance, 102–103; founding of, 15; patient care in clinic, 86

Surgical education, 228

Utilization: and the physician, 197; England vs. the United States, 156; and health insurance, 152–153; and hospital costs, 101

Visiting Nurse Association, 316

Vollan, Douglas D., 242

Voluntarism, 125; and health agencies, 316; and hospitals, 133–140

Wagner, Mayor Robert (NYC), 119

Wellesley Project, 279

West End Project, 286